Mercury Poisoning

and

"Health Care"

Lessons Learned From a
30-Year Battle
For Health

by
Tim Stanley

2 Timothy Publishing
Irvine, CA

Mercury Poisoning and "Health Care":
Lessons Learned From a 30-Year Battle for Health

ISBN # 978-0-9842391-3-9
Library of Congress # 2013910663
First Printing, September, 2013

2 Timothy Publishing
P.O. Box 53783
Irvine, CA 92619-3783
USA
www.2timothypublishing.com

Printed in USA

For a copy of this book by mail, order online or send a check or money order to the P.O. Box above. Shipping and handling are included in the amounts stated. Total cost: $24.00 (CA mailing addresses, add $2.25 sales tax); Canada: $40.00 total.

See website for discounts on bulk purchases.

This book is not intended to diagnose or treat any disease or medical condition, nor is it to take the place of professional health care guidance. Use of any of the information in this book is the sole responsibility of the reader.

To our children

"My people are destroyed for lack of knowledge."

Hosea

"Buy the truth and do not sell it."

Solomon

Preface

The purpose of this book is to share information—to share something of what we have learned about caring for ourselves and for our family with the hope that it may be helpful to others. To do this, I will tell you the story of my wife's thirty-year battle with mercury poisoning. The details of her story are unique because we are all different, but the principles behind her return to health are the same principles behind a potential return to health for countless other people.

My wife, Deborah, is not a rare case. She is only one of a large and ever increasing number of people whom our medical system cannot help. Had we followed the advice of her doctors, Deborah could long ago have been institutionalized and become yet another drugged-up, personality-void, waif pining away in some mental ward. Thank God, she has been anything but that! In the midst of her adversity, she did a wonderful job raising our children, has since had a successful career, and has been an inspiration to many.

From the time we discovered Deborah's mercury problem, we have been asked many times, "How do you get mercury poisoning?" The answer is not so simple. Every time we tried to answer this question, we felt that our short answers were not only woefully inadequate, but in fact missed the mark. The reason is that *any* short answer to the question will almost invariably be hung on a faulty framework of understanding. In most cases, the better question is: How can we keep exposure to mercury from becoming mercury poisoning?

In the process of solving Deborah's health problems, we found out that the accumulation of metals in the body can be a major underlying component of ill health and disease. But it is not that simple. There are other major factors as well. We also found out that there are enormous conflicts of interest when it comes to what is called "health care" rendering an enormous amount of it useless, if not downright harmful.

I originally intended to merely tell Deborah's story and to list resources where the reader could find additional practical information on mercury poisoning and related matters. However, in the process of doing my research and compiling the book, I did not find any single source, or even a collection of several sources, that covered the subject close to adequately. I realized that if I stayed with my first intent, the amount of time it would take the reader to get a good overview of the subject matter would be unacceptable. So, I set out to write the most helpful book on the subject that I could, and that is why the book is in the form in which you have it.

The book does three things: It tells our story, it gives comments on the lessons we learned, and it provides backup information in the form of references, notes, and resources which enable the reader to expand his or her own investigation.

Deborah's story and the stories of some of the other people I will tell you about put a human face on the widespread, if not prevailing, condition of ill health in the US population, and shows how we can be delivered from it. What we want to address is this: How did we get into this condition of ill health, and what is our way back to wellness?

Regardless of where you are in the pursuit of healthy living—whether you are a novice or someone who has been earnest in the endeavor for decades—there is something in this book for you. If you have allergies, blood sugar problems, adrenal or thyroid problems, recurrent infections, any autoimmune condition, a bipolar condition or any mental instability, Parkinson's, MS, or if after describing your symptoms your doctor told you, "I've never heard of that before," this book could be invaluable to you. If you have young children, I know of no better example of how to care for them than that of my wife.

Sometimes our health challenges are overwhelming. But if we get on the right track, we have a good chance of arriving at better health and getting away from "health care" that isn't. By telling Deborah's story, it is our hope that many people will be encouraged and empowered to embark on precisely that kind of journey of discovery.

We humbly offer what we have learned.

Tim and Deborah Stanley

WARNING
This book is largely anecdotal in nature and contains the opinions of someone who is not in the medical field. It is the story of how some people have taken responsibility for their health care and what they have learned in the process. It is not intended to diagnose or prescribe anything, to make any scientific claim, or to take the place of your health care practitioner. It is intended only for the thoughtful consideration of people who take full responsibility for their actions. If you do not fit into this category, <u>please do not read the book</u>.

Table of Contents

**Mercury Poisoning and "Health Care":
Lessons Learned From a 30-Year Battle for Health**

Part I
The Setting and Going Another Way

Part II
Mercury!

Part III
Let Your Food Be Your Medicine and
Let Your Medicine Be Your Food

Part IV
More Lessons Learned, Conclusion

Introduction

As of this writing, what is commonly called "health care" accounts for between seventeen and twenty percent of the US Gross Domestic Product. With a large population bubble approaching old age, even the most elementary understanding of mathematics will tell us that there is zero possibility that our increasingly expensive approach to "health care" in the US can be maintained in any way resembling what we have been accustomed to. That is good news. From the standpoint of prevention and treatment of chronic illness, it may be hurting us more than it is helping us. Even if we could continue to pay for all the bypasses, joint replacements, transplants, and drugs that people want, we would be better off having a mindset of preventing disease rather than trying to treat it.

There are different means of maintaining health and of becoming healthy, but there are certain principles that cannot be ignored. Unfortunately, in our "health care" system the most foundational of those principles, as a matter of course, have been relegated to a secondary status, if not ignored entirely.

In earlier days, it was common for coal miners to take a canary into the mines with them. They did this because a canary is more sensitive to toxic gasses such as methane and carbon monoxide than people are, and the canary would become sick before the miners did. By observing the health of the birds, the miners could escape from the mine before a buildup of toxic gasses overcame them.

I have lovingly called my wife our canary for a long time. She is more sensitive than most of us and has been an early warning system not only to our family, but to other people as well. The things that have bothered her and have made her sick are the same things that make others sick—she just became sick with less exposure. I have written this book because I think a great many people can benefit from listening to this "canary."

Although this is largely Deborah's story, also included are the stories of many other people we know. To protect their identity, their names have been changed as well as insignificant details of their stories.

In order to tell Deborah's story, I must address certain issues in detail such as diet, alternative care, and even how to talk to your doctor. What is written here is not theory; it is life practice. I am not passing on secondhand information but only that which we or others we know have experienced or seen firsthand. We were given a set of circumstances, this is how we handled them, and this is what we learned in the process.

We live in a society where we are constantly bombarded with sensory information about everything—including health matters. So great is this bombardment that our thinking can be tossed about like a small sailboat in a storm. The storm rages so loudly that many of us cannot hear our intuition that was given to protect us. Although our bodies are talking to us a lot of the time, few people know how to listen to theirs. Our minds, which stand between our intuition and our bodies, are confused. The purpose of this book is to right the ship.

Through the decades that we have been attempting to live a healthy life, many people have come to us seeking some specific advice. We have been glad to help when we can, but in short conversations we can only discuss the immediate need, and that is almost always woefully inadequate. Our hearts ache to see that so many people simply do not know how much damage they are doing to themselves by going against the fundamental principles of healthful living. In many—if not most—cases, what may be necessary is a complete change in lifestyle, and that thought takes time to develop.

Deborah's story is mostly in chapters 1-6 and 8-13. Chapter 7 is the story of a friend, and chapters 14-24 give further understanding to the preceding chapters, although some of our story is included there as well. The appendices and resources can be very helpful, and the book contents are backed up by more than 300 references. Hundreds of notes add to and complement the main text. The index is great for quick reference, although I do not recommend it if you are not reading through the book. The value of the book as a whole is much greater than the value of the sum of its parts.

Part I

The Setting
and
Going Another Way

Chapter 1
The Setting

I loved my wife very much, it was our anniversary, and I wanted to do something special for her. So I asked her if I could take her out to dinner. For most people, going out to eat is no big thing—you just go, and you have a nice time. But we had not gone to a restaurant for more than a decade. You see, beginning many years back, whenever we went out to dinner, she would get sick. Sometimes violently. She always seemed to react to something, and it was always something different. So, over the years, she eliminated more and more foods from her diet.

It was obvious to us that we were dealing with a serious health issue, but we had no idea what it was. Eventually, we found it impossible to eat out and be able to avoid foods that she reacted to, so she fixed all of her own meals at home. That being the case, for me to ask to take her out to dinner was risky. But there was a hotel that had a restaurant that overlooked the coast, and I thought that maybe she could just order a plain green salad with nothing on it and take the rest of her food with her. We could sit there and enjoy the view together just like we had in times past before she lost her health. What harm could there be in that? After all, she had made a lot of progress. She was no longer bedridden, and by this time was able to function pretty normally except for the dietary limitations.

She hesitantly agreed, we got all dressed up, and after I picked up the baby-sitter for the children, we went out for the evening. We were so happy to be going on a date, and she even sat "girlfriend style," close to me in the car on the way to the restaurant.

We were seated at one of the best tables in the place—right next to the window—and we just sat there watching the surf crash on the rocks below. After sending the waiter away a couple of times, we finally ordered—and got the usual puzzled, disappointed look when we declined the appetizers and she just ordered a simple green salad. By this time we were well accustomed to the puzzled, disappointed looks when it came to eating in public. For years, if we went somewhere for dinner, or if someone came to our home for dinner, we had at least a somewhat awkward time.

It was quite different in the late 1970s than it is today. At that time, severe food allergies were not common. Today, most people know someone who has multiple, serious food allergies, and therefore they have at least a little empathy. But it was not so then. Deborah was always the "odd woman out," and many people would quiz her about her health all through dinner and even afterwards. They just could not let it go, and more than a few people were accusing. Since we did not want to spend our evenings that way (and we didn't think it was pleasant for others either), we greatly limited having social mealtimes.

That night, thankfully, the waiter was gracious and did not make a scene.

But we did.

About halfway through the meal, Deborah suddenly became very ill. She told me, "Tim, you better get me home right now." I got up, left some money on the table, and helped her out. We barely made it. She was completely white and collapsed as soon as I got her to the car. The next morning she was still pale and greatly weakened but was definitely on the mend. Though this kind of physical reaction had occurred several times before, this time we had no idea what had caused it.

And it would be another twenty years before she ate *anything* that she or I did not prepare.

We soon discovered what had happened: The green salad "with nothing on it" in fact did have something on it. Just as with all green salads at nearly every restaurant, a product called Stay Fresh[1] was sprayed on the lettuce leaves to keep them from wilting, and she had reacted to the chemicals in that compound.

By this time, we had become very careful to stay away from foods with additives, but this one was new to us, and it taught us a big lesson. That is, with very rare exceptions, you can't stay away from additives if someone else is preparing the food.

Now days, more and more people are adversely affected by the various poisons that we put on, or in, our food. Some people know it; most don't.

By the time of her collapse at the restaurant, many foods had been eliminated from Deborah's diet. They included tomatoes, eggs, cantaloupe, all processed foods, and almost anything that anyone else prepared. Her reactions varied depending upon the culprit. Often it was migraines; more frequently it was light-headedness or feeling faint. At times eczema broke out, usually on her hands and arms. At other times, she had diarrhea. But she always became very weak.

Sometimes the reaction was mild, sometimes severe. Sometimes it was so severe that all she could do was lie on the floor and wait until I got home. At those times she couldn't even pick up the phone.

In their early years, our children grew up around a mother who was frequently lying on the floor, unable to do anything. Some kids grow up with a parent who has this kind of reaction to drugs or booze. Deborah never indulged in those things; her reactions were to normal foods.

In the Beginning

Deborah was born into a middle-class family that was on the rise. Her father had grown up as a poor country boy in the South, but following World War II, and thanks to the GI Bill, he became an aerospace engineer in the early 1950s. Consequently, he and his family received the best "health care" available. All the latest technology was available to them.

During the time when we were learning how to overcome the limits of gravity and put a man into space, many medical advances had taken place too. Consequently, many people got the idea that now that we understood so many things, we could easily overcome the limitations of our bodies through science.

So Deborah was a DES daughter. That is, her mother, like two million other pregnant American women during the 1950s and 1960s, was prescribed diethylstilbestrol under the mistaken notion that it would reduce the risk of pregnancy complications.[2]

But Deborah was born with jaundice[3] and had a digestive problem that made her vomit frequently. As a toddler, she had adverse reactions to foods, low appetite, repeated worm infections, sore throats, and outbreaks of eczema.

The doctors gave her injections of gamma globulin to boost the immune system and liquid B vitamins to increase her appetite, and gave her mother ointments to put on the eczema.

When she came down with a common cold and her tonsils were enflamed, her parents followed the modern thinking of the day and had her tonsils removed. What need could there possibly be for these "unnecessary" parts?[4]

Like countless other middle-class American families who were relatively well off during the 1950s and early 1960s, her family could also afford the new processed foods that were so easy to fix—five minute rice, macaroni and cheese in a box, snappy breakfast cereals, and of course, sweets.

Deborah's family delighted in the new "fast food" restaurants. (This was before junk food became the bane of the lower classes.) And her family rarely, if ever, turned down any tasty food.

It was all so easy.

If they did not feel well, they took whatever the doctor prescribed in the way of medications. If they had minor ailments and something advertised on TV looked like a good idea, they took that too.[5]

The down side with all the new foods (that was immediately apparent) was an onslaught of dental cavities. But the cavities were really not a problem—they could easily be filled by the dentist, and you could go right on eating the same tantalizing foods.

Smoking was quite in vogue in those days—just about all the movie stars and entertainers smoked—and her family, with Deborah the only exception, fit right in.[6] In short, they were a thoroughly modern family. They were well to do and living "the good life."

At a very young age, Deborah had allergic reactions to eggs, and sometimes tomatoes bothered her, but those problems seemed to go away as she grew up, and she seemed to her doctor, to herself, to her family, and to those around her, to be of average health. Much later, having something to compare that time with, she told me, "Actually, as a child I was dull, lethargic, and unmotivated. Looking back on it now, I realize I lived in what was essentially a stupor. It was the result of a sugared-up diet that eventually led to hypoglycemia."

However, the burst of life force that comes with puberty overrode Deborah's underlying physical condition, and when I met her, when she was sixteen, she seemed to be of normal health. Also, in high school, she started to care about her weight, and that meant eating a little better, so that probably helped as well.

Throughout our courting years we had no hint of what was to come.

Early on, I was concerned about her diet. She told me that sometimes she would eat a whole box of Oreo cookies in one sitting. I thought that my diet was much better and cautioned her. After all, when I came home from school, I would eat a large dish of ice cream or maybe a can of peaches (packed in heavy syrup). At the time, I thought I was eating dairy and fruit, and certainly that was better for you than cookies and candy. Right?

Shortly after we got married, Deborah began to react to cantaloupe and citrus fruits. Eczema would break out on her hands if she even touched the juice from one of these. She told me that when she was a young child that had happened some, but she never thought anything of it.

But when Deborah became pregnant everything changed. The body that had been taxed to the breaking point began to break. Deborah had wanted children, but neither she nor I had a clue as to her actual physical condition, nor of the price that we were about to pay.

Early in her first pregnancy, she lost her coloring and was very susceptible to sickness. Something was obviously wrong. She miscarried in the first trimester. The doctor dismissed any concern by telling her, "That happens sometimes," and we remained ignorant of what was going on with her physically.

After about a year, Deborah got pregnant again—this time with our son. The same thing happened. She became pale and generally did not feel well. "Oh, sometimes it's that way," the doctors told her. Regardless of what they said, we knew something was very wrong, but we did not know what to do about it. "Young and dumb" describes perfectly our state at that time. Unfortunately, those we were around who were older, including the physicians we saw, were no wiser. We cared very much for her health and for the health of the child, so if anyone gave any kind of warning, it certainly was not clear.

Deborah did the best she could to take care of herself at that time, and her diet was much improved. In fact, by that time, we thought we were eating in a very healthy manner. But that did not make up for past abuses of the body or for a ton of ignorance.

Our dear son was born two months premature and was a sickly child from the beginning. Also, after he arrived, Deborah stopped eating wheat because that was determined to be the cause of new outbreaks of eczema. Both of them were pale, and neither of them had much strength.

Shortly after our son was born, we heard about another kind of doctor, who we were told had a very different approach. Since we were certain that Deborah's case was serious, and all the medical doctors we had seen had been no help, we determined to go see him. His name was Bernard Jensen, and he was an expert iridologist. An iridologist is someone who is trained to look at the iris of the eye to "see" the condition of the different systems of the body. This all sounded like science fiction to us.

There was no Internet in 1974, and at that time, the term "alternative medicine" may not have existed. However, the term "quack" did exist, and had we not been so desperate to get a better understanding of what was going on with Deborah's body, we would not have spent our hard-earned money to go see Dr. Jensen. But we *were* desperate, and since we were taking a trip to Los Angeles anyway, we made an appointment to see him while we were there.

I had never been to Los Angeles before, and (sorry Angelinos) at that time LA was a Festival of Smog. The décor was concrete and asphalt, and we could hardly imagine an uglier place. Dr. Jensen's office was right downtown in the middle of it, and as we came close to his office, it seemed to me like a strange place to be seeking anything to do with health.

Dr. Jensen's office looked more like the sergeant's office on the military base where I had been stationed than any doctor's office we had seen before. The waiting room was full of people sitting in straight backed wooden chairs, the floor was asphalt tile, and there was a simple wooden desk in the corner where the receptionist sat. Other than that, some books were on the desk and an eye chart was on the wall. That was about it.

The exam room was essentially the same. There was no examination table. The patient sat on one of the same straight-backed chairs, and Dr. Jensen sat on a typical office chair with wheels. His tools were a flashlight and a magnifying glass.

He first explained that the eye was "the window of the body," then he came close and with the magnifier looked into the patient's eyes and began to describe what he saw. The whole exam and consultation took about thirty minutes.

Without her telling him anything, in a very confident way, Dr. Jensen told Deborah all the problems that she was having. He also described exactly how she felt. This surprised her, and she knew that his assessment was accurate.

There was one thing, however, that we just could not get a handle on. He told her that her bowel was impacted with putrefied material. I was examined by him too, and he told me the same thing. Since we both thought we had good bowel movements and did not feel any abdominal discomfort, we thought this was at least weird, if not just plain "off."

Dr. Jensen prescribed pretty much the same thing for both of us: alfalfa tablets for cleansing, vitamins, and enzymes. For Deborah, he added some minerals that he said she was deficient in.

He must have also said something more about dietary matters, because we started growing alfalfa sprouts at that time and probably made some other changes, but that appointment was nearly forty years ago, and we don't remember much. What we do remember is that we had never heard of any kind of dietary "cleansing" before, and we could not imagine how we could be deficient in vitamins—after all, we took a multivitamin.

We purchased and even re-ordered what he prescribed.

In the following months, Deborah did not seem to get worse, but there was no measurable instant change for the better either. So, since I was only making a subsistence living at the time and our health insurance did not cover the prescribed products, we did not continue with them.

Our largest difficulty, however, was that we simply did not know how to deal with the new information. What Dr. Jensen had told us was too different from anything we had ever heard. He might as well have been speaking to us about life on Mars. At the time, we could not link up an overall picture. The whole experience was just too shocking.

But we had medical insurance, and later, when Deborah became pregnant for the third time, she went to see a doctor again. She told him of her allergies, of her miscarriage, and of the troubles with her previous pregnancies and with our son's birth. All this doctor's medical training only enabled him to tell her, "Well, it was just meant to be."

I am glad we did not have to pay for the visit. But then we got exactly what we paid for.

Sorry to say, the medical clinic where our insurance was accepted was, *at best*, worthless. It was an early Health Maintenance Organization, and to put it bluntly, they simply didn't care. All the staff expressed the same attitude. Their patients were a burden to them in that they had come to the clinic, and the staff missed no opportunity to let them know that that was the case.

But they did "help" us when our baby was sick. He was frequently sick and had multiple ear infections. So, they gave us Ampicillin, an antibiotic, and Dimetapp,[7] a decongestant, and in a few days the symptoms cleared up. However, in six weeks he was sick again. The doctor told us to use the same treatment. This happened a few times, and the doctor still insisted on the same treatment. We began to think that the whole thing was stupid. The kid just became sicker and sicker. We became convinced that the medications depleted his system and set him up for the next bout. And, like clockwork, a few weeks later it would surely come.

One day while Deborah was sitting in the rocker holding our son, she asked me to bring the medications to her. I opened the refrigerator door and began to reach for the pink and purple bottles that were sitting there on the shelf, but something stopped me. I withdrew my hand, closed the door, turned around, and told her emphatically, "No more. That's it."

She agreed, and though we did not know what to do, we were determined to take another way.

Chapter 2
Collapse

At the time we quit the prescriptions, we did not know what it is that fundamentally causes illness. We were still almost entirely under the influence of that system that disempowers us and makes the matter complicated. We were under the system of "health care" that in its nature is so often contrary to health.

About two years after our son was born, Deborah gave birth to our daughter. When she did not have the vitality to produce breast milk—which had been flourishing after our son's birth—her doctor was not the least concerned. He told her the standard line of the day, that is, that the new baby formulas were better than mother's milk anyway.

The births of both of our children were crisis births. As mentioned earlier, our son was born two months premature. He was born at the University of California, San Francisco Medical Hospital, and that was a wonderful experience. The staff was very interested in him because he was not the usual "preemie" for that hospital. Most of the premature babies born there at that time were the children of drug addicts and weighed no more than two pounds. These children had little chance of developing normally, ours did, so in this sense he was the best textbook that the medical residents could get, and we were treated like royalty.

By the time our daughter was born, I had changed jobs and our insurance had changed. We could not go to UC San Francisco, as that would not be paid for by our insurance. We needed to go to another hospital, which also had a clinic for pre- and postnatal care. Though it was a private hospital, that HMO (referred to earlier) was a good preview of what socialized medicine on a limited budget could be. The attitude expressed by staff for Deborah's prenatal care and postnatal care could be summarized simply by saying, "Gee lady, I'm not getting paid to solve your problem."

When Deborah was pregnant with our daughter, she lost feeling in her arms and started having contractions at the beginning of the seventh month. The doctor told her, "Get yourself a good bottle of wine and go to bed." In those days, for the most part, we still followed doctor's orders. The effects of the wine, however, eventually increased to the point where she could not sleep for 36 hours straight. The wine was intended to calm, but the opposite occurred. We would not know why for some time.

Looking back, we are fortunate that our daughter was not born with Fetal Alcohol Syndrome.[8]

About three months after our daughter was born, we moved to Southern California. Before we moved, and because we would be losing our dental insurance, Deborah decided to have her wisdom teeth pulled. They were slightly impacted, and it had been recommended that the procedure be done. After the teeth were extracted, she was given codeine for the pain and reacted to it. She completely lost her equilibrium, and it was all she could do just to hold onto the bed while the whole world spun around.

The stress of the birth, of the move, and of the removal of her wisdom teeth with the complications proved too much. She began to have frequent migraines, her allergies escalated, her stomach was upset, and she broke out with hives and eczema. On at least one occasion, she was completely covered with hives and spent all night in and out of a vinegar bath to obtain some relief.

We did not know how to term it at the time, but her toxicity had reached a high level of severity. But we did not understand toxicity and had no idea what to do.

Within a few months of our move, Deborah completely collapsed and was bedridden for three weeks with a low-grade fever. For about six months after that, her routine consisted of getting up to feed the babies, then lying back down to gather the strength to be able to do it again.

It was a tender scene to see our son lovingly drive his little plastic cars over his mother while she lay sick in bed. But I had no idea what to do or how to help her.

As time went on, Deborah slowly gained strength. About a year after her collapse, she felt well enough to go to a potluck dinner with some friends. There she ate some creamy soup and reacted very negatively to it. She told me to stay, but she was going to go home and she would take the kids with her. After getting home, with difficulty, she got the kids into bed. By the time she did, she thought she was going to pass out and remembers being on the floor and forcing herself to stay awake until I got home.

More and more foods were being added to the "don't touch" list. A little later she began having environmental and chemical allergies. Smoke from cigarettes and from wood fires was particularly a problem. If she was exposed to one of these, she became highly agitated and literally had to run away from the source.

With my new job, we had better insurance and were able to see some doctors who at least had the concept of care, but all were at a complete loss when it came to the allergies. They did not link her miscarriage with anything either. Nor did they link the cysts and fibroids that grew in her breast, the hormone imbalances, and the migraine headaches with anything.

The doctors ordered a skull X-ray to try to find the cause of the migraines, but it revealed nothing. Deborah found the cause by trial and error on her own: broccoli and the cabbage family of foods.

But our progress was slow. Painfully slow.

After our daughter was born, and knowing that another pregnancy would likely kill her, Deborah took birth control pills for about three months.[9] While on the pill, she felt bad all the time. In her words, "My body was just whacked."

She learned later—on her own—that among other things, birth control pills deplete the B vitamins. Many of her symptoms were classic of vitamin B deficiencies, but apparently none of the physicians she saw understood this. And we didn't yet either.

All the while, Deborah's food allergies grew progressively worse. She had splits and cuts on her hands, and they were cracking and bleeding. The doctors (as they nearly always do) treated the symptom, and prescribed cortisone cream. The cortisone made her skin thinner so that it tore easily. But she wrapped her hands at night so that they would heal enough in order for her to make it through the next day. For years, on and off, she put ointment on her hands and wrapped them in plastic wrap before going to bed.

And night after night she cried herself to sleep.

Chapter 3
Diagnosis: "Nuts"

Seemingly, Deborah was an oddity outside the realm of "normal" medicine. Because of this, and because they did not understand her case, her doctors became accusing and even attacking. This was especially the case when she told them about her food allergies and sensitivities to chemicals. They did not believe her and gruffly asked, "Well, what happens?" She would then explain that she got migraines, would lose all her strength, and sometimes would go into vomiting fits. This silenced them, but they showed no interest whatsoever in what she had said.

She saw several MDs, and as her condition worsened, they increasingly treated her as if she were the problem. If she asked questions, she was out of line. If she mentioned anything about what she had read in an alternative health book, she got a good tongue lashing. It was basically, "Everyone else is a quack besides me—I'm the doctor!"

The medical professionals seemed to take it as a personal affront that Deborah's ailments were not according to what they had learned in medical school. "How dare you have a condition that I cannot treat! I paid a lot of money for med school, and now I'm in a great deal of debt. You're supposed to have something I can prescribe a medication for, and then you're supposed to get better— you are not cooperating!" Of course they didn't say exactly that, but some came close, and the attitude was common enough.

Eventually, one of her doctors took me aside and told me that Deborah was not able to do simple arithmetic, and it was her assessment that Deborah had a mental problem.

So her hands were cracking apart, she had violent reactions to many foods, she was so weak she could hardly function, and the diagnosis was that she was nuts!

As it is, many people with Deborah's condition are diagnosed as having different forms of mental illness.

Thankfully, we did not believe that doctor and did not pursue a course of treatment along those lines.

How many people are in mental institutions today simply because of poor nutrition! It is too depressing to go into the details of this, so I will not. But if you or someone you love is suffering with mental problems, know that there could well be a very simple physiological reason for it. And there are alternatives to going into the endless downward spiral of more and more powerful medications that destroy the person and can eventually require them to be institutionalized.

The formula is very simple. Go after the main culprits: sugar, refined foods, and artificial ingredients added to foods. Detoxify and fortify. In other words, get the poisons out, and get good nutrition in. Although we have seen many people suffer terrible consequences from taking prescription drugs, we have never seen anyone harmed from detoxifying and fortifying the body.

I want to tell you of two similar cases to underscore this point. What is written here is not theory. We did not read about these nor did we hear about them secondhand. Both are stories of people we know, and we were involved in both cases.

Jimmy was about five years old. He was in a Sunday school class I taught, and I knew him quite well. He had a sweet disposition, and I enjoyed being with him very much. But sometimes he had an absolutely horrible personality change. If he ate a hot dog, he would go berserk and become a monster. He became disoriented and violent. Eventually, it was discovered that the condition was triggered when he ate foods with nitrates, nitrites, or certain other non-food additives. His mother caught on and removed all artificial ingredients from his diet, including food colorings, preservatives, and the like. The episodes stopped.[10]

Mark is a young man we know. When he was in his early twenties, he began to show signs of a bipolar[11] condition. He was a young professional, had a great job, and most of the time was fine. But the condition worsened, and he was put on medication. The medication affected his personality negatively, and he did not feel like himself. (How many times have you heard that?!) Eventually he quit the medication, preferring the risk involved over feeling "off" all of the time. After a while he became greatly depressed, deranged, and delusional. He lost his job, his marriage, and his sanity and ended up on the street. Thankfully, his mother did some research on the web and found someone who claimed that the bipolar condition could be effectively treated by nutrition and vitamin supplementation.[12] Eventually she was able to convince Mark— which by that time was no easy thing to do—to begin the nutrition and vitamin program. Mark has been fine now for years, has resumed his career, and is in harmony with himself and with others. His condition is controlled simply by proper diet and vitamin supplementation. [13] [14] [15] [16]

Do you think such cases are rare?

Keep reading.

Resources
Our Daily Meds, by Melody Petersen, 2008
Pharmaceutical advertisements and industry-positive press gives one side of the story. This book gives the other side. It is well-researched and documented.

Additional resources are in the notes that accompany this chapter.

Chapter 4
Set on the Right Path

"Try diet first."

"The fundamental principle of true healing consists of a return to natural habits of living." Jethro Kloss

The big turning point for Deborah came when she met Viola. Viola grew up on a homestead farm, and as such she was connected to the earth in a way that few of us are. After she married, she moved to the suburbs where she grew vegetables and raised rabbits in a small yard to feed her family. Her concept of health was nutritionally based.

At the advice of a friend, Deborah went to see her. At the time, Deborah was on the ropes physically and mentally, but Viola talked to her and gave her a plan. Viola's goal was to get Deborah on her feet so that she could understand how to take care of herself and her family. Her plan was very simple: proper diet and vitamin supplementation. This seems elementary to us now, and may seem so to some readers, but at the time we did not know *how* improper and destructive the typical American diet is, nor did we know how nearly all-encompassing is its way of death.

Deborah remembers that time in this way: "Viola was not spoon feeding me; she was giving me the tools I needed so I could learn how to help myself. I started reading the list of ingredients on the foods I bought at the grocery store. That was quite revealing.

"In the mid-1970s, health food stores were still a new concept, and vitamins and supplements (for the most part) were groundbreaking. Nutritional therapies were not well known as they are today, and there were few practitioners. It was not at all like it is today. Now, more and more people have become fed up with the AMA, and almost everyone knows people who are taking another way. But at that time we had very little, if any, exposure to alternative medicine."

When Deborah was well enough and was able to handle it, Viola gave her resources to learn from on her own. She referred her to a few books: *Let's Eat Right to Keep Fit*, by Adelle Davis; *Low Blood Sugar and You*[17], by Carlton Fredericks; *Back to Eden,* by Jethro Kloss; and *Kitchen Medicines,* by Ben Charles Harris.

From that time, Deborah began to learn about the nutritional requirements for wellness. So that you will understand what I mean by this statement, I will point out that before then we had made a lot of progress and thought we ate pretty healthy—certainly healthier than most people! The problem was we were comparing ourselves with what other people did, not with a truly healthy standard.

Gradually, Deborah regained some strength. What motivated her was that she had to keep going for the sake of the children. Within six months after seeing Viola, she had greatly improved.

Hypoglycemia, Hyperinsulinism, and Glucose Intolerance
Deborah told me, "In one of our talks, I remember asking Viola, 'What's wrong with me?' She told me, 'You have hypoglycemia.'"

Today, nearly everyone has heard of hypoglycemia, and some people know something about what it is. At that time, in the mid-1970s, it was not so.

Viola asked Deborah to, when she could, read Carlton Fredericks' book. To Deborah's surprise, there in that book was a description that matched her condition. She put it this way: "Fredericks' book brought order to my thinking where previously there had been chaos. Everything made sense. I had something to pin the symptoms to, and I could trace these things all the way back to my childhood. I was so stunned—there was a logical reason behind all this. There was finally a name."

It is important to tell you here that none of the physicians Deborah had seen, or was to see for a long time, ever diagnosed her with hypoglycemia. For this reason, and because of the commonness of the condition, I will for the most part suspend Deborah's story here and discuss hypoglycemia and related conditions for the rest of this chapter. The discussion that follows will explain what was going on inside of Deborah at the time and is also going on in about one out of ten Americans. **You will undoubtedly find someone you know in the pages that follow.** The condition, though denied by current mainstream American medical practice, is as serious as it is common.

It may seem odd in a book about mercury poisoning to talk about hypoglycemia—especially in detail. No so! The two often go hand in hand.

> **Hypoglycemia is a metabolic disorder in which the body does not process sugars *and carbohydrates* properly, leading to a condition of low levels of sugar (fuel) in the blood. It is frequently caused by the excess production of insulin. In such cases, the condition can more accurately be called hyperinsulinism with secondary hypoglycemia.**

We have seen people with hypoglycemia become dizzy and nearly pass out. More commonly, we have seen hypoglycemics go into almost a stupor and be unable to think clearly or do anything. Others have become so cross and agitated that their behavior was far from socially acceptable. Some have gone into shaking fits, and still others have gone into near panic attacks. **Yet, not one that we know of was ever diagnosed by their medical doctor as hypoglycemic.** As a matter of fact, some of these people were told explicitly by their MDs that they were *not* hypoglycemic. However, in each case, after these people ate, the symptoms disappeared and they returned to a normal, or at least a somewhat normal state. Depending upon how far the condition had progressed, some were revived within minutes or hours. Those who had a low blood sugar condition for a longer period of time or were more depleted in a particular incident often did not feel that much better until the next day.

You may well ask, "Why didn't their doctors diagnose them?" The simple answer is that, unlike the very lucrative diabetes industry, there is no money in treating hypoglycemia. It is controlled entirely through diet.

The cases of hypoglycemia I just described, medical doctors call "functional hypoglycemia," and they insist that everyone has that condition at times. Yes, everyone may have a somewhat similar condition at times, but when the condition becomes a way of life, that is another matter.

The secretion of too much insulin by the pancreas is usually the result of that organ being stressed by habitually having to deal with more glucose than it safely can. When a stressed pancreas responds by excreting too much insulin into the bloodstream to neutralize the excess glucose, the result is commonly a low blood sugar condition. When the pancreas cannot produce enough insulin and the excess glucose continues to get dumped into the bloodstream, the result is a high blood sugar condition. But in both cases, it is not nearly that simple. The pancreas does not act alone but in concert with the rest of the body.

I added the term "glucose intolerance" to the subheading of this part of the chapter. By "glucose intolerance," I am NOT referring to "Impaired Glucose Tolerance," a term used to describe a form of "pre-diabetes." I am using the term to mean exactly what it says— bad stuff happens when you ingest sugar.

For the sake of convenience only, I will frequently use the word "hypoglycemia" in this chapter and ask the reader to understand that I am also referring to hyperinsulinism and the related glandular problems of someone who is glucose intolerant.

Symptoms

Symptoms of hypoglycemia vary from one individual to another. Also, in some people, the condition has progressed far more than it has in others. Further, in any individual the symptoms are not static in any one day, let alone over a period of years or decades. Sadly, very few people who are in the beginning stages of the disease recognize non-diabetic hypoglycemia for the serious condition that it is. For one thing, a chronic, or recurring, hypoglycemic (low blood sugar) condition can turn into diabetes (high blood sugar) very easily.

Both Deborah and I have seen diabetes up close and personal in our families and want nothing to do with it. We also know very well that **"the hypoglycemia of today is the diabetes of tomorrow."**[18] This understanding has kept us vigilant through the years.

Some common symptoms of a low blood sugar condition, of hyperinsulinism, and of glucose intolerance are:

* If we need to eat (not, "if we are hungry") and are abnormally low on energy, irritable, edgy, or confused, then hypoglycemia or hyperinsulinism are almost certainly a factor.

* If we repeatedly find ourselves suddenly needing to eat NOW, we likely have a low blood sugar condition. When a person with a blood sugar condition (diabetic or hypoglycemic) says they need to eat, they commonly mean that they need to eat within the next 60 seconds, not that it is time to start looking for a restaurant.

* If we find that at times we become withdrawn in social situations, seemingly for no good reason, and are just trying to survive, we may have an insulin or low blood sugar related condition. At those times, it is likely that we waited too long to eat or did not eat correctly.[19]

* If we notice an increasing craving for sweets and feel like we can't make it through the day without them, it is likely that the condition has progressed. The condition can be arrested by switching to a proper hypoglycemic diet that consists of slow-burning fuels instead of fast-burning ones. Basically, this means proteins with vegetables instead of sugars with simple carbohydrates.

* If we crave sweets and can't stop nibbling on them, we can be certain that we are on the blood sugar roller coaster. This is a serious condition.

* If we simply lack energy, are dull, or are fatigued too much of the time;

* If we are easily irritated, have temper flare-ups, have a sense of panic for no good reason, have unreasonable anger or an intense feeling of needing to just survive;

* If we have light-headedness, dizziness, vertigo, shakiness, frequent headaches;

* If we have multiple food allergies or asthma, hypoglycemia or hyperinsulinism may be a large part of the problem.

* Forgetfulness, poor concentration, confusion, unexplained nervousness, anxiety attacks, mood swings, crying spells, or depression are also common symptoms of hypoglycemia. Many hypoglycemics, including my wife, are diagnosed as neurotic, psychotic, or simply as having "a mental problem."[20] There is no rocket science required to understand this. If the brain is not getting a proper fuel supply, it cannot function well.

* If you have the yo-yo syndrome you probably have a blood sugar disorder. A typical hypoglycemic is frequently "strung out"—just like a drug addict—with chemical reactions that he cannot control. His emotions are all over the map. Though he may "hold his mud" the best he can, the chemical reactions within him can be so severe he may think he is going insane.

* If you have multiple sclerosis, you just might want to switch to a hypoglycemic diet. The symptoms may be completely relieved.

If some of the above symptoms look too familiar, you may find it helpful to read this entire book carefully and mark it up to use as a reference tool. I am not an "expert," but we do have in our immediate family—my wife and I and our children—more than 120 years of combined experience in dealing with hypoglycemia. We have also observed diabetes closely on both sides of the family for four decades.

Note: I am not a health practitioner and am not qualified to tell you what to do in your case. I am merely telling you of our experiences and observations and the conclusions we have drawn from them.

Testing

In all the years that Deborah had a low blood sugar condition, **she never tested low when she went to the medical labs to get blood drawn for her fasting glucose tests. Why?**

One of the problems with blood sugar tests in general is that they do not tell you where you are getting the sugar from. Is the current level of blood sugar due to an adrenaline surge? Just going to a doctor's office or getting poked with a needle can trigger an adrenal response that can nullify the accuracy of the test. Deborah does not like being poked with a needle and likes the sight of blood even less. Undoubtedly her body reacted to this stress and raised her blood sugar level, thus distorting the tests.

Adrenaline responses can be subtle and unrecognizable. Stress, anxiety, and a host of other conditions can also make blood sugar tests unreliable. **Several glands are involved in the blood sugar equation, not just the pancreas. The engineering is far more complex than simply the production of insulin.**

Once Deborah started testing her blood sugar at home, she found that she usually tested close to 58 mg/dl. Normal levels are between 80 and110. For decades, Deborah tested low. Then her levels gradually began to go up. Now, she commonly tests in the 80's— normal for some people, but quite high for her. Does that mean that the condition went away? Far from it. Most likely she is either producing less insulin or now has a greater resistance to it. The organs are damaged, and she must be as vigilant as ever. She knows very well that she could become diabetic at any time. This is one reason why it is necessary to understand what I have called "glucose intolerance" in this chapter.

Someone with several of the symptoms of hypoglycemia may find it helpful to purchase a blood sugar test kit. However, **just because blood sugar levels test in the normal range, that does not mean you are in the clear. The problem is much trickier than that. Therefore, assessing the symptoms of hyperinsulinism or hypoglycemia is commonly more accurate than blood tests**. I think it is wise to do both, however, because blood testing (as stated below) can solve the mystery for many people.

If a blood sugar problem is suspected, we have found it helpful to perform two tests:

1. If you are feeling lousy or having an episode, a lot may be learned by testing your blood sugar right then.

2. Under more normal conditions, we have found it helpful to test the blood sugar before breakfast (and before brushing teeth), then test it again an hour after breakfast, two hours after, and again four

hours after breakfast. If there is a tendency to low blood sugar, a physician's "complete checkup" will not reveal what testing in this manner often does. Repeating this kind of testing on multiple occasions will give a good indication of what is going on. Testing is discussed in more detail in Chapter 14.

[If you have several of the symptoms of hypoglycemia or hyperinsulinism, and proper diet does not stabilize the condition or if allergies remain prolific, you may want to test for mercury. See Chapter 9.]

A Complex Condition and Sad Statistics
If you have a low blood sugar condition, it is likely that you also suffer from **adrenal problems** and/or **food allergies**. In addition, a sugared-up diet—which is almost always the culprit[21]—frequently brings on **yeast infections**. All these things, and more, can bring about serious health issues that may not show up on standard blood tests. The glands and hormones can be going absolutely haywire trying to balance the body and you can be in very bad shape, yet all the tests can read "normal."

There is a way out of this quagmire: "Let your food be your medicine." If you suspect you have a blood sugar problem, you may want to switch to a hypoglycemic/diabetic diet for a few months. If you feel better, you have likely confirmed a glucose problem of one kind or another. The diet is discussed in Appendix II.

Although non-diabetic hypoglycemia is denied by mainstream US medical practice, those who understand the condition consistently estimate that about ten percent of the US population suffers from hyperinsulinism, hypoglycemia or a form of glucose intolerance that has not _yet_ developed into diabetes or into what is now called pre-diabetes.[22] Severity of the condition in different individuals varies greatly, and in all likelihood most of these people bungle along day after day, year after year, without getting to the root of their physical problems.

The American Diabetes Association now tells us that about 8.3 percent of the US population suffers from diabetes, which is high blood sugar. They also tell us that a little over 25 percent of the population is in a classification that is now called "pre-diabetes."[23] In other words, even by the most conservative of estimates, more than a third of the people in the US have a blood sugar disorder.[24] **This is because we are eating a grotesquely abnormal diet and our pancreas and other organs and glands cannot keep up with the assault of nutritional obscenities we are hurling at them.** Most pointedly, the average American consumes close to a half-pound of sugar every day, seven days a week, 365 days a year.[25]

What Your Doctor Will Say, and Why

Unfortunately, the medical textbooks, and consequently those who are trained in the US medical system, deny the most common forms of hypoglycemia. This was not always the case.[26] But it is now, and this is what medical doctors will routinely tell you:

First, they will tell you that those who talk about non-diabetic hypoglycemia are quacks and that there is no "scientific" basis for their statements.[27] [28]

Second, they insist that hypoglycemia is a reaction response in diabetics. Yes, hypoglycemia is commonly a reaction in diabetics. When a diabetic's blood sugar goes high, it often drops low. That is a low blood sugar condition; I agree. But that is not the whole story. Low blood sugar affects many non-diabetics as well. This was well understood before the highly profitable diabetes industry came into being. For the history, please see this note.[29]

Third, a typical MD will tell you that everyone has low blood sugar at times. They may even use the words "idiopathic," "functional," or "benign" hypoglycemia. If you are having some of the symptoms of low blood sugar, almost all physicians will tell you, "Just eat some sugar" or "Have a candy bar."

If your blood sugar goes really low[30], *too low for other foods to help*, you had better take some sugar. You do need to get your blood sugar level up. But I do not agree that you eat a whole candy bar! According to our experience, if you have a low blood sugar condition, eating candy bars is a very bad thing to do. If you eat too much sugar, it will likely cause your blood sugar level to spike and then drop again. That practice will eventually leave you in a worsened state.

[It is strange, but telling, that the suggestion from medical doctors, and in the books they write, is always to "eat a candy bar" or "have some sugar." I have yet to hear or read of an MD saying or writing in this situation: "Eat an apple," or "Have a bite of fruit."]

You can tell immediately if a physician has any understanding of non-diabetic hyperinsulinism or hypoglycemia by how he or she treats the sugar issue. Also, books written by hypoglycemics are a world apart. These people have suffered with the condition and they know better. They get sugar out of their diet, and they eat right (according Appendix II) in order to live. Period.

Again, I will remind the reader that I am only a reporter, telling you of the things we have learned through experience. **We have found nothing close to as valuable for understanding hypoglycemia, hyperinsulinism, and glucose intolerance as the testimony of those who have suffered with the disease and have learned how to control it.** They alone understand the condition.[31] Though their experiences are different, the principles they have found, and by which they can live a normal life, are very largely in agreement.

Deborah told me that the problem with the doctors is that, "Nobody believes you. They say, 'Oh yeah, I have that reaction too. I just eat a candy bar and I'm fine.'" Yes, that's you, but your advice can be a disaster for others.

It is amazing to me that the same doctors who tell a diabetic that a blood sugar spike is unhealthy, or even dangerous, somehow cannot understand that a blood sugar spike is also unhealthy for someone who is *not* a diabetic. In fact, spikes in blood sugar stress the organs and can be dangerous whether we are diabetic or not. They can be avoided by those who have an abnormal blood sugar condition simply by eating a proper hypoglycemic/diabetic diet. Unfortunately, it is highly unlikely that your doctor knows what that diet is.

It is probably _not_ in your best interest to use the word "hypoglycemia" with your doctor. If you do, more than likely he will think you are nuts and "turn off" to anything else you have to say. However, if you show him your log of blood tests and test kit, he may respond in a more professional way.

Although I have met several people who understand non-diabetic hypoglycemia, I have only met one medical doctor who does. That is because he suffers from it himself. He was a client of mine, and one day I saw him pull out a bag of sunflower seed kernels just like I had seen my wife do for many years. He looked pale and weakened, and I knew exactly what he was getting the seeds out for—he needed fuel. I asked him if he was hypoglycemic, and he nodded. As he munched on his sunflower seeds, I told him that my wife was hypoglycemic also and that she carried around a bag of sunflower seeds for emergency fuel too. Even though he was in a low blood sugar state, this doctor lit up—someone understood! We talked about the dangers of eating candy at such a time—how it will pick you up, but if your case is chronic, you will crash shortly afterwards and may be worse off. He told me how he had learned to control his condition by timing his meals and eating correctly. He also told me that though he timed his medical procedures with great diligence to coincide with his meals, sometimes if he felt he was "in trouble" (any hypoglycemic knows exactly what is meant by that), he would lick some hard tack candy to help get through a procedure. At such times he did not have a choice. He needed to get his blood sugar up immediately. He also knew how much sugar he should take at such times.

This doctor understood the need to keep the blood sugar at close to a constant level, and he understood the difficulties of someone with high or low blood sugar to do that. He also understood the importance of eating only the proper wholesome foods.[32]

I said something to him about the standard medical industry response to hypoglycemia. As he chewed his sunflower seeds slowly, he just rolled his eyes and shook his head. He obviously had had his battles, and like every hypoglycemic I have spoken with who has overcome their problem, he knew the uselessness of combating that one.

The point is this: **if you have this condition, do not expect your doctor to understand it.** To understand would be to go against his or her medical training, and they are not going to do it. If you have the condition, you may want to do what we did and take charge of the problem yourself by getting your diet straightened out. For one whose condition has become a repeated or continual problem, I don't believe there is a good alternative.

Unfortunately, people often let their blood sugar condition get so bad that by the time they switch their diet, there is a lot of damage to repair. The body cannot repair itself that quickly, and there is no wonder drug to heal a damaged pancreas, damaged adrenals, a damaged thyroid, a damaged liver, or an endocrine system that is out of whack.

Hypoglycemia, hyperinsulinism, and glucose intolerance are huge subjects, and by necessity we have gained a practical understanding of them. Once any of these conditions becomes chronic, there are no quick fixes. For a person with any of these conditions, the only protection is a good understanding of exactly what they are dealing with, because only they can make the adjustments needed in order to maintain a normal life.

The Glucose Tolerance Test
We need to talk about the Glucose Tolerance Test, which is recommended by mainstream medical practitioners to test for diabetes and reactive hypoglycemia. The test is very simple—you consume enough sugar to kill a horse, and if you have a bad reaction to it, if your pancreas can't handle it, you have "scientific proof" that you have a problem. Well, if your pancreas was on the verge of collapsing before you submitted to the test, by the time you have ingested all that poison…

Perhaps a reasonable alternative to subjecting yourself to such madness would be to simply change to a healthy diet and see if you feel better. Of course, this is criticized as being "unscientific" by those who claim to be so much smarter than we common folk.

I am not making this "scientific" and "unscientific" stuff up. We have heard this over and over again for decades. It is the standard medical industry line. The prevailing attitude is that they are scientific and that everyone else is a quack or just plain stupid.

More needs to be said about the Glucose Tolerance Test, and again what needs to be said is best told with a true story. This is the story of a friend of ours.

Sally came from a well-to-do family. She was a college student when we met her, and when Deborah found out that she was also hypoglycemic, the two became close friends. Sally told her that sometimes her blood sugar would go so low that she would pass out. This had happened so often that her roommate was accustomed to it and knew how to help her if she found her in that state.

Sally had taken the Glucose Tolerance Test and performed well. No problem, she was not diabetic.

Why didn't the test show her low blood sugar condition? Because Sally's body did not behave in a "scientific" way. It did not always react the same. And so it is. It is too bad that the medical establishment will not acknowledge this.

And I find it amazing that the test did not kill her.

There are a lot of factors when it comes to blood sugar, and the body will not always respond in the same way. That is not unscientific, it is life.

Dr. Julian Whitaker, MD, in his *Guide to Natural Healing*, does not give much credibility to the Glucose Tolerance Test and related tests. By related tests, he is referring to testing the epinephrine (adrenaline). He then goes on to say that, "The most useful measurement of diagnosing hypoglycemia is often a more old fashioned method: assessing symptoms."[33]

It is not only we who object to the Glucose Tolerance Test, and Dr. Whitaker is not the only MD to state its unreliability. Many medical doctors are very much against it. But they are in the minority and are, in effect, shouted down.

The Diabetes Doctor and "A True Hypoglycemic"

The complete inability of American mainstream medical doctors to deal with non-diabetic low blood sugar, however, may best be illustrated by the story I will tell you next.

Having a long family history of blood sugar problems, I too developed a low blood sugar condition. A client of mine, who was a diabetic, told me I should go see his doctor. I did. I filled out all the forms, took all the tests, told him the trouble I was experiencing, and he examined me.

After the test results came in, I went back for a consultation. This doctor was probably in his late sixties, was a diabetic himself, and had spent his entire career treating diabetes. I was his last patient of the day, and he was quite interested in my case and in what I had learned up to that point.

But I was an enigma to him. He told me that I was not hypoglycemic and that in all of his practice he had only encountered four "true" hypoglycemics. By that time I was accustomed to Deborah being called a nutcase for saying she was hypoglycemic, so I did not press him for an explanation, and he did not offer one. But he seemed at that time to be grasping the concept that there in front of him was someone who had a definite blood sugar problem but was neither diabetic nor what he called a "true hypoglycemic." My condition did not match what he had been taught. I had all the symptoms of low blood sugar, yet my glucose test did not reveal it.

This doctor knew that he was dealing with a pancreas problem and that it could lead to diabetes. I knew that too. But all he had understood to be true did not fit the patient before him. He sent his office help home and pondered in silence for quite a long time. I waited patiently for him to sort out what was going on in his mind. Eventually he came out of his contemplations and told me something like, "I'm sorry, I don't know how to help you. **You know your body better than anyone else can; do what it tells you to do.**" Then in a very unsatisfied voice, with a forced half-chuckle to ease his discomfort and mine—though he knew it did neither—he added, "And if you ever become a diabetic, come see me. I can help you then."

He retired within a year or so and died from diabetic complications shortly thereafter. Up until my appointment with him, he was the only medical doctor we had met who could at least somewhat see beyond his training to the obvious.

"A true hypoglycemic." We have heard that term since and can only conclude that Deborah, Sally, and I, and so many others we know, are false ones. Sorry, but this is so ridiculous it is not worth commenting upon further. Or at least that is how I was going to end this paragraph. While writing this book, however, I learned what he probably meant by "true hypoglycemics." It is that the blood sugar count is below 40 mg/dl. I read this definition in *Total Nutrition*, edited by Victor Herbert, MD, and have since seen this number in other sources. I suppose that definition must have been put in the medical textbooks. Normal levels are 80-110 mg/dl. At 40 mg/dl, you are close to a coma.[34] If this is what medical students are taught, no wonder our physicians have no understanding of the condition![35]

I want to go back to the statement made by the doctor mentioned above: "You know your body better than anyone else; do what it tells you to do." There is no wiser statement that can be made. We have a God-given intuition, and it is wise to pay attention to it. The caveat is that if sugar is in the diet, it is commonly making so much noise that it is unlikely that anything else can be heard.

The difficulty that American medical practice has with non-diabetic hypoglycemia is that there is no money in treating it. It is taken care of simply by proper diet. I would like to think that simple ignorance is behind this stance, but when you follow the money and see the huge revenue stream in the diabetes business that would be cut off by addressing this correctly…

But the Good News Is,
If you have hypoglycemia, or if the list of symptoms earlier in this chapter looks too familiar, take heart! Hypoglycemia, hyperinsulinism, glucose intolerance, and even diabetes can be managed. Everyone's case is unique, but certain common principles

apply, and by understanding those principles, we can figure out how to manage our own condition. And if we stay on it, it may not be that difficult. Thankfully, many people have gone before and have figured out a lot of it for us.

Blood Sugar Mechanics and Band Practice
The mechanics of blood sugar and the intricate function of the pancreas with the other glands and organs are so complex that no one will ever be able to understand them. On the other hand, the basic principle of this function is quite easy to grasp. If the pancreas is continually overworked—and eating the way the great majority of us do, it is overworked—it will ask the adrenals to help. The adrenals step up and demand more insulin. So your pancreas secretes more, and now you are overloaded with insulin. If this goes on too long, the pancreas starts shutting down, and instead of producing an excess of insulin, now it will not produce enough. In some cases the pancreas shuts down too much, and to stay alive you may now need to take insulin for the rest of your life. **In other words, the creditors are at the door**, your pancreas is failing, and now you are a full-blown diabetic. **And in most cases, it could have been prevented**.[36]

It's worse than that. In the process just described, **other glands and organs are involved too.** They work in concert, not as individuals, and now they are out of whack too.

The principle behind this malfunction is as simple to understand as band practice at school. The liver acts like the bass drum and lays down the beat. It processes the sugars we ingest, converts them into different forms, and is supposed to release them in the right timing. The pancreas, like the snare drum, fills in some of the details of the rhythm that the bass drum establishes. The adrenals are the trumpets who sound the call to arms, all the other instruments join in at their appropriate times, and it all works very well when they play in concert.

But a little kid finds a feather duster (refined sugar) in the janitor's room (your grocery store), gets into the band room, goes over behind the bass drum player, and starts tickling his ear with it (you eat that sugar). Now the bass drum player (the liver) is distracted by the added stimulus and can't keep the beat, so the snare drum (the pancreas) takes over. But the kid keeps tickling the bass player's ear (you ingest more sugar), so the bass player nods to the trumpet players (the adrenals) and they move over behind the snare drum player and blast away at his head. The snare player goes berserk and starts pounding away (secretes too much insulin). The piccolo player (the thyroid) now gets into the act, because he's supposed to manage this section of the music (the rate of metabolism), but by this time all the other instruments (organs and glands) have gone off and are playing according to their understanding of what they are supposed to do. What comes out is not smooth jazz, but rather a highly irritating jumble of noise. The music that the whole school (your body) was enjoying now sounds so bad that everyone is distracted and set on edge. No one can concentrate, all profitable work ceases, and everyone is ticked off.

In such a case, only a deaf band conductor ("health care" professional) who is paid by the hour, and not by his performance, would try to instruct (write prescriptions for) the various instruments on how to play better. A wise conductor, on the other hand—and one who must get results—would simply go over to the little child who is tickling the bass drum player's ear, take him by the hand, escort him out of the room, and lock the door.

Whether I have presented the functions of the organs adequately or not is immaterial. The point is, get the brat out of the room!

The problem is it's not funny. Many of us have damaged organs that have forgotten how to play in concert with the rest of the body and have taken the lead in telling us of their unhappiness.

This is why hypoglycemia is at the same time difficult, yet easy, to understand. The only one who can't figure it out is your doctor. He is still looking at the music sheet and thinking, "No, that French horn *was* playing the wrong note."

Living with Hypoglycemia
Once you have developed a blood sugar abnormality, there are no quick fixes. Hypoglycemia or glucose intolerance is not one condition; it is a set of conditions which involves the adrenals, the

thyroid, the liver, and the other glands and organs. But, as I said, take heart—there is a way to lead a normal life. The solution is quite simple: Turn the diet around.

Later in the book, I will discuss in detail why your doctor does not tell you about the diet imperative, but for now let me just say that some of the better physicians do—but they tend to be too mealy-mouthed about it. Very few, if any, will get in your face *at the early stages* of a blood sugar problem and tell you in no uncertain terms that you must get sugar and refined carbohydrates out of your diet or the consequences can be disastrous. I believe there are two reasons your doctor will not do this:

1. He or she could lose their medical license if they did. (Much more on this later.)
2. They know full well that most people will go get a second opinion and hear what they want to hear. And your doctor—just like you and I—has bills to pay.

Many doctors genuinely believe that their patients cannot control themselves or act responsibly concerning their health. This is part of their training, and in fact there is plenty of evidence to back up that thought. Many people will not be responsible, period. The problem is that every time a physician or patient gives in to this behavior they reinforce the premise.

The point is this: We need to take responsibility for our own health. We cannot expect others to keep our best interests in mind when there is so much money involved in the business of keeping us unhealthy and dependent. As with a diabetic who does not want to go on the medication roller coaster, a hypoglycemic needs to understand his or her condition inside and out. They must listen to what their bodies are telling them and make the necessary adjustments.

One who is hypoglycemic, and particularly one who also has adrenal abnormalities, must learn to accept the fact that he or she cannot live as other people live. Drinking coffee, soda pop, and alcohol may be for others, but not for him. Eating sweets and fast-burning carbohydrates may be what others do, but he does not dare do so. Living a careless life, lacking in self-control, others may—but not him. Furthermore, he must always reserve at least a little energy. He cannot afford to run out or he will be sick. With that reserve, he or she can function normally and live a fulfilling life.

Many have gone before and proven it.

The "Why" Behind the Disease

The biggest health problem in the US is that we Americans are long accustomed to a diet that is killing us. Someone who drives over the speed limit as a matter of course has no right to complain if she eventually gets a speeding ticket—even if at the time she was only going five miles an hour over the speed limit. It is the same with someone who eats refined foods. There are consequences. It does not matter if "everyone is doing it." We may seem to get away with it for decades, but actually it is not so. For many of us, it's time to pay the piper. Neither hypoglycemia nor diabetes are strange things that happen to us. We just got pulled over. And now we cannot "get away with it" anymore.

Unfortunately, the seriousness of diabetes is downplayed. It is portrayed by a **hundred billion dollar industry**[37] as manageable. Just keep "smoking their dope" and you can eat anything you want.

I wish I was exaggerating.

"Do you have a sweet tooth? With a little planning, you can go ahead and enjoy your favorite desserts." So says the American Diabetes Association.[38]

A Hypoglycemia Summary:

Hypoglycemia is a metabolic disorder that involves the pancreas, liver, and other organs and glands. The pancreas itself is both an organ and a gland, and is one of the least understood parts the body. It is a part of the digestive system, and it is also a part of the endocrine system. As a gland, the pancreas produces several hormones, and insulin, which regulates the blood sugar, is one of them. As an organ, the pancreas secretes pancreatic juices that contain digestive enzymes that assist in the absorption of nutrients—carbohydrates, fats, proteins, etc. These functions are highly complex and have been compromised in a person with any kind of blood sugar problem, whether it is hypoglycemia, hyperinsulinism, diabetes, or any kind of glucose intolerance.

Here is a brief sketch of what we are dealing with in hypoglycemia:

1. The condition, as described in this chapter, is denied by the medical profession due to enormous conflicts of interest.
2. Medical tests for the condition are woefully inadequate or are even misleading, because there are simply too many factors involved with the condition.
3. If the pancreas is not functioning properly—and this is the case with any blood sugar disorder—then the adrenal glands are not functioning properly either.
4. If that is the case, the endocrine system—which functions in concert—is compromised.
5. If that is the case, any number of ill health issues can be brought on.
6. And it all goes back to a blood sugar problem.
7. And that goes back to excess consumption of sugar.

Back to Deborah's Story

All this discussion of blood sugar problems gives the reader a better understanding as to why, after twenty-three years, Deborah's body was telling her, "Enough! You are not going to abuse me anymore."

But there was a lot more to Deborah's ill health than low blood sugar or hypoglycemia. Hypoglycemia was just the tip of the iceberg. Unfortunately, in this she is not a rarity.

Caution!
I must remind the reader of the warning that follows the preface at the beginning of the book. I am only a reporter, telling you of our experience and observations, and the conclusions we have drawn from them. I am not telling anyone what to do in their situation. Everyone's situation is unique, and all of us need to be responsible for caring for our own body.

Resources

The resources given here are decades old. Even so, I have found no better information anywhere.

New Low Blood Sugar and You, by Carlton Fredericks, 1985
In our opinion this is **a "must read"** for anyone who has several of the symptoms described in this chapter.

www.fred.net/slowup/hai185.html
This is from the Adrenal Metabolic Research Society of the Hypoglycemia Foundation and is the work of Dr. John W. Tintera, MD. He and his wife both had the condition. They know what they are talking about.

Is Low Blood Sugar Making You a Nutritional Cripple? By Ruth Adams and Frank Murray, 1970

Banting's Miracle, by Seale Harris, MD, 1946
This is the biography of the discoverer of insulin written by a medical doctor who specialized in diabetes and who, after the discovery of insulin, identified non-diabetic hypoglycemia. A large medical clinic in the South is named after the author, but his extensive work on non-diabetic hypoglycemia has been all but destroyed. If you want to see how far current medical practice has departed from common sense when it comes to diabetes and non-diabetic hypoglycemia, read this book. It is out of print, but can still be obtained. Ask your librarian to get it for you, or better yet try online used booksellers such as abe.com.

Chapter 5
Taking Care of the Children

"An ounce of prevention is worth a pound of cure."

In this chapter, I want to tell you what propelled Deborah to take care of herself. It was the needs of our children. She was determined that she would have healthy children, and her resolve was in the midst of her own physical adversity. She was not, and is not, a superwoman—just a normal one.

Deborah did not have much strength. What she did have was a clear vision, or understanding, of how she was going to care for her children, and the result of that vision was hope. We are certainly not the only ones who have proved repeatedly that where there is willingness to do the right thing, there is also divine guidance and strength to carry it out.

It was our son's needs that started us on the road to alternative medicine. As mentioned in the first chapter, he was born in physical distress. He was sickly as a child, and after his birth, the medical doctors we saw were of no help whatsoever. After we gave up on the doctors, the antibiotics, and the decongestants (see Ch. 1), Deborah discovered that she could "turn the corner" on our son's illnesses faster than the antibiotic could, and could do it with no downside.

What she did was make a food-medicine in a base of plain yogurt. It consisted of desiccated liver, cod liver oil, vitamin C, and a vitamin B complex tablet squished up. The cod liver oil and vitamin C are both natural antibiotics. Her goal was to fortify the immune system as powerfully as she could. She put it this way: "With the prescriptions, it had taken about 24 hours before we started to see the effect. I figured I could beat that time, and did. Within 24 hours, the children were coming out of their illnesses. I determined that if that didn't work, I'd go to the doctor.

"We never had to."

Deborah's best resources at that time were two "folk medicine" books: *Back to Eden* by Jethro Kloss and *Kitchen Medicine* by Ben Charles Harris. She learned to treat all the illnesses and maladies we had naturally—usually with things that we already had in the pantry or spice cabinet.

Our children, like all children, are different. Our daughter had different inherent weaknesses than our son had. So they needed to be cared for individually. Our daughter had food allergies and an asthma-like condition. Our son was obviously hypoglycemic. Deborah learned early on that, "All foods do not agree with everyone, but everyone should eat the nutritional foods that agree best with them."[39]

Deborah only fed her family with natural foods. She made yogurt popsicles, hearty breads, and nutritious meals, and the kids loved it all. She also made various teas—both to drink and to apply to the body.

At the same time that she was learning what was good for us, she learned what was not good for us. She avoided mineral oil-based products, because they can deplete stored vitamins, and alcohol-based products, because of her allergies. She eliminated unnecessary household chemicals, such as most cleaning products.

Our children grew up without a pediatrician, and we had no family doctor. Our family took no medications. Our medicines were the food we ate, supplemented with vitamins, minerals, herbs, and enzymes.

Not only have we not had any antibiotics in the house, our children never had a cough drop or throat lozenge in their mouths. They rarely had a pimple, and still may not know what an antacid is. They never had a bite of junk food and never had a cavity.

Concerning junk food and cavities: Perhaps the biggest help was that we did not own a television during their early years. Countless temptations of body, soul (mind and emotion), and spirit were avoided. Without that distraction, our children became very good readers at a young age. They had no trouble concentrating in school. Our biggest challenge was running fast enough to put good educational material in front of them.

My reason for telling you this is to state emphatically that it can be done. Many parents have proven it. Frankly, life is hard enough; why add to the burden by undermining the foundations of health?

Three Interesting Notes:
First, our children did get sick every year, and it was always right after school started. Some years they got sick more than once. It was usually the same kind of illness—a snorky nose with a slight infection. At the time, we did not know how to counter this. All we knew was to fortify them with the food-medicine I told you about earlier, but that alone did not prevent them from getting sick.

Second, both children came to us (separately and at different times) when they were young adults and told us how thankful they were that we did not have a television during their early years. By the time we bought one, they were too well-adjusted and had very little interest in it. Even when the best sporting events were on (that is what we bought the set for), none of us had the patience to sit through an entire game. We all had better things to do.

Third, when our daughter went off to college, she proved for herself where cavities come from. After quickly earning a few, she went back to the way she was raised and eliminated sugar from her diet.

Time, and Choosing Life
I know a lot of readers are thinking that the way of life described here takes time. Yes, it does. A new way of life needs to be learned; and we can pay now or pay later. But look what we gained. The health of our children today is a direct result of all that effort. Furthermore, they know how to take care of themselves and are a help to others also.

A side benefit we are receiving from this is that our children now share what they observe and learn with us. In many cases the students have become the teachers. We learn from each other.

And I think that's the way it should be.

Much later, when our daughter was an adult and having lunch with some work associates, the conversation turned to the evils of sugar. I seems everyone at the table was aware that eating sugar was not a good thing to do, but one of the ladies shrugged and said, "Well, you can't keep kids from eating sugar." Our daughter's reply was, "Oh, yes you can! My momma did it!"

I have a lot more to say about healthy eating in later chapters, but here it is sufficient to say this **concerning food: "If God made it, it's good; the more man messes with it, the more unhealthful it becomes."**

For Deborah to take the way of a healthy lifestyle was not a philosophy she bought into. It was a matter of survival. For her, it was as clear as, "I have set before you life and death... therefore choose life."[40]

Use of Vitamins

I mentioned our use of vitamins with the children, and although I have a lot more to say about the subject later, I need to address two matters here: Many people have been told by their doctors that vitamins are a waste of money, because they get all the vitamins they need from their food. Some people have also been warned about overdosing with vitamins. They have heard that this is possible, and they are afraid to use dietary supplements because of that. I will address both issues briefly.

First, it is an amazing thing that those who say that vitamins are a waste of money always seem to be those who are charging a lot more than the cost of vitamins for their services.

Second, with the basic vitamins needed—the B *complex* and vitamin C—it would be difficult to harm yourself if you used any common sense whatsoever.

An overdose of vitamins and *food* supplements is quite different from an overdose of a powerful medication. As long as you use moderation and don't make things too complex by adding too many items, it is easy for your body to tell you how you are doing, and you can respond accordingly.

Deborah told me, "Overdosing of a vitamin or supplement was pretty easy to identify. I knew when I had reached the tolerance level, because a headache would be the result. So, at that point I backed off. The kids got fish liver oil two times a week instead of every day."

In our home, bug bites and bee stings received a similar yogurt treatment as that mentioned earlier in this chapter, just applied to the skin. The liquid would dry into a film, and the treatment worked just as well topically as it did orally. I mention this here because it is important to know the value of topical applications.

Professional Help and Wise Counsel

As stated earlier, we did not have a family medical doctor during this time. If Deborah felt she needed some help, she went to see Dr. Bundy.

Dr. Bundy was a chiropractor.

I know very well that many people freak out when they hear the term "chiropractor." They have been told by their medical doctor that chiropractors are quacks and that they will hurt them. There are probably some people who picked up this book, saw the word "chiropractic" in the Table of Contents, immediately put it down, and would read no further. From our experience in speaking with such people, the overwhelming majority of them have had no personal experience with chiropractic whatsoever. They have simply been instilled with fear by the AMA folks who have a great dislike for competition. (See Appendix IV.)

I am not claiming that all chiropractors are good or that some people have not had bad experiences with them. Far from it. I am saying that it should stand to reason that long-standing proven alternatives such as chiropractic, acupuncture, herbal remedies, etc. have a legitimate basis.

Many people have come to realize the deceptive nature of the quick-acting medications that our medical system is built around. They have begun to understand that too often these medications do nothing more than mask symptoms—symptoms we are given so that we will know that there is an underlying cause of ill health.

Dr. Bundy was an extraordinary man who understood the ability of the body to heal itself. He was not presumptuous, although he had as good an understanding of the human body as anyone we have ever known. And, although he knew it well, he was not limited to the standard Palmer School method of chiropractic. He was very intuitive, he listened, and his attitude was to work with you to help you understand how to care for yourself.

There is a discussion of chiropractic in Chapter 8, and I tell of several cases from our experience in Chapter 22, but Dr. Bundy needs to be mentioned here because it was he who helped us during the time we were raising the children.

In taking the responsibility of caring for ourselves and for our family, we do need the help and counsel of others. Which others is the question.

At the top of that list Deborah and I put our Creator. We, and millions of others before us, have proved the veracity of the words, *"Trust in the Lord with all your heart, and do not lean on your own understanding. In all your ways acknowledge Him, and He will direct your paths."* [41]

Chapter 6
Living and Dying

I use the word "living" in the chapter title because a few years after her collapse, Deborah was able to function somewhat normally. She was on her feet again, was able to work from the home, and took care of her children and husband. This was a huge improvement over where she had been.

I use the word "dying" in the chapter title because the list of foods and chemicals that she reacted to grew with each passing year. So did other sensitivities.

The sensitivities that Deborah suffered from are experienced by many people. Deborah, like the canary in the coal mine, simply experienced them under milder conditions than most of us do. So, canaries like Deborah serve as an early warning system for the rest of us.

As you read this chapter, it is *highly* likely that you will gain some insight into one or more factors that negatively affect you or someone you know. For that reason, I will briefly discuss some of Deborah's ailments here.

Deborah's **sensitivity to noise** was acute. The clanging of dishes or of silverware—however slight to someone else—was excruciatingly painful to her. Sometimes she would inadvertently yell, "Stop that!" when someone else was the responsible party. Moderately louder talk was piercing, so she often wore ear plugs. She loved it when I played the piano but always wore ear plugs to cut the edge off the sound.

She had **elevation sickness.** Deborah was sick on every vacation we took. She almost always had migraines, often had heart palpitations, and sometimes could not breathe very well. It took us a long time to understand that this was often due to a change in elevation. We usually went up to the mountains for our vacations, but not always, so the problem was difficult to isolate.

Eventually, a client of mine who was a physician explained this to me. She explained that just like most people will experience elevation sickness at 10,000 feet or so, some people have the same symptoms at lower elevations. The cause is the same—pressure on the internal organs and brain. But why did Deborah experience this at considerably lower elevations? The answer was to elude us for decades. One thing we did understand after talking to my client, was that many of her other illnesses were due to changes in atmospheric pressure. It was not just a matter of elevation, but of pressure. That is why she always felt good when it rained.

Deborah also developed **arthritis.** She had joint pain, first in her elbows and knees, and later in her hands. Arthritis is a condition in which toxins accumulate at the joints. The need, she learned from reading her books, is to purify the blood. She used chaparral (which later was removed from the market) and burdock root, which in time alleviated the problem. If she goes off burdock supplementation for too long, the condition will return. Taking it *as part of her regimen* has made the arthritis easy to manage.[42]

From time to time Deborah would complain about feeling "**pins and needles**," sometimes in her joints, sometimes not.[43]

When Deborah was in her early thirties, she had some dental work done and **reacted to the Novocaine.** When she got home from the appointment, she collapsed on the floor and was unable to hold her head up. She had no strength in her muscles or spine. When she finally had enough strength to call the dentist, he told her not to worry, it would wear off. Thankfully, after a few days it did. He told us what we had become well accustomed to hearing: "I've never heard of that before."

We have since learned that Deborah's reaction is not rare at all. The dentist merely had been taught what all dentists are taught—that there are certain risks with Novocaine and all other anesthesia and to keep his mouth shut. Regardless, it was clear to us that we were not going to get any further help from him.

At the time, we were still naïve and thought that doctors first and foremost wanted to help people. Now we understand more and can only think that his concern was not Deborah's health, but his own liability. It is a pity that we live in a society where the one who speaks the truth or behaves properly so easily becomes a prey.

By that time, we knew better than to go to a medical doctor concerning Deborah's reaction. That they knew nothing other than to medicate had been proven to us too many times before. If we took her to the doctor, we knew that they would want to medicate her, and there was no possibility that they would believe that Deborah was as sensitive as she is.

There was no World Wide Web in the early 1980s, and in the many health books we had, there was nothing about reaction to Novocaine. What Deborah did know to do was to flush with vitamin C. How effective that was, we don't know. She was in a collapsed state for several days, and it was quite scary until she began to come out of it.

One of the take-home lessons here is that the eating of sweets that leads to tooth decay is not a minor thing. Dental work can have very serious complications—even decades after the initial tooth decay is dealt with. I have much more to say about this in Chapters 9 and 10.

Food Allergies[44]
Deborah saw an **allergist**. However, in the late 1970s and early 1980s these specialists were not checking for foods but only for hay fever and the like. Mentioning reactions to chemicals or anything else got a blank look. Concerning reactions to foods, their treatment was abstinence. But it was becoming increasingly difficult to find foods that Deborah could eat that she would not react to.

During all this time, Deborah prepared two dinners every evening—one for herself, and one for the kids and me.

In the mid-1980s, Deborah found a medical doctor who was treating allergies by purifying a person's urine and then injecting it into their muscle tissue. His technique was "off the wall," but we had a referral from a patient who had been helped, and we felt that the theory might have some merit. More to the point, we had to try something.[45] But the treatments were ineffective.

As time went on, other foods, including beef, wheat, corn, and soy were by necessity eliminated from Deborah's diet. By the way, either wheat, corn, or soy, or a combination of them, are in just about every processed food.

Deborah still had oats, rice, nuts, carrots, onions, and dairy in her diet, but all these and many more foods were to eventually drop off of the list of foods she could tolerate.[46] Since she could not get the necessary nutrients from foods, Deborah stayed alive with the help of dietary supplements. She reacted to many of them too. She read up on them, but what would work and what would not eventually came down to trial and error.

Through her food allergies, Deborah learned a life of discipline and gained a depth of self-control that I have seen in very few people. There was no good alternative. Although she was a lot better off than she had been, and the crisis state was alleviated, the overall decline of her health kept progressing. All she was doing was slowing it down.

Reactions to Chemicals

In the mid-1980s, about a decade after her food allergies had begun in earnest, Deborah began having reactions to chemicals. About this time we went to visit her mother, who lived nearly 400 miles away. Before we left to return home, Deborah washed her vegetables off in the water at her mother's kitchen sink. Her reaction to the soft water on the vegetables was so severe that she vomited nearly all the way home.

Deborah had had a few chemical sensitivities before, but now they came with a fury. It even got to the point where, when we were traveling, she could only use two kinds of bottled water without having a negative reaction. To water!

She reacted very negatively to cleaning products, so she learned how to use vinegar, borax, and baking soda to clean with. She reacted to commercial deodorants, so began using baking soda. (And she still smells sweet. ☺)

The negative reactions to environmental factors were accumulative and often got worse. She could not tolerate the off-gassing of plastics. Once we purchased a new bed that was a top-of-the-line model by a major manufacturer. After it was delivered, I took off the plastic wrapping and began to set up the bed. The mattress was so fumy *I* could hardly stand it. I was shocked. Apparently, the mattress in the showroom that we had seen had already off-gassed. By the time I realized there was a problem, the delivery people were gone and had taken our old bed with them. We could not return the new one. We spread baking soda on the mattress and covered it with layers of sheets and blankets. For months, every day we aired out the room for as long as we could. We renewed the baking soda. Deborah took plenty of extra detoxification products and did regular enemas. Neither of us got sick—at least not in a way that was immediately noticeable—but fighting the potential toxicity was war.

In the late 1990s, Deborah commuted to Long Beach for her work. When she passed the oil refinery between Carson and Long Beach, she would instantly become extremely drowsy. She fought it off, but at least one time she thinks she may have fallen asleep at the wheel. She bought a high quality air purifier for her car, and the problem ceased.

Thyroid

In the late 1980s, Deborah got a referral to a medical doctor whom she decided to try. This doctor believed that **thyroid deficiency** was responsible for a myriad of problems. In his mind, if the thyroid was off, everything was off. He tested her for thyroid function, determined she was deficient, and prescribed natural thyroid supplementation.[47] The thyroid he prescribed is derived from the thyroid glands of pigs.

This physician was different from the other medical doctors Deborah had seen. He would listen to her. She told me, "To some extent we were peers sharing information." (By that time Deborah was a wealth of proven health information, and one would have been foolish not to listen to her.) This physician helped her understand her blood tests, gave her the customary examinations, and introduced her to colonics. Eventually, he confided in her that he knew that the direction that American medical practice was going was not in the best interest of the people they were serving. He also told her that he spent a lot of his time reading "alternative" health publications.

Deborah believes that going on the thyroid was the right course of action to take. Some of her health conditions did seem to even out, at least a little. But the doctor could not help her much.

Referrals

I should point out here that we have always tried to get a personal referral from someone who has been helped by a health practitioner before we go see them. Advertising is absolutely the worst way to select a washing machine repairman, let alone a health professional. And those lists of medical specialists given out by a clinic or by your doctor may be nothing more than advertising.

There is nothing like a *patient* referral—hence the necessity of developing a network of friends and contacts. That is what this book is about—the sharing of information. There is no substitute for it. The most help we have received has been from reading health-related publications[48] and speaking with people who themselves have had some challenges and are pursuing a healthy lifestyle. We follow no one blindly.

In our opinion, health professionals can only help us so much. If we are not managing our own health the best we know how, the value of their help may be minimal and can even be a net negative.

Electronics and Electromagnetic Fields

With the advent of cordless phones, cell phones, and now Wi-Fi, traffic transponders, and GPS, the amount of potentially harmful electromagnetism and electronic waves we are subjected to has increased dramatically. These threats to health continue to increase at a feverish pace.

When the cordless and cell phones arrived, we were not aware of electromagnetic fields (EMFs), or if we were, we certainly did not know of their harmful effects. By that time, in the late 1980s, Deborah had started a new career and was using a cell phone for her work. Early on she had pain in her hand and arm. She thought she was pinching a nerve when holding the cell phone, because her hand would tingle. Later, her ear and the base of her skull started getting numb when she used the phone. With the cordless phone, she experienced a piercing pain in her ear and across the base of the skull. When using a corded phone, it was painful, but not nearly as bad. We tried everything—we got rid of the cordless phones, put cotton in the other telephone receivers, used ear plugs, and bought special earpieces. I researched the problem as best I could and came up with nothing. I called the phone company on the off chance they might offer some help. The response I got was not a surprise—"Uh, we don't know. We've never heard of anything like that." Again, this was an untrue public stance, no doubt because of potential lawsuits. It is not true that the telephone industry is unaware of the health problems related to electromagnetic fields, or EMFs.

This kind of response—and we have met it everywhere for decades—was, and is, difficult to take. Nevertheless, this is the world we live in, and we must be the ones to adjust.

Eventually, we found out that Deborah's condition is not rare at all.

In the year 2000, an ear specialist confirmed that Deborah had hearing loss in her left ear. Deborah's job required heavy telephone work, and eventually the pain got so bad that she had to quit her job. We decided not to file a workman's compensation or disability claim. From our research, we understood that if something happened to my income, Deborah could be greatly limiting her future employment if she filed either kind of claim.[49]

Telephones were not the only problem. High voltage electrical transmission lines became troublesome too. We could no longer walk along the bike path near our home because of the power lines. The severity of her reaction increased as time went on. Eventually, she could no longer drive on certain streets where there were high voltage lines. When she got near the power lines she would have tremors from her forehead to her chest. Sometimes it also tingled down her arms.[50]

Deborah began to notice that her face would tingle when she was in front of certain computer monitors. The same happened if she got too close to a television. This hit a crescendo when laptop computers came out. The waves given off by these devices are several times more powerful than those given off by a conventional monitor.

The good thing about this problem is that by the late 1990s, information was much more readily available. Actually, it is not a good thing. The reason that the information is now available is because many more people are suffering from the effects of electro-magnetic fields. Although neither the industry that manufactures these devices nor our government[51] will advise us of the hazards of the products, there are many people who are sounding out the warning. All are called quacks or neurotics by the medical establishment. I call them canaries. My canary and the other canaries in the mine are giving their early warnings. Can you hear them?[52]

What to do? We live in a deep sea of electromagnetic waves, and it is not possible to eliminate exposure. But we may not have to live next to a cell phone site, we don't have to put a TV dish on the roof above our bed, we don't have to wear a "Bluetooth,"[53] and we can turn off our cell phone at least sometimes.

Thankfully, some people have also come up with what are called EMF modifiers. These devices, which themselves give off a charge, are made to cancel the waves of EMFs.[54] Deborah wore a Teslar watch and a copper coil EMF interrupter called a Q-link. She also placed diodes (small electrically charged pieces of stone or metal) on our cell phones. At least some of these devices work. With the aid of the diodes and Q link, Deborah can use a laptop computer now without any problem. She uses her cell phone only in a pinch—perhaps a few times a year.

Those who say that EMFs are no problem deride all this as quackery. They will probably continue to do so until they or someone they love has a problem. Hopefully some readers will listen to the canaries and make adjustments if they are called for.

Before leaving off discussing EMFs, I will tell you a (somewhat) humorous story about EMF modifiers. We have an electrician friend who has been zapped a few too many times. His body became charged, and he suffered for years because of it. Then he found out about EMF modifiers. He uses some very strong ones (they are made with different charges) and he is fine now. The funny part of this story is that one time he accidentally left one of his small, polarized, charged, glass modifiers on his wife's dresser, which is close to her side of the bed. The next morning she complained that she hardly slept that night. She never had sleep problems, so our friend thought that was a little odd. This went on for a few nights. She simply could not go to sleep. After a few days she was worn down and very cross. Then our friend remembered what he had done. He removed the seemingly innocent piece of glass from his wife's bedside, and the next morning she woke up greatly refreshed after a good night's sleep. He wouldn't tell me if he told her what the problem was, and I am not going to ask her.

Depression

Deborah told me, "Early on, I learned that depression is a very real component of physical illness—it relates directly to blood sugar and many other maladies.

"Depression can be brought on by things in our environment that we cannot control. It can even be too many things going on with friends or too much housework. If I find myself overwhelmed, I have to break back and start over. It is necessary to do something to snap the cycle and release the tension. Crying helps. It releases the tension. Then, thinking about it, I identify what it is that is bothering me, and I give myself more time. I cancel an obligation or do something to break the cycle.

"I've learned that there are certain triggers for depression. The first is exhaustion. Even if you think you are not that tired, you may in fact be. Your mind says it's not that bad when actually you are already "over the top." A good example is commuting on the freeway. Commuting is extremely exhausting and stressful.

"Another trigger to depression is hurt feelings. In our interaction with others, we can have conflict. Don't hold grudges. Let it go. Most things are not that big of a deal. And play straight up—with no hidden agendas."

Depression can be food-related. Specifically, depression can result from blood sugar highs or lows, from food sensitivities, which bring about a state of toxicity, or from a combination of the two. Straightening out the diet may solve the problem. This is trial and error, but by following the intuition the error factor is greatly reduced. We were, after all, given an intuition to protect us.[55]

Depression can also be brought on by various environmental toxins. If we are exposed to toxins (of any kind) faster than we can dispose of them, depression can result. Just being in a stuffy building or otherwise breathing bad air can affect us long after we have left the source. On the other hand, being in good, fresh air is uplifting.

The first discussion of depression that Deborah had with a doctor was with the one who put her on thyroid medication. Since she was going through early onset menopause at the time, he talked about natural body hormones and suggested that she try DHEA, and if that didn't work, to try Pregnenolone. With DHEA, Deborah experienced two weeks of euphoria, then she crashed and became very depressed. With Pregnenolone, she didn't feel a thing.

Deborah's comment? "I don't want the euphoria—it is despair waiting to happen. Just as surely as you go up, you will come down. What I want is a base line—an even keel. Even if it is low, that is better than the ups and downs."

Depression is often related to stress, and although stress is usually spoken of in negative terms these days, Deborah and I are convinced that we need enough stress and challenging work to help maintain a healthy mental outlook. What is needed is a proper balance.

Further Narrowing
As the years went by, Deborah's system was becoming more and more sensitive, but we could not figure out the reason. Her body was fighting against her, but why? She bled very little during her menstrual cycle. She was dizzy, fatigued, and frequently tense. Her muscles tired easily, and walking uphill was exhausting. Her skin was always dry, her teeth felt loose, and she could not eat food oils without getting a migraine.[56] She could not tolerate fragrances. If

someone had perfume or cologne on, Deborah would frequently have to stay away from them, or she would immediately feel a headache coming on. She had occasional intestinal cramps. When she had routine physical exams and the doctor tapped the usual places on her abdomen and asked if it hurt, she always answered "yes." It never mattered. The physicians always ignored her and went on to check something else.[57]

From the early 1990s through 2006, Deborah was down to five foods that she could eat. She also had a whole host of chemical allergies. Among them were alcohol, wood and cigarette smoke, auto exhaust, chlorine cleansers, and almost all household chemicals.

In one sense, the narrowing down of the diet was okay—she could remain relatively healthy if she avoided the things she reacted to. But eventually she was beginning to react to one of the five foods that she *could* eat. As she had gone through the cycle many times before, she knew that it would be just a matter of time and she would be down to four foods.

She started eating more tuna—it was one food that agreed with her system very well. The other foods she ate were chicken, romaine lettuce, sunflower seeds, and asparagus.

In all of her affliction, and because she could not eat what other people eat, Deborah was often the "odd person out" socially—especially for the first two decades or so. Today, some of the health conditions she has suffered with are more common, but twenty to thirty-five years ago it was not so.

Added to this, she was frequently treated with disdain by physicians from whom she had sought help. We now understand why she was treated in that way—medical doctors are taught to think of people with multiple "unexplained" symptoms as neurotic.

Thankfully, however, through her systematic experimentation, Deborah was continually gaining confidence.

Resources:
EMF Modifiers
https://www.ewater.com/
This was Deborah's best source for EMF modifiers of various kinds. The devices come polarized and non-polarized. You can read the articles on the website and even talk to Fred, who Deborah says is a wealth of knowledge on the subject.

http://www.teslar.com/ Deborah bought a watch from them which was very effective until her mercury was removed. She does not need to wear the watch now.

http://www.qlinkproducts.com Deborah wore a Q-link necklace for years before her mercury was removed. She does not use it now.

http://healthline.cc/ Dr. Bob Marshall's site.

Note: About three years after mercury removal, Deborah felt better without the watch, the Q-link necklace, and a diode that she used to carry in her pocket. We still use the diodes on our computers and cell phones, however, to create a "safe zone." For Deborah, this makes the difference of being able to use the devices or not.

Government Agency:
The Center for Devices and Radiological Health is the branch of the US FDA that will tell you that there is no "scientific basis" for saying that EMFs can cause physiological problems.

Chapter 7
Raised From the Dead

This chapter and the one following it are parenthetical. Finding the missing link to Deborah's health problems would take decades, so to write of that at this point in the book would be premature. What I want to do in this chapter is tell you the story of a dear friend of ours whom I will call Larry.

Larry was on his deathbed and had a miraculous recovery. His story mirrors Deborah's in many ways, so I have placed it here in order to introduce some important principles that are common in both of their stories of recovering health. These principles and some alternative means of care are discussed in the chapter following this one.

Larry's story underscores two very important points. First, we need to get at the root, or source, of our health problems. Second, sometimes—as in Deborah's and Larry's cases—finding that root can take a very long time, and we need to survive and remain as healthy as we can in the meantime.

Larry and his wife, Ann, used to come over sometimes on Sunday afternoons after church, and we would have lunch together. During one of these times, Larry told us the story of how he was, as he put it, raised from the dead. Before we knew him well, Larry had been on his deathbed for years. He was literally hanging between life and death.

I'll let him tell you his story here. To protect his identity and the identity of some other persons, I have changed his name and some insignificant details of his story; otherwise, what is written here is directly from the notes I took while interviewing Larry.

"In the early 1970s, I had a couple of attacks of hepatitis. One of them was severe, but it seemed that I was over it. Years later, health trouble flared up again, but neither I nor the doctors I went to were sure what it was. Eventually, I was diagnosed with hepatitis C. Later, the diagnosis was that I had hepatitis A, B, and C all at the same time.

"As time went on, I ended up very ill and was on my back nearly all the time. For long periods of time I could not walk very far at all.

"I was admitted to the hospital and after a while was dismissed, no better but having been told that there was nothing more they could do for me. The medical people who discharged me were quite concerned and didn't think I would make it. I was very gray in appearance and extremely weak.

"But I gained some strength and eventually was able to attend some business meetings. I had not been working for years, but felt I should try to do so, and did. The business I was involved in was in dire straits, and the work turned out to be horribly stressful. It hit hard, and I collapsed.

"I then went to _____, a famous research hospital. Their only course of treatment was to use steroids. But I had seen what steroids had done to a friend of mine who was put on them, and I didn't want any part of them. That man really suffered!

"An 'alternative' doctor I knew also advised me not to take the steroids unless it was absolutely a matter of life or death. From what I had seen in this friend, death would have been preferable. So I lay in bed.

"During that time, some Chinese-American friends helped me. They gave me various Chinese foods such as red rice, etc. After some time, a Chinese doctor from _____ came to the States and visited some of my Chinese friends. They told this doctor about me, and he wanted to see me.

"This man was one of the top doctors in _____. He would come over to the house and treat me with massage and acupressure. That was all he could do as he was not licensed to practice medicine here. He told me that he had become a medical doctor simply because he wanted to help people, and he could not understand the condescending methods of medical practice in this country. That really mystified and upset him.

"In China, he told me, medical doctors are required to study both traditional Chinese medicine and what they call 'American medicine.' He would say, 'I wish I had you in China, I would do this and that.' But I was in no shape to travel, and the doctor could not practice here.

"What he could do was recommend certain treatments to a Chinese American physician who in turn could write prescriptions for certain herbs. Those herbs fell into two categories: those that were to support and those that were to detoxify the body.

"The herbs did gradually help, but I was still on a roller coaster. When I would have a bad attack, a doctor would come over and give me a massive dose of vitamin C intravenously. Before the injections, my liver enzyme levels would be in the 4,000s, 200 times higher than the normal range. With the vitamin C, the levels would plummet like a rock. Although some people have been cured from various diseases and ailments by vitamin C, I was not one of them. Even during my best days after the IVs, I never got back to full strength. But I was improving.

"At that time, my treatment consisted of herbs, diet, and the vitamin C injections.

"For the next years, I was led to try a number of alternative medical treatments. I drank juices, saw a doctor in New York who gave me some medications, and even went to the Gerson Institute clinic in Tijuana. A lot of things seemed to help a little, but nothing was close to a cure.

"Besides the vitamin C injections and juices, coffee enemas seemed to be the most effective. I do coffee enemas to this day. They are very beneficial to release toxins.

"I went through a lot of things. What I'm telling you here are the major steps. The thing is, we refused to give up. We went from one thing to another as the Lord brought them into view.

"I went through this kind of process for about seven years. There was some improvement, but still it was a roller coaster, which is typical of that disease.

"I'll jump to the last thing. At the Center for Advanced Medicine in Encinitas, there were two founding doctors. Both were Christians. One was a fellow by the name of Bill Kellis, who when he was in his twenties was told he would never walk again. He began to study and cured himself. He and a fellow by the name of Mark Drucker founded the institute.

"They tested me with some machine made in Germany [probably a Rife machine or similar]. They had you hold electrodes and would touch pressure points—tiny areas on the body where certain nerve control centers are. Medical doctors in this country scoff at the practice. What they found, however, was that I had a number of viruses still with me even though I was somewhat better.[58]

"The first thing they did was start me on a further detoxification of the body. They gave me a powder and some things to start with, and I had to be very careful in what I was eating. After three months of a more intense detoxification, they told me that they had a combination of South American herbs that they believed would kill the hepatitis viruses. I started taking those herbs in 1991 and took them for two months. They tested me after that and couldn't find a trace of hepatitis. From that time on, I have not been on the roller coaster.[59] The entire treatment of herbs cost us a whopping $90.00 a month for the two months.

"Since that time—and it's been twenty years now—I've been tested with some of the most sophisticated tests and no one has found a trace of hepatitis. My liver enzymes have also continued in the normal range.

"I should tell you that some of the doctors along the way became very angry with me, especially those who wanted me to go on the steroids. But we did what we thought was right, and we know that the Lord had a hand in the whole process. He led us all the way.

"I should add that I think as more and more people from various backgrounds find out firsthand the value of abandoning the typical American diet, it will be greatly beneficial."

That was the end of my interview with Larry. But I want to tell you one more thing. After that time, for about fifteen years, Larry was strong enough to have extended speaking engagements in many places around the world.

Chapter 8
Detoxification and Alternative Treatments

*"The most complex of processes are governed by simple
natural laws."*

At the heart of both Deborah's and Larry's stories are two guiding
principles: Detoxification and fortification. Get the poisons out, and
get good nutrition in. This is the basic understanding behind the
success stories of tens of thousands of people who have learned a
healthier way to live. They are the fundamental principles behind
much of what is commonly called "alternative medicine."
Discussing these principles here provides an essential base of
knowledge for understanding Part II of this book, which deals with
mercury poisoning.

Sadly, virtually all of what is stated in this chapter is either denied
by, or scoffed at, by our medical system. That system is built upon
different principles, some of which by their nature are contrary to
the principles of detoxification and fortification. Our modern
medical system is also very expensive, whereas the methods
covered in this chapter either cost very little or nothing at all. It is
no wonder, then, that there exists more than a little friction between
the two camps.

In many instances, it is impossible to draw a line between
detoxification and fortification. Certainly this is true when it comes
to proper diet and exercise. It is equally true when it comes to some
vitamin and herbal therapies. I discuss fortification in detail in Part
III, but must point out here that these two—detoxification and
fortification—are often inseparable. If we do not discharge the
poisons that naturally (or unnaturally) build up in our system, all
good nutrition is for naught.

The Principles of Detoxification
Our bodies are being assaulted daily with poisons. The number and
magnitude of environmental toxins we are subjected to defies our
ability to quantify, let alone understand. This assault is steadily
increasing, so detoxification needs to be addressed on every front.

Like our friend Larry, Deborah got the concept of detoxification from herbal books. By reading in the herbals about food allergies, Deborah became aware that some foods were leaving a lot of debris in her system—especially in the bowel and in the blood. This was a huge step.

Before I address alternative treatments we have used, I want to cover several fundamental points concerning toxicity. **Most of these are so simple that they are often ignored**, which can be to the great detriment of our health.

First, toxicity is not only physical in nature. It can be mental and spiritual as well. We do not need a scientific study to tell us that certain kinds of thoughts poison us—even physically. We need to turn away from such thoughts and reject them. Anger, bitterness, deceit, contentiousness, envy, hatred, holding a grudge, thinking ill of other people, proud thoughts, covetousness, etc., all need to be rejected and turned away from, because they tear down our overall health. We are composed of spirit, soul, and body, and any one of these affects the other two.

I regards to this, if we need to apologize or otherwise make things right with someone, let's do it. We will reap the benefit, and at least our little sphere of the world will be a better place for it.

Second, the transit time of waste products through the body is crucial. The bowel is not a pipe; it is part of the digestive system, and nutrients and toxins are being absorbed from it into the bloodstream. A tremendous amount of health is lost because of a toxic bowel. From the time food is ingested to the time it is *fully* discharged should be no more than 24 hours—preferably 12. The longer waste products stay in the system, the more we are poisoned by them. If our bowel movements are not full evacuations, we are storing toxins. That requires our filtering organs to work harder, and that eventually tears down our health. For proper elimination, think of foods in terms of fiber, lubrication (oils), and moisture.

Most people think they eliminate adequately. Few do. Actually, if we don't eat right and exercise sufficiently every day, we probably *cannot* eliminate adequately. A certain amount of undigested food—usually the result of a diet without enough fiber—will stay in the bowel and putrefy. This highly toxic matter will frequently accumulate for decades. The proof of this we will give later in this chapter.

Third, sufficient intake of water is crucial. That's water. Not tea, not sodas, not fruit juices, not milk. Water. The highest quality we can get. Most of us do not drink enough water, and countless health problems are simply due to this lack. Water cleanses the inside of the body as well as it does the outside. It is impossible for our bodies to filter out toxins adequately without a sufficient supply of water. Drinking an adequate amount of good quality water can also cure a great many ailments and diseases. Some specific examples we know of firsthand are given in Chapter 22.

Fourth, the exercise imperative
Exercise is valuable for far more than muscle tone and cardiovascular health. Exercise is a necessary means of detoxifying not only the body, but the mind as well. Deep breathing of fresh air allows the lungs—the largest filters in the body—to expel waste and be recharged with that which sustains life. Muscle movement works out more than the "kinks"; it works out accumulated waste materials. Enough good cannot be said about adequate daily exercise; and enough ill cannot be said about the lack of it.

When I was in my teens, I worked for an old farmer who liked to say, "You can't have a good day until you sweat." He had a very good point. Whether we are "working out" or working in the garden, both can be highly beneficial.

The California Indians intuitively knew the value of sweating. They even built special structures called sweat houses. They were old-fashioned saunas. The people sat around a fire, sweat, and scraped the sweat off their skin with sticks. They would then go jump in a river or lake to wash off. They were refreshed, and so are we when we "sweat it out." What is the "it"? Accumulated toxic matter.

Sometimes I hate exercising as much as anyone. But like others with the same problem, I always feel better afterwards.

And by the way, fat cells are the body's prime storage site for toxins.

All the preceding points about exercise are equally valid when it comes to mental exercise. How many ills are cured simply by working physically and mentally! And there can be a huge difference between working and having a job.

Fifth, general detoxification is a must. The blood, liver, kidneys, bowel, skin, and the rest of our bodies appreciate a good cleaning and being kept clean. Many times we can wonder what it is that makes us feel so bad. Usually it is not one thing, but many. Often we will never know what "it" is that makes us feel so bad. So, to ask what "it" is may be to ask the wrong question. We live in a soup of toxins—a lot of which we cannot avoid. So, general detoxification is a necessity.

Sixth, in a specific detoxification regimen, we will sometimes feel worse before we feel better. This is normal. Consider what a detoxification regiment is: We are stirring up poisons and bringing them to the surface. Until they are expelled, we will not feel well. Therefore, the expelling is vital or we are just re-poisoning ourselves.

Detoxification needs to be gradual, and overloading the system needs to be avoided. Deborah realized early on that to be mildly sick in order to discharge toxins is needful. If she made herself too sick while detoxifying, she drew back on treatment. It is our thinking that any illness from detoxification should be mild and should not be for more than a day or two. If it is, we believe we are overloading our system.

Seventh, there are layers of toxicity and there are layers of healing. Often when some acute health issue is relieved, the body expresses its thankfulness in the form of euphoria—all is well! Then, after a short while, that levels off, and we may feel just as bad as we did before. At such a time we can incorrectly think that our treatment of the condition did not work. Not so! We just peeled off a layer of ill health, and the body is now demanding us to take the next layer off. This is precisely the same reaction that many people experience after an automobile accident.

I'll give you an example of a friend of ours. Immediately after his auto accident, Mike's shoulder was very tender; then when the shoulder finally eased up, his lower back began to tell him of its discomfort. Then, after the lower back had calmed down, his foot began to complain. Were not all three injuries there from the beginning? Of course they were. The brain was simply telling him what to address first.

Eighth, moderation is a virtue. There is no sense in any detoxification program that floods the system with poisons and compromises the immune system. We do not want to stir up (internally release) more toxins than we can safely eliminate. We do not want to do something in a fast way, but in a safe way. Detoxification should be a way of life, not a binge.

> **"Treat the body as a whole, not as parts, and allow it to heal itself."**

Alternative Treatments

The first thing to say about alternative treatments is that, unfortunately, our medical system has for the most part opposed them to the best of its ability. A brief history of this opposition is in Appendix IV.

The second thing to say about alternative treatments is that there are often many ways to arrive at healthfulness. One example is that merely having a cheerful and positive attitude can frequently cure what any number of various treatments cannot.

The alternative methods listed here follow the principles of detoxification and fortification as previously discussed at the beginning of this chapter. They are based upon the premise that the body will heal itself if certain obstructions to health are removed. Although impossible to prove with the kind of certainty that some folks foolishly insist upon, the methods described in this chapter work too much of the time for me to get involved in a fruitless academic debate over them.

Enemas

The benefits of an enema, or flushing the bowel with water, have been known at least since the time of the early Egyptians. Usually, people have an enema to relieve severe constipation, and they are very effective for that purpose. But enemas are equally effective for far more than that. We, and many other people over the centuries and around the world, have proven repeatedly that if we are simply not feeling well, giving ourselves an enema frequently sets us aright again. Grandma was right when she said, "You will feel better." Many people give themselves an enema when they feel a cold or flu coming on and thus avoid those common sicknesses.

Do you think an enema is gross? An enema is not gross. When millions of people needlessly take so many antibiotics that they compromise their immune system—*that* is gross! And when we spend billions of dollars annually on those antibiotics and call it "health care"—*that* is disgusting! Is there a place for antibiotics? Sure. In my opinion, and in the opinion of a small yet growing number of medical doctors, antibiotics are a reasonable *last* resort.

If you think giving yourself an enema is crude or uncivilized, consider it again when you are tired of feeling sick. You will quickly become a proponent of the treatment. A $10 enema bag purchased at the local drug store may prove to be one of your best friends.

If you have a good first aid book, follow the instructions given in it. If you don't, and Grandma is not available to help you, you can ask your doctor or look in Dr. Jensen's book for specific instructions.[60] If you are still not comfortable after looking into those sources, you may want to do what I do.[61]

Just like any other skill, it takes practice to learn how to effectively give yourself an enema. But if you feel bad enough and appreciate the results, you will learn very quickly.

We only use water for an enema. In our opinion, a considerable amount of knowledge is necessary, and good common sense must be exercised, if using anything else. Part of common sense is not following the fads. We let someone else make all the mistakes.

Colonics

A colonic is a deep enema—one that flushes the entire bowel, not just the last portion of it. Now reader, if you thought the discussion of enemas was tough, before you completely freak out at the mention of colonics or colon irrigation, bear with me and allow me to tell you the story of **Kellogg's Corn Flakes.**

John Harvey Kellogg (1852-1943) was an American medical doctor who ran a large sanitarium, or medical clinic, in Battle Creek, Michigan. Observing the condition of thousands of patients who came to the sanitarium, Kellogg became convinced that much, if not most, of the ill health that he saw was the result of improper diet and an unhealthy lifestyle.

Dr. Kellogg recommended abstinence from tobacco and alcohol, a regimen of exercise, which included deep breathing, and a well-balanced, mostly vegetarian diet, which favored laxative and high-fiber foods. He stated repeatedly and emphatically that the bacteria in the intestine could either help or hinder the body. Dr. Kellogg went on to say that a poor diet favors harmful bacteria, which can infect body tissues and lead to a diseased condition. He believed that most disease is alleviated by a change in intestinal flora. He could hardly have been more right. Even many modern doctors are beginning to come around to understand this.

Though Kellogg personally devoted much of his time to patients lacking financial means, the sanitarium was largely for the well-to-do or middle-class. In the late 1800s the typical breakfast for the wealthy and middle class American was eggs and meat; for the poorer city people, it was usually gruel, porridge, or some other form of boiled grains. Neither of these was satisfactory to Kellogg. Because he had tremendous success treating patients with coarse ground yellow cornmeal,[62] he developed a breakfast cereal composed of it. Dr. Kellogg and his brother, Will, started the Sanitas Food Company in 1897 in order to produce flaked cornmeal and some other cereal products.

Will was the financial guy. He had been John's bookkeeper when John took over as superintendent of the sanitarium.

Will wanted to add sugar to the corn cereal to make it more palatable. Dr. Kellogg strongly disagreed. He believed that the addition of sugar would be most harmful. This resulted in a personal and business rift between the brothers that would last until the end of their lives.[63] Will went out on his own, established the Battle Creek Toasted Corn Flake Company, the sugar sold, and the rest is history. Dr. Kellogg became the target of a lot of criticism in medical circles, his work was forgotten, and millions of people were helped down the road to diabetes and countless other serious health problems. The money was in selling sugar, not in suggesting discipline.

This leads to my point of mentioning Dr. Kellogg in this section on colonics. To make the progress he needed to with his patients, Dr. Kellogg not only changed their diet, he also insisted that every patient be routinely flushed with water. Besides drinking a proper amount of fresh water, the patients were given what was commonly called a high enema. A high enema is an enema that irrigates the entire colon, not just the last portion of it. The high enemas, or colonics, or colon irrigations, as they can be called, were followed up by administering (*unpasteurized*) yogurt. The patients also ate yogurt, so they received the healthy intestinal flora from both ends. And you can bet your last dollar that Kellogg did not give his patients sugared-up yogurt.

Colonics have come a long way from the days of Dr. Kellogg's "high enemas," but the principle is the same—detoxify by flushing out the colon. It is worth noting that colonics were a standard part of medical treatment, and colonic equipment was in most American hospitals until the mid-1960s, when drugs were developed to "do the same thing."

They don't do the same thing.

Some medical doctors today are proclaiming loudly all over the web that colonics are entirely unnecessary, that the bowel empties well on its own. Oh? The colonic tube doesn't lie. Everything that comes out of you can be clearly seen by means of a viewing tube that is built into the machine.

Some doctors also say that colonics are dangerous. Oh? Do the same people tell you that the puncture rate on colonoscopies is about one in 1,200 and that complications resulting from colonoscopies are several times higher than that? Do they tell you what those complications are, what will happen if something goes wrong, and what the statistics are for the various complications?[64]

[In talking to your doctor, if you insist on scientific data concerning these risks, he will squirm as if he has just had the colonoscopy device inserted into his rear end. He cannot give you an honest answer and cannot honestly tell you why. I will explain why later.]

In summary, colonics can be a valuable part of a detoxification program, because old, putrefied material in the bowel that is very toxic—and can be causing significant harm—can be removed. Colonics are inexpensive (about $80.00), safe (when performed by a qualified tech), and when combined with proper diet and other detoxification methods, can be a boost to better health. Again, I am not talking theory in this book—only things we or someone we know has experienced firsthand. Our family has benefited greatly from these treatments, and we know many other people who have as well. I only wish that everyone could know the value of colonics as a means of bettering health. See Chapter 22 for specific colonic stories.

Vitamin C

Not feeling well? You may want to do what we do. When we don't feel well, we take 500-1,000 mg of vitamin C and stir it in a glass of water. More often than not, within 45 minutes, we are much improved. We use a product with rose hips if possible. I don't know what vitamin C does, and I don't know that Linus Pauling[65] really did either, but it frequently works very well.

Treatments with massive doses of vitamin C should not be ignored either. See Chapter 7 and Resources at the end of this chapter.

Herbs

Deborah got her help with herbs, not from the Chinese who have understood the healing power of herbs for millennia, but from those who learned from the Native Americans. In many respects, the

Native Americans were not lacking in understanding either. Though there are some notable exceptions, many of these peoples lived in harmony with their environment for hundreds of years. We would do well to learn from them in this regard. The Native Americans knew something of their connection with the land. They may have had many superstitions, but at least they had respect for the land they were living on. They were part of it, and they knew it. Man was formed from the dust of the earth. These "roots" are deep, and we should have great respect for them.

Practically speaking, people of Chinese ancestry, who are to some degree physiologically made up of Chinese herbs, might do better to stick with Chinese herbs. In our opinion, those of us who are not of that ancestry may do better sticking with local herbs whenever possible. Typically, Chinese medicinal herbs are stronger in potency than traditional American herbs. All should be used with caution.

From our experience and observation, medicinal herbs are nothing to play around with. Before taking them, we think it is prudent to get a couple of good herbal books written by different people and learn all you can.

Besides using local herbs or herbs that are hereditarily part of us, another important principle in the use of herbs for healing is that herbs are activated by heat. In many cases, they can be more effective taken as a tea or applied as a poultice than simply eaten fresh or taken in dried form.

The strength of an herbal tea can have everything to do with its effectiveness. In some cases, a mild tea is what is needed while the same tea in stronger concentration can be counterproductive. In other cases, a strong tea is necessary. Our children received only the mildest of teas. Read the herbal books.

A word about spices: Most spices are herbs and are not just for flavoring food. They are also frequently used to aid digestion and to guard against pathogens. It is helpful to think of spices in that way. Mexican food utilizes a lot of chili peppers. Historically, this is not for flavor so much as it is to kill pathogens. Garlic does the same and is one of nature's super medicines. Garlic and other "hot" spices are stimulants, so moderation may be a good idea.

For more on herbs, see Chapter 20, Herbs, Guidelines; and Chapter 22, Herbal Treatments and Remedies.

Chiropractic

There is a place for chiropractic just as surely as there is a place for any proven medical treatment. There are also unsubstantiated claims made concerning this profession just as there are in the medical profession, or, for that matter, in the claims made by the fellow who sold you your washing machine. We humans have a common problem when it comes to selling things. Also, just as with medical doctors, carpenters, accountants, and gardeners, some chiropractors are more skilled than others. Before hiring anyone (and we should look at any health care practitioner in those terms), it is wise to first get a strong personal referral. It is much safer to deal with people who have something to lose.

The basic principle behind chiropractic is that the body has a tremendous ability to heal itself if the flow of nerve energy is not impeded. This is highly logical and a good reason to consider this alternative.

Our AMA friends are correct when they state that there are unsubstantiated claims about the effectiveness of chiropractic made by some individual chiropractors and chiropractic associations. But to deny that hundreds of thousands of people have been greatly helped by chiropractic treatment is to purposefully turn a blind eye to a tremendous amount of personal experience.

Perhaps the basic controversy is over whether spinal manipulation can be effective for *any* medical condition. I think a little common sense goes a long way here. If we have back or neck pain, or a pinched nerve that we cannot take care of ourselves, we see a chiropractor. If we were to have pneumonia, we would be more likely to visit a naturopath, osteopath, or medical doctor.

By stating the above, I am not saying that there is no validity to the claim that spinal manipulation can cure or at least control many other kinds of aliments and promote general health. I think the logic is sound enough even if the "science" is probably impossible to prove. But this book is about firsthand knowledge, and our experience is limited in this regard, so, other than a few stories in Chapter 22, I will withhold further comment on those claims.

I need to say something here about the AMA's longstanding battle with chiropractic. Until 1983, the AMA held that it was unethical for medical doctors to associate with an "unscientific practitioner" and labeled chiropractic as "an unscientific cult." In 1976, five chiropractors sued the AMA, several nationwide health care associations, and several doctors for violation of the Sherman Antitrust Act. They lost the case but won on appeal. The judge ruled that the AMA had violated Section 1 of the Sherman Antitrust Act and had engaged in an unlawful conspiracy "to contain and eliminate the chiropractic profession." From that time, the AMA Principles of Medical Ethics was changed to state that a physician "shall be free to choose whom to serve, with whom to associate, and the environment in which to provide medical services." The judge's ruling makes very interesting reading. The judge declined to "pronounce chiropractic valid or invalid on anecdotal evidence." In the ruling, the judge stated, "I do not minimize the negative evidence. But most of the defense witnesses, surprisingly, appeared to be testifying for the plaintiffs." Concerning the boycott, the judge stated, "There are too many references in the record to chiropractors as competitors to ignore ... The AMA obviously was not successful in defeating the licensing of chiropractic on a state by state basis, but that failure does not mean that they had to resort to the highly restrictive means of the boycott." The case was cross-appealed from both sides and was confirmed by Wilk v. the American Medical Association (895 F.2d 352; 7th Circuit, 1990.) The court gave the opinion that the AMA had engaged in a "lengthy, systematic, successful, and unlawful boycott" designed to restrict cooperation between MDs and chiropractors in order to eliminate the profession of chiropractic."

I have included a few chiropractic stories that I know firsthand in Chapter 22. They may be "anecdotal" and not based on "scientific" evidence, but people who have been simply and safely cured from horrible back or neck pain don't care. They—and I am included among them—are happy to be on with their lives without having resorted to dangerous surgeries or to heavy doses of pain pills. Thankfully, we had a choice. It could have turned out otherwise.[66]

Many chiropractors may dislike me for saying this, but either a doctor of chiropractic sees the key to your particular ailment or he or she does not. I have recommended chiropractic since shortly after injuring my back 35 years ago, and have not a little experience with it. The other members in our family have also received treatments for nearly three decades, which we have monitored closely. Added to this, I have also received a large amount of feedback from the many people to whom I have recommended chiropractic. I have come to the conclusion that if a particular chiropractor does not make *very significant* progress on your ailment within two or three visits, it is probably best to get another personal referral and try someone else. I am well aware that these practitioners only make about $50 a visit, so that's a tough thing to say when most medical doctors charge a lot more than that and are often not as helpful. But it's your time, your health, and your fifty bucks.[67]

If we get helped by one chiropractor and not by another, it is not necessarily that one chiropractor was "good" and another was not. Oftentimes, one individual will be able to address a certain issue that another cannot. Experience tells me that chiropractic, like any form of treatment, is as much an art as it is a science.

Experience also tells me that without an adequate knowledge of acupressure and therapeutic massage techniques, a chiropractor's toolbox is too limited to be very helpful in many cases. Frequently, constrictions or "knots" in the muscles will not allow a chiropractic adjustment to "hold." If that muscular problem is not addressed adequately at the same time, you may be wasting your time and money.

I am very thankful for the Palmer School of Chiropractic. That method may be the best technical chiropractic training. But I will quickly add that I have been fortunate to be the patient of skillful practitioners who also understood acupressure and therapeutic massage, had a sensitive touch, and were intuitive as well as technically competent with that standard method.

As stated earlier, many times a chiropractic adjustment does not "hold." That is, as with a "feel good" massage, we can feel better for a short time and shortly afterward have the same nagging discomfort. Sometimes additional treatments will clear up the problem, but I have never seen anyone get lasting help from going to the same chiropractor every week for months. In my opinion, in that kind of case, the cause of the problem has not been found and such visits are likely a waste of time.

If a chiropractor gives you exercises or self-treatments to do, it may be a good idea to do them. He is telling you that he cannot do what you can do for yourself at home. In dealing with any health professional, we should not expect miracles and think that we do not need to be proactive to help ourselves.

We have to be practical about hiring any health professional. It is just like getting our taxes done or having our car repaired—we need to gain an adequate understanding of the job, and if we need help, we should hire the best person for the work that we can.

One last thing: If you have found a chiropractor who understands your body and can effectively treat you, perhaps a "tune-up" now and then is a good idea. I base this statement solely on personal experience.

Acupuncture

According to our AMA friends, this is another "unscientific" means of health care. But as far as I can tell, the Chinese (who brought us acupuncture) are not a stupid people. At least they are smart enough to be a creditor nation and not a debtor nation. (Ouch!) It seems to me that the chief mistake they made was that in earlier years they used gunpowder merely for entertainment (in the form of firecrackers) and did not go on to develop it to propel cannonballs.

Due to the intelligence of these people, perhaps their system of medical care—mostly herbs and acupuncture—should not be scoffed at.

Acupuncture has been around for more than 2,000 years. The principles are very similar to that of chiropractic, although chiropractic, as we know it today, came much later. The fundamental principle behind both is to put the body in balance that it may heal itself.

Deborah has had several treatments from two acupuncturists. Some were for detoxification, were too strong, and made her ill. Other treatments helped greatly with a pain issue. Some treatments seemed to make no difference whatsoever.

A friend of Deborah's had a horrible neck problem, which had caused her to suffer severe headaches for more than a year. She would have had surgery, but even the surgeon admitted, *when asked if he would do the surgery on his mother*, that it would be too risky. After rejecting the idea for months, but continuing to suffer greatly from the pain, she went to see an acupuncturist she had been referred to. She woke up the next morning without a headache for the first time in more than a year.

Most of the points mentioned previously in the discussion of chiropractic can be applied to acupuncture as well.

Acupressure
Deborah and I are far more familiar with acupressure.

If you don't already have one, you may want to go to the web or to a health store and get yourself a good reflexology chart. They are very inexpensive. If you are real ambitious, you might pick up a book on the subject too. Keep the chart in a handy place where you and other family members have access to it. The next time you, or anyone in the family, have a particular ailment, you can try acupressure on the related pressure points on your hands or feet. You may be pleasantly surprised. I will give one example here.

One day I woke up with a horrible neck ache. Maybe you know the kind—it was so bad I could hardly function. I had an important business day ahead of me, and I had a few choices:
1. Cancel everything, go to bed, and be miserable.
2. Go to the drugstore and buy a high-powered pain killer (we don't keep any in the house).
3. Call the chiropractor and wait (in pain, doing nothing) until I could get in to see him.
4. Get out the reflexology chart and see if I could help myself. [68]

I chose option four. By firmly pressing on a "pressure point" on my hand, and holding it for about ten seconds, the pain was eliminated. I had to repeat the procedure two or three times during the day, but at the end of the day, I had forgotten all about the neck ache. I got my work done that day by using an "unscientific" method. How foolish of me not to have proven the science first!

Osteopathic Physicians

We have very little experience with osteopathic physicians. Deborah saw one early on who confirmed the natural route she had taken but who added nothing further to her knowledge. Nevertheless, at the time it was comforting to her that someone with extensive medical training understood her, agreed with her, and did not tell her that she was nuts. For more on osteopathy, see Appendix IV, A Brief History of the AMA.

Naturopathic Physicians

The first thing that should be said about naturopathic physicians is that their training varies immensely. Some have extensive medical training; some have little training at all. It is probably for this reason that, at the present time, they are only allowed to practice in seventeen states.

We have some experience seeing naturopathic physicians. The ones we have seen have been helpful. Unfortunately, however, the concept of "giving you something" in the way of a medication for your ailments is deeply engrained in our society. The naturopathic physicians we have seen have this leaning. The products they recommended, although usually not prescription drugs, were nevertheless potent. For the most part, these products have fallen into the classification called "nutricuticals" and are typically vitamin, mineral, amino acid, and/or herbal compounds.[69] The term "nutricutical" is new; you probably will not find it in your dictionary. A few of the products recommended were somewhat helpful. For the two of us, who are not accustomed to strong, fast-acting medications, the recommended dosages for the products we tried were too high. Sometimes far too high. If we are going to try one of these products, we start with greatly reduced doses.

Integrative Medicine

"Integrative medicine" is a new term that is used to describe practitioners who use a blend of "alternative" and "traditional" medicine. I only mention it so that the reader will be familiar with the term. Many MDs have joined "integrative" associations.

Massage

There are several different types of massage—from deep tissue massage to very light lymphatic massage—and the skill of the practitioners varies greatly.

My wife and I give each other a back massage on occasion using a machine, which is usually effective. (See Resources.)

Taking it up a notch, my wife used to see a masseuse once a month. It helped her greatly. It reduced stress, and in her work environment at the time that was very needful. Then her massage lady moved away. The new masseuse could not do what the previous one did. This is a common story. Like chiropractic, acupuncture, and medical practice, massage is largely an art. There are very logical principles involved, and people can have the same training, but some practitioners will have a better touch and be more intuitive. And that can make all the difference.

There is a tremendous difference between what I would call a "feel good" massage and a massage that addresses a specific problem such as localized pain. If a muscle becomes constricted and tightens up, those tight spots—sometimes called "trigger points"—need to be dealt with. Many times the source of the problem is not where the pain is felt but quite a distance away. For example, **carpel tunnel** or tendonitis in the hand is often caused by muscular knots in the neck or shoulder. In such a case, you can treat the wrist until the cows come home and not get to the source of the problem. Trigger point massage for the specific purpose of solving a pain problem is an art in itself and is quite different than a typical massage. See Resources.

I will say something about another kind of massage: lymphatic massage.[70] Very little is known about our lymphatic system. The more the experts write about it, the more you realize they don't know much. But one thing is certain—the flow of lymph is vital.

Deborah found lymphatic massage as well as other massage treatments helpful during her heavy metal detoxification.

NAET

NAET stands for Nambudripad's Allergy Elimination Techniques. The techniques were developed by a person who had even worse allergies than Deborah. The treatments are almost too weird for me to try to write about. I will simply say that they involve "energy balancing" and testing is with applied kinesiology. The NAET webpage will tell you a little more. Other than the fact that some of these kinds of treatments work, and Deborah was probably helped by them, I would say it is all snake oil.

Deborah has had several sessions administered by two different practitioners. The second group of sessions was administered by the trainer and certifier of the technique. The jury is out on this one. Because Deborah had different kinds of health treatments at the same time (massage, acupuncture, and NAET), it is impossible to know what worked and what did not, or if it was a combination of the treatments that was helpful. We can say that for Deborah, most of the NAET "clearings" were unsuccessful. However, Deborah is able to eat many more foods now, and NAET could be partly responsible for that improvement.[71]

The treatments for allergies offered by the medical community, such as inhalers, cortisone, etc., come with serious side effects, which even those who prescribe them admit are contrary to health. It is doubtful that NAET can cause harm. So, what are you going to do if you have a debilitating allergy problem? NAET treatments are inexpensive, and someone who cannot solve allergy problems through diet and lifestyle adjustments may find help with them.

Aromatherapy, Etc.

I know that some readers will think that this is a lot of bull too. Well, who isn't happy when an apple pie is cooking in the oven?

Aromatherapy can be like the reset button on your garbage disposal. I am not suggesting that you are a garbage disposal, but I am saying that you and I need to be reset sometimes. And aromatherapy can help. If nothing else, it can help eliminate toxic thoughts, which if allowed to linger, can produce toxic chemical reactions in the body.

There are many ways to use aromatherapy. Deborah usually uses essential oils; I bring in flowers from the garden.

Aromatherapy, listening to classical music, or getting up early to see the sunrise and hear the birds sing probably won't cure appendicitis. But any one of these may relieve the stress that could lead up to it.

Quacks

In closing this chapter, I need to say something about quackery and the tendency of some people in "alternative" medicine to go too far, or to simply go into what we call "la-la land." This is common enough, but when compared with the countless dangerous treatments practiced by mainstream medicine, the "alternative" methods mentioned here are harmless enough, and all have proven effective to one degree or another.

By the way, our "alternative medicine" friends do not have a monopoly on quackery. They just don't have the economic and political muscle to call everything they do "science."

It is a good thing to have a choice, and in everything we need to use common sense.

Resources

Natural Detoxification: A Practical Encyclopedia, by Jacqueline Krohn and Frances Taylor, 2000
Deborah highly recommends this book.

Tissue Cleansing Through Bowel Management, by Bernard Jensen, DC, PhD, 1981
A "must read."

The Way of Herbs, by Michael Tierra, 1998
This is the best herbal we know of.

Reflexology Hand, Foot Chart, CR Christopher Shirley, Pacific Institute of Reflexology, 2002

The Trigger Point Therapy Workbook: Your Self-Treatment Guide for Pain Relief, 2nd Edition, by Clair Davies with Amber Davies, 2004

Primal Panacea, by Thomas E. Levy, MD, 2011
A good book on the use of high dosage vitamin C. I do not agree with all of Levy's statements. Like many other health writers, in this book Levy tends to promote one solution for all health problems, a concept I reject. However, if one tenth of the information in the book is valid, what he has to say is well worth looking at. And I can vouch for much more than one tenth.

V.E. Irons, www.veirons.com, PO Box 34710 N. Kansas City, MO 64116
Irons has excellent supplements to help with a fast or intestinal cleanse.

Massage machine:
We use a HoMedics, model PA 100A http://www.homedics.com/
A vibrating device that helps most of the time; sometimes greatly.

Colon hydrotherapy (colonics):
For practitioners in your area, contact the International Association for Colon Hydrotherapy, www.i-act.org

If you are in Orange County, California:
Embrace Health, Costa Mesa CA (949) 642-3424

Intravenous vitamin C infusions:
Institute for Progressive Medicine, Irvine CA (949) 600-5100. Many other clinics on the periphery of the medical establishment also do the infusions. (You may search under "integrative" medicine.) I don't know of any hospitals that do the treatments. Would like to.

Part II

Mercury!

Chapter 9
Discovery

In the last chapter, I discussed briefly several forms of "alternative" treatments that Deborah and I have used in caring for ourselves and for our children. In this chapter, we will return to Deborah's story.

Although Deborah had exercised the utmost diligence, had tried many different means to solve her health problems, and had been to several doctors and other health practitioners, it was obvious that we had not found the root of her health problem. As I said at the end of Chapter 6, she was down to five foods that she could eat. There was a reason behind it all, but it eluded us for decades.

In the late 1990s, warnings began to appear on grocery store shelves next to the canned tuna about the possible mercury contamination of fish.[72] One of those notices caught Deborah's attention, because tuna was one of the few foods she could eat without having a headache, feeling woozy, or simply feeling ill. As a matter of fact, tuna agreed with her very well. Her other primary source of animal protein, chicken, at times caused problems, so we switched to "organic" chicken. That helped but did not solve the problem entirely. Sometimes she would still feel somewhat sick after eating chicken—especially chicken breast meat. So, her intake of tuna had increased considerably. It was tuna for lunch, chicken for dinner.

Deborah talked to her doctor about her concern that she was eating so much tuna. He told her that "the good outweighs the bad" and not to worry about it.

But the matter kept coming back to Deborah's mind, and at her next visit with the doctor, two years later, she asked to be checked for mercury. He dismissed it outright, told her that mercury was not the problem, finished her exam, and sent her away.

After this time, a friend of ours and his wife began coming over to our home with some regularity on Sunday afternoons. He is the friend I have called Larry who is the subject of the story in Chapter 7. On one of those occasions, he told us his story and mentioned the doctor and the clinic he had gone to that had helped him.

By the time Larry related his story to us, Deborah's reactions to chicken breast meat were becoming commonplace. One day I spoke with her along these lines: "You are only fifty-four years old, you are down to five foods, and now it looks like it will soon be four. You need some help. I don't care how many times we have tried and failed to find help, we need to try again. It's not going to get better. Why don't we go to the clinic that helped Larry?" She was cautiously receptive, but insisted that first she was going to be tested for mercury poisoning.

She already had a routine medical exam scheduled, and while with the doctor she told him that she needed to be tested for mercury poisoning. He tried to push it off again, but she told him that she was not leaving until he helped her get the test. He told her, "You call the lab, I don't even know how to have this tested." [73]

Deborah did the research necessary and got the test. The results showed that the amount of mercury in Deborah's blood was twice the level that was considered dangerous. Eventually, we were to find out that she also had very high levels of nickel and cadmium, [74] and high levels of lead and some other lesser-known metals. Simply stated, Deborah's body was the equivalent of a Superfund site. When discussing her lab results, one of the first things the doctor told Deborah was, "Don't donate your organs."

The doctor did not know much about metal poisoning, but he did know someone who did. He also told her that there was a process called chelation, whereby specific substances could be taken that would attach to heavy metals and remove them from the body through the urine and feces.

Actually, there are a lot of people with heavy metal poisoning. But it is seldom checked for, because our medical doctors are taught not to look for it unless there has been an "industrial" exposure. [75] I put quotes around "industrial" because we think of industrial exposure as being smokestacks and waste pipes from dirty factories. In fact, much of our industrial exposure may be from what we commonly perceive to be among the cleanest of industries—the medical and dental industries. I will address this in detail later but here need to state that mercury, cadmium, nickel, lead, aluminum, and other metals are often major contributors to, if not outright causes of [76],

Alzheimer's disease[77], Parkinson's[78], chronic fatigue[79], multiple sclerosis[80], autoimmune diseases[81], arthritis[82], Meniere's[83], kidney problems[84], digestive disorders[85], and many other diseases.[86]

Mercury is the most toxic non-radioactive element on the planet. Damaging concentrations in the blood are measured in parts per billion.[87] It is a neurotoxin of the worst sort that can damage or destroy the brain and nerve cells that control motor and communication skills. It is highly soluble and easily passes through the placenta into a developing fetus.[88] When mercury and lead are combined in the body, the effect is exponentially more toxic. Ditto when it is combined with aluminum.[89] Though our bodies need many trace minerals, mercury is not one of them. In the body, mercury, lead, arsenic, and aluminum are *always* toxic.

Perhaps most disturbing of all, mercury poisoning commonly sets in slowly as the metal gradually builds up in the body. Symptoms often do not appear until months, years, or even decades after exposure. By that time, the mercury is embedded in the tissues and can be very difficult, if not impossible, to extract.

How Do You Get Mercury Poisoning?
This is the first question nearly everyone asks. We eventually realized that to ask this question is to ask the wrong question, and that any short answer to it is misleading. The fact is that some people with high mercury exposure don't get sick, while others with much less exposure do. So the better question is, "How can we keep mercury exposure from becoming mercury poisoning?" The answers to both questions are in the next five chapters. Arriving at them explains why I said in the preface that, when it comes to mercury poisoning, **short answers are not good answers**.

For those who parachuted into this portion of the book: If you have, or suspect that you have, a chronic mercury poisoning condition, it may be a very good idea to slow down and understand well what you are doing before allowing anyone to treat you. Dealing with mercury that has become imbedded in the body can be dangerous, and you can damage yourself greatly by not taking proper precautions.

Naturally, we too wanted to find out how Deborah was *exposed* to mercury. In doing our research, we realized that it might be easier to say where or how we are *not* exposed to mercury. In times past, mercurial antiseptics, such as Mercurochrome, were common.[90] In the 1950s, we grew up well acquainted with a red-orange liquid that we put on our cuts and scrapes with a glass dropper. Some kids even painted their faces with it to look cool. Mercury has been used as a fungicide for more than a hundred years.[91] Some ointments, skin creams, and salves still contain mercury compounds, though many of the compounds in these products have recently been banned. "Silver" dental fillings are in fact half mercury. The composition of amalgam fillings is approximately 50% mercury, 30% copper, 10% silver, 9% tin and 1% zinc.[92] Obviously, to call them "silver fillings" is misleading. They should be called "mercury fillings," shouldn't they?

Mining operations have used mercury as an amalgam for gold for thousands of years.[93] [94] The burning of coal releases mercury—all around the globe.[95] Mercury was (and in some places, still is) used in the production of chlorine[96], paper pulp, and paint and dye pigments.[97] Thimerosal, a preservative used in vaccines and many other medical products since the early 1930s, contains mercury. Some lesser-known preservatives do too.[98] Our new "green" light bulbs (CFLs) contain mercury vapor.[99] The list of mercury containing products commonly used is long enough to be nauseating.[100] Looking at the list of products makes one amazed that due to the highly toxic nature of mercury anyone is alive today. We have mined so much of the stuff that now our oceans and most of our waterways have dangerous levels of it.[101] For this reason, we cannot eat fish without the risk of increasing our exposure.

Low level chronic (constant, continual) exposure to mercury can be dangerous, because the metal can accumulate in the body. By looking at the list of sources just given, one can safely infer that our exposure is invariably from multiple sources. Further, our exposure is to multiple forms of mercury molecules, some of which are more toxic than others. The molecular forms of mercury can also change within the body. As sure as liquid balls of mercury are difficult to pick up when spilled, because they easily break apart, within the body mercury can also break apart, combine with other substances, and go just about anywhere—and consequently cause all kinds of problems.

Mercury exposure is far more common than people are aware of, and depending upon the kind of exposure, the concentration and rate of exposure, and how well the body's filtering organs are functioning, the unfavorable health consequences can be significant. Infants and small children are particularly vulnerable.

Classifications of Mercury[102]

Mercury is usually classified into three main groups: elemental mercury (aka metallic mercury), inorganic mercury, and organic mercury. Elemental mercury is the form we are the most familiar with. It is the liquid used in thermometers, the gas used in fluorescent light bulbs, and the largest component of the metal alloy that the dentist put in your mouth. Though extremely toxic, liquid mercury is poorly absorbed by the body, so it is not nearly as dangerous in small exposures as many of the other forms of mercury.

Mercury vapor from this liquid is entirely another matter. Mercury vapor is readily absorbed through the mucus membranes and lungs, and because it can cross the blood-brain barrier[103], it commonly accumulates in the brain.[104] Liquid mercury easily evaporates and becomes mercury vapor, thus making indoor spills dangerous.[105] [106]

Inorganic mercury is a category of mercury compounds, or salts, the most common of which is mercuric chloride. Other common forms are mercuric sulfide and mercuric acetate. These compounds are commonly found in (some) batteries, disinfectants, and body creams.[107]

Elemental mercury and mercury compounds are highly soluble and highly diffusible. As such, if they enter the bloodstream, they typically change into forms of inorganic mercury that are usually, but not always, excreted out of the body.[108] Over time, mercury and other metals can slowly accumulate in the body, especially in the central nervous system, the kidneys, the liver, the bowel, the pancreas, and in various glands.[109] **Hence the importance of the previous chapter and of Part III of this book.**

Organic mercury is different from elemental mercury in that it also contains at least one carbon atom. Organic mercury comes in three common groups: methyl mercury, ethyl mercury, and phenyl mercury. Methyl mercury is what we hear about in fish, ethyl mercury is what we hear about in vaccines, and phenyl mercury we don't hear about much, but is used in fungicides.

For thousands of years, mankind has found mercury very useful... and harmful. And it is not only miners, scientists, and hat makers of past centuries who have suffered its effects. In 1956, 1960, and again in 1971, grain treated with ethyl mercury killed hundreds of people in rural Iraq.[110] Thousands more were poisoned but did not die. They mistakenly ate treated grain that was supposed to be used for seed, not consumption.[111] In the mid-1950s, Minamata, Japan was struck with an epidemic of mercury poisoning. The source was eventually traced to discharge from a chemical plant that poisoned the fish in Minamata Bay. Nearly 2,000 people died from that exposure, and many more thousands were seriously injured—for life. In the former Soviet Union, so many thousands of industrial workers were poisoned by the use of mercury that Soviet scientists took the lead to learn how to chelate, or extract, mercury from the body. In the mid-1950s Soviet scientists developed dimercapto-1-propanesulfonic acid, or DMPS, which remains the preferred means of chelating mercury.

Mercury has many useful chemical properties, but it is a super-concentrated neurotoxin that can cause havoc in the body in seemingly infinitesimal concentrations. The metal, because it is a conductor, is attracted to the central nervous system, which is electrical in nature.[112] The thyroid gland is a common collection site. Mercury may induce high blood pressure, because it can alter (harden) the cells that line the interior of the blood and lymphatic vessels.[113] Digestive problems often have heavy metals, including mercury, as a major component because their presence can alter the structure of, or inhibit the action of, enzymes.[114] **Mercury poisoning is a great imitator. It is commonly associated with compromising the immune system to the extent that it can manifest itself as many diseases and conditions of ill health.**[115]

Because both the sources of mercury exposure and the compounds of mercury toxicity are so varied, it is wise to **think in terms of the total burden of mercury on the body _as well as_ the total toxic burden on the body from all toxins.** Based upon that, I will now discuss some of the most common sources of mercury exposure.

Dental Amalgam, Amalgam Illness
Other than mining operations and "industrial" exposures where mercury is used, high on the list of sources of exposure are mercury or "amalgam" dental fillings. [For a history of mercury used in dentistry, see these notes.[116 117 118]] With mercury fillings, there are a number of ways that mercury can find its way into the bloodstream and from there into the tissues of the body. First, when the product is being placed in your mouth, mercury vapor is released. When breathed in, mercury vapor easily finds its way into the bloodstream. Second, you can obviously swallow some of the metal. Third, when you chew on a mercury filling, mercury vapor is released.[119] Fourth, bacteria in the mouth act on the mercury in the filling, converting some of it into **methyl mercury**. Methyl mercury is fifty times as toxic as elemental mercury. Fifth, the fillings, like the teeth, wear down. But unlike teeth, this is not merely from friction; it is partly by dissolving.[120] Sixth, if decay forms under a mercury/amalgam filling, mercury, as well as the other metals, can leach directly into the bloodstream. And **dental X-rays do not show decay under a filling made of any material** unless the decay is severe.

The dental industry is strictly regulated when it comes to handling mercury. The EPA is in charge of this and classifies mercury as a highly toxic substance. Therefore, there are stringent guidelines that your dentist must follow when storing and handling the substance before he puts it into your mouth. Your dentist and his assistant are also warned by the governing authorities to protect themselves while they work on you. When mercury is *removed* from your mouth by your dentist, he or she is again required to follow certain guidelines, because it is once again classified as a highly toxic substance. Also, after it is removed, mercury must be handled and discarded in the prescribed manner. However, when mercury is in your mouth, the EPA has no jurisdiction; our public health authorities do. And they tell us that mercury used in the dental trade is perfectly safe. **In other words, according to the law of our land, the only safe place for the stuff is in your mouth!**

Most Americans have, or have had, at least a few mercury/amalgam fillings, and many of them are on the molars where it has been standard dental practice to cover as much of the grinding surface of the tooth as possible with the metals that can make people sick.[121] Therefore, it is not difficult to understand why our health authorities are in denial about mercury/amalgam toxicity. The way our legal system works, it is not possible for your dentist to say much about it either. If monetary awards were given out for all the harm mercury fillings have done, it could bankrupt the entire dental profession many times over. That would not be good for anyone. It is sad that we can have warnings about fish consumption due to methyl mercury, yet we are not warned about the same stuff in our mouths. Regardless, if you have mercury/amalgam fillings and have a metallic taste in your mouth, you can be certain where it is coming from. Likewise, if you have both a number of mercury fillings and a laundry list of "unexplained" health problems, it is highly likely that these two are related to one another. Dealing with dental amalgam is covered in the next chapter.

Eating Fish
Eating fish—especially large predator fish—and eating shellfish is also high on the list of sources of mercury exposure. The public health warnings about fish consumption are at least somewhat contradictory, so I will address several of the issues involved.

When elemental mercury is ingested by fish, it changes its molecular structure and becomes a far more toxic substance—the methyl mercury referred to earlier. Fish do not expel methyl mercury; they store it in their tissues. Therefore, the big fish that eat the little fish typically contain higher concentrations of mercury. According to the FDA, shark species, king mackerel, swordfish and tile fish have the highest levels of mercury. For a chart of mercury levels in various fish and shellfish species, you can go to this FDA website.[122] Please understand, however, that individual fish do not read our charts and may or may not comply with them. Also, the studies that this chart is based upon are over a very wide geographic area, so the averages can be misleading. You can have one hand on a block of ice and the other on a stove burner and have an average temperature that would be considered in this kind of chart as quite comfortable.

Probably the biggest debate is over the most commonly consumed fish in the US—tuna. Tuna fish sandwiches have been an American staple for generations. When the EPA hammer came down on fish, the tuna and albacore industry, facing certain ruin if they did not do so, fought back. Both sides of the issue have weighed in with their "science," but financial interests (on both sides) tend to distort the "findings" and "studies." So, as the politics are being worked out, shrapnel from the fight has caused a lot of confusion for the consumer.

Many government, industry, and health writers have gone to great lengths discussing what amount of methyl mercury ingested from fish is safe. Most of the discussion, however, I believe is flawed for four reasons:
1. Mercury can easily change form within the body, so a discussion merely of methyl mercury can be misleading.
2. It is the total burden of mercury on the body that is important. For example: A person who has no amalgam fillings and eats fish occasionally is one thing; a person with a mouthful of amalgam fillings who eats a tuna fish sandwich every day is another.
3. People expel mercury at different rates. Some people's bodies hoard it; others seem to expel almost all of it. I discuss the reasons for this in the chapter on mercury detoxification.
4. The effects of methyl mercury poisoning follow a long latent period between the time of ingestion and the appearance of symptoms.[123] Relying upon charts or upon blood tests to determine a safe rate of exposure does not take this into account.

Unfortunately, abstaining from eating fish does not mean you will not ingest methyl mercury from fish. Ever wonder where the "junk fish," the "non-commercial fish," that are caught end up? About half of the world's fish catch is converted into fishmeal and fed to livestock or is used as fertilizer.

Methyl mercury—whether ingested or produced in our bodies—is one of the most harmful forms of mercury exposure because it can easily be absorbed by the tissues. It has a half-life of about 50 days, which means it typically takes that long for methyl mercury in the system to be reduced to half of its original concentration.[124] What remains can accumulate in the body not only of adults and children, but also in the developing brain of a fetus.[125]

Mercury Vapor

Exposure to mercury vapor may be as harmful as any kind of mercury exposure, because it readily enters the bloodstream through the lungs and commonly settles in the brain. So much for our new "green," [126] florescent coil light bulbs. If one of these breaks in the house, that is not good. The EPA warns as follows: Get out of the room and air the room out for 10-15 minutes before cleaning up. Don't vacuum! That just throws the vapor all over. Clean up thoroughly with wet towels, seal the remains of the bulb and any cleanup materials in an airtight container, and dispose of all of it at the nearest hazardous materials collection site. See this note for more specific EPA instructions.[127]

Is this overreacting? Maybe. It is easy to say it is, but having known mercury poisoning up close and personal, we don't use the bulbs.

Vaccines

Some vaccines, such as flu shots, are commonly preserved with a compound containing **ethyl mercury**. If the vial contains more than one dose, you can be almost certain that it does.[128] Ethyl mercury, like methyl mercury, is a form of "organic" mercury and is also absorbed by the body, though not as easily as methyl mercury. That these are some of the most toxic substances known to man is undeniable. Toxicity of these substances is measured in micrograms, or millionths of a gram.

At the advice of government, manufacturers began to phase out thimerosal, the most common of the preservatives, in 1999. Nevertheless, as of 2012, the substance has not yet been removed from all vaccine products in the US.[129] Some multidose vials of flu vaccines, tetanus vaccines, and some meningococcal vaccines still contain the product.[130]

Before the phase-out of thimerosal from childhood vaccines was completed in 2003, however, thimerosal was in the great majority of the vaccinations administered in the US. When the number of childhood vaccinations "recommended"[131] by the US Centers for Disease Control and Prevention (CDC), and hence by physicians, increased greatly in 1988, all hell broke loose. Children routinely received 12.5 to 25 micrograms (mcg) of mercury in a single vaccination. If vaccinations were combined—and they usually were—the dose was considerably higher. If they were given multiple shots, the total was higher yet. If they got the dregs off of the bottom of a multidose vial (many vials contain ten or more doses, and the instructions on the vial say "shake well"), they got a lot more.

According to the FDA, 1.5 mcg in a day was, until 1997, considered harmful to an eight pound baby.[132] If the baby was small, the concentration was proportionally more dangerous. If Mom got shots while she was pregnant, the baby got a dose before coming out of the womb.

Unfortunately, until the "thimerosal scare," it appears that nobody did the ninth grade algebra required to convert the percentage of thimerosal in the vials into micrograms and thus realize that our vaccines contained far too much mercury. Eventually, testimony got to the bottom of the matter: If our health officials noticed at all, they saw thimerosal listed as .01%, and thought, "That's an insignificant amount." Turns out it's not. Not even close.[133]

Hundreds of top health officials, physicians, and scientists had a lot of egg on their faces. And countless others suffered much more than embarrassment. In Chapter 11, I tell the story of someone we know who has suffered enormously, probably due at least in part to thimerosal.

Regardless of the outcome of the thimerosal fiasco and the commonness of fluorescent bulbs, mercury dental fillings, and other mercury containing products, no exposure to the metal is healthy. Even cinnabar ore, from which mercury is derived, can be toxic. Early California Indians painted themselves with the red pigment from the rocks and became ill by doing so. They passed the mercury on to their offspring through the placenta due to this unhealthful practice, and over generations, in all likelihood, genetic weaknesses developed in their children.[134]

A Toxic Soup

To complicate the matter, where mercury is, other metals are usually present. Mercury is a good amalgam—it attracts other metals, especially heavy ones, and as far as our bodies are concerned, that is not good. **For this reason, mercury poisoning, or toxicity, should not be looked at alone, but instead as heavy metal poisoning.**

I should mention here that now that mercury is being phased out of vaccines, the use of aluminum has come into vogue.[135] Aluminum is undoubtedly less toxic, but perhaps we should consider the total toxic burden on the body—especially when it comes to babies and young children! To understand what I am referring to, please compare the 1983 and 2010 CDC vaccine charts in Chapter 11.

The bottom line on mercury exposure is that the fish have taken the rap. The CDC and the other public health agencies under them have placed the blame for our mercury problems squarely on the one party that can't be sued: the fish.

Mercury Poisoning Symptoms

Because of its highly diffusible nature, mercury can travel all over the body, and the symptoms of this toxin will depend upon its form, what elements it is combined with, and what kinds of cells are penetrated. Therefore, the symptoms of mercury poisoning can be "all over the map." However, there will be certain patterns, and by looking at these patterns, an educated guess can be made if a metals toxicity problem exists. Look at the symptoms of hypoglycemia in Chapter 4. The two conditions can have nearly identical symptoms. Also, read Chapter 6 and Chapter 11.

Symptoms of mercury toxicity come and go. We are living organisms, our bodies are adjusting constantly, and the problem is both chemical and electrical. For additional symptoms, see these notes.[136] [137]

The Mercury Syndrome and Environment
When our natural filtering organs cannot eliminate it adequately and mercury becomes established in the body, it sets up a self-perpetuating environment. This unhealthy environment acts like a magnet and attracts more mercury. Thus Deborah's "positive" reaction to tuna mentioned previously. Furthermore, tissue cell walls become thickened, not allowing the natural flow of fluid to cleanse them. In effect, mercury poisoning creates an environment in the body where the metal is stored and kept safe from being diluted or washed away. And all the time it is calling for more.

If that is not enough, this unhealthy environment is a prime host for fungi, yeast, and other parasites. Nearly all health practitioners will tell you that once any of these becomes established, it is no easy job to get rid of them or get them back into control.

Mercury poisoning can look like many other diseases, especially autoimmune diseases and hypoglycemia, when in fact it may be the underlying cause.[138]   For this reason, if you have MS, Parkinson's, fibromyalgia, lupus, arthritis, or any autoimmune condition, we think it is prudent to get your metals checked. Your doctor, as Deborah's, may very likely say that you don't have metals poisoning and that testing is unnecessary. The problem is probably with the medical textbooks, which have scary stuff about the worst heavy metals poisoning cases in which people have been exposed to "industrial" mercury and are about ready to drop dead. But the same books neglect "toxicity," where metals poisoning happens through more common exposures and the sufferers are not quite ready to drop dead. Apparently "toxicity" *is* "poisoning" everywhere but in the medical profession.[139] Anyway, if you suspect mercury or any heavy metals problem and your condition is worsening, you may not want to wait until you are ready to drop dead from it. A blood serum test will cost very little, and you just may find the culprit. Your insurance may not pay for this test because your doctor will typically say you don't need it. So, you have a decision to make: Are you going to take care of your health, or will you let your "good insurance" deter you from doing so? In our opinion, people should take charge of the care of their own bodies.

Testing

Heavy metals are a "hot potato" in the medical industry. Few practitioners want to touch it, and most labs don't either. So your doctor, like Deborah's, may not even know where to go to get the testing done. See Resources.

From our experience and according to our understanding, we think a serum blood test for mercury *and* a red blood cell test for copper should be performed first. According to Cutler, the symptoms for copper poisoning are indistinguishable from those of mercury poisoning.[140] Copper is an essential trace mineral, mercury is not. We don't want any mercury, and we don't want copper in excess or out of balance with the other necessary trace minerals.

If mercury is in the blood, we either have a current exposure, we are saturated, or both. Mercury from an exposure may leave the blood relatively quickly, but that does not mean it has left the body.

If you have or have had amalgam dental fillings, besides testing for mercury and copper you may want to check for silver, tin, and nickel also. If you have high levels of all or most of these metals and don't have other metal parts in your body, guess where those metals are coming from!

If you have smoked or been around a lot of secondhand smoke, you may want to be tested for cadmium and nickel. If you are ill, you may want to check for lead and aluminum too. Also, it may be a good idea to get your necessary trace minerals tested. Deficiencies in healthy minerals can cause the body to attract the unhealthy ones.

If nothing shows up in the blood, you may, or may not, want to get a hair analysis test. Mercury concentrations in hair can be about 250 times that of blood concentrations.[141] With the hair test, we think it is wise to get the other metals tested too, especially lead, aluminum, copper, nickel and cadmium. The US Centers for Disease Control (CAS 7439-97-6) says that "long-term exposure of mercury can be estimated from levels in hair." However, it is not that simple. Hair analysis also has its limitations. For example, in the Holmes, Blaxill and Haley article in *International Journal of Toxicology*, July-August, 2003, hair testing of autistic children showed little mercury while non-autistic children of the same age group showed significant to high concentrations of mercury. The hair analysis shows what is being excreted, not what is in the system. Autistic children commonly cannot excrete mercury sufficiently because they may not have the metabolic mechanism to do so.[142] With hair testing, if you have abnormal levels of other metals and very low levels of mercury, it could in fact be indicative of a mercury-related problem.[143] In Deborah's case, we saw no need for a hair analysis test.

Because mercury imbeds itself in the tissues, it is difficult to test accurately without being provoked. In some cases, a urine test provoked by DMSA or DMPS may be helpful. Please see all the warnings about DMPS in this book *and elsewhere* before submitting to this drug.

The CDC says, "Blood and urine mercury levels are useful to confirm exposure, but there is no definite correlation between blood and urine mercury levels and degree of mercury toxicity." I believe this statement is accurate. The urine test, however, is useful for tracking *changes* in discharge rate.

Interpreting the meaning of the test numbers requires some understanding. For example, the Agency for Toxic Substances and Disease Registry (the ATSDR is a part of the US Department of Health and Human Services) has a paper titled: *Evaluating Mercury Exposure: Information for Health Care Providers*. In that paper, in the section called "Laboratory Tests," it states that if a person has a urinary concentration of *elemental* mercury that is less than 20 µg/L (micrograms per liter, or mcg/l) there will be no signs or symptoms of poisoning. The paper states that this is "useful for the assessment of acute and chronic exposures." For acute exposures of *elemental* mercury, maybe. For chronic exposures, I don't think so. For organic mercury, which is 50 times as toxic, no way. The body will typically have both elemental and organic mercury in it, so to talk about one without talking about the other, in my opinion, is misleading. Deborah and many others have made marked improvement after getting mercury out of the body but never tested as high as 20 µg/L. A medical doctor I interviewed for this book who has treated mercury-toxic patients with DMPS for thirty years did not remember seeing a case higher than about 50 µg/L, even when the test was provoked by a chelator.

Some medical professionals who perform chelation say that levels under 10 µg/L in *provoked* tests done correctly indicate that it is likely you do not have a toxicity problem at the present time. Others put the number lower. But numbers can be misleading. They are averages, and we may not be average. Some people are much more sensitive than others, and no amount of mercury in the body is safe. Also, total toxic burden on the body is what counts most, and mercury, or all metals for that matter, is just part of the equation.

The fact is, no one knows what level of mercury is toxic to someone. It largely depends upon the individual's sensitivity and upon the presence of other metals. It is easy to say that counts of *elemental* mercury under 100 µg/L are not causing significant problems, as the ASTDR website states, but in fact there is nothing to back that statement up with. And we are inevitably dealing with other forms of mercury as well.

The bottom line? The value of testing is limited to specific circumstances. For diagnosis, in some cases, looking at symptoms may lead to a more accurate assessment.

Understanding at Last!
When we had the confirmed results from the laboratory concerning Deborah's heavy metal poisoning, I took her to the clinic where our friend, Larry, had been helped. We were not able to see the same physician that Larry saw, so another doctor saw her and looked at her test results. She described some of her ailments to him, which I told you about in Chapter 6. She went on to tell him of some of the (seemingly) less tangible ailments. She told him that she could often feel a crying "jag" coming on. She said she realized at those times that something physiological was happening to her and that she needed to stop it, but it was like a wave that engulfed her and she could not. She told him that at some of those times she experienced despair, and if it was not one of those two feelings, that her thoughts at those times were just empty—there was nothing there. He told her, "Oh, that's just emotions."
I am surprised we got out of there before that man got a black eye—from my dear wife. I was sitting right there with the two of them and remember thinking, "Uh-oh, this is not going to be good!"

But Deborah "held her mud" and we all got out of the appointment without anyone receiving bodily injury.

Our "just emotions" friend knew very little about mercury poisoning, but he did correctly tell her to get her amalgam dental fillings removed.

By this time, we had done our research and understood that **the removal of mercury-containing fillings can expose the patient to a great deal more mercury**—especially through vapor while the drilling work is being done. With a mercury count as high as hers, and knowing the sorry condition that many people with mercury poisoning are in, we knew the risks of having this done at all, let alone having it done without the utmost of safety precautions in place.

After we left Dr. "Just Emotions," we went to see a dentist he recommended because we could see him on the same day, and supposedly he had a protocol for safely removing mercury/amalgam fillings. The appointment was a fiasco. The office manager was so pushy and arrogant it is a wonder that the office had any patients at all.[144] The dental appointment itself went okay, but when it was time to go back up front and get some idea of the cost, it was like pulling teeth. It eventually became apparent that they wanted a blank check. No thank you.

That same day, however, we received the most significant insight into Deborah's health problems since Deborah met Viola, the woman who helped her get on her feet.[145]

As Deborah was coming down the stairs from the dentist's office, she struck up a conversation with a lady who was also leaving the medical building. I was sitting at a picnic table in a small park-like area across the way reading a book and saw them talking. They talked for quite a while, and then Deborah brought the woman over to meet me. They acted like old friends as she introduced me to Mary. In fact, they were old friends—linked firmly in the common bond of the attempt to be free from mercury poisoning. With utter amazement Deborah had heard Mary describe ailments which mirrored her own, and the two of them repeated most of their conversation to me. [146] It was the first time we had met or heard of anyone who had the same sensitivities that Deborah had to the telephone, to computer monitors, to noise, to high voltage lines, to a great number of foods, and most of all to the over-treatment of doctors who simply did not believe that she had the sensitivities that she said she had. And yes, Mary had low blood sugar as well. The sense of wonder and of joy for the three of us was overwhelming. It was a remarkable day, and we thanked our heavenly Father the whole way home.

Until she met Mary, Deborah never put metals together with the electrical problems she suffered. Now everything made sense. With metals in her central nervous system, Deborah was in effect a big conductor. Her sensitivity to electromagnetic fields—a condition denied by the electrical and electronics industries and the American medical establishment—was more than understandable. Deborah and Mary (and who knows how many thousands of others) are not nuts; these industries are not forthright. Deborah was not unscientific in her attempt to be freed from this plague; the scientific data has been locked away out of the sight of an unsuspecting public. [147]

Resources are at the back of the book.

Chapter 10
Amalgam Removal

Through further research on the web and with what the doctors told us, we were convinced that the first step in combating Deborah's mercury poisoning should be the removal of her mercury dental fillings. But in an industry that insists that mercury is not a problem, who could we trust to do it, and what protocol should be followed to minimize further exposure?

[The dental industry will not address chronic illness caused by amalgam.[148] Their position is probably best stated in a 2006 issue of the *California Dental Association Journal*: "Amalgam-related complaints are often an expression of underlying psychic problems..."[149]]

We also had the huge question of anesthesia. Deborah had had horrible reactions to anesthesia (see Chapter 6) and had done without it for more than twenty-five years. The last fillings she had done, about twenty years before, were done without anesthesia.[150] We knew very well that Deborah's current sensitivities were far greater than they were when she had reacted so violently to Novocaine decades before.

We ended up going to a dentist whom we had known for years. We knew his family and knew that he would be honest with us. By the time we saw him, he had also begun to get heavily involved in alternative medicine and was researching and experimenting with a method of testing body sensitivities. He respected Deborah's sensitivities and tested her for a few different anesthesias. He recommended Citanest for the upper jaw and Septocaine for the lower jaw.

This dentist was well aware of the dangers of mercury exposure and took it seriously, so we felt he was the right man for the job. One of the telling ways that we knew we could trust him was we asked him what he did to protect himself. That was a good question, and when he told us, we were convinced he understood the danger involved.

It is important to note here that the dentist did <u>not</u> tell us that mercury is toxic; we told him it was and that we wanted it out of

Deborah's mouth. By that time we had learned the reason why, when you bring up the mercury issue with your dentist, he acts like he just found half a worm in an apple he was eating. Your dentist must play according to the rules, and the rules are these: 1) To this day (March, 2013), the American Dental Association has held to its position that "no valid scientific evidence has shown that amalgams cause harm to patients with dental restorations, except in rare cases of allergy."[151] It goes on to say that for a dentist to remove amalgam for the "alleged purpose of removing toxic substances from the body, when such treatment is performed solely at the recommendation or suggestion of the dentist, is improper and unethical."[152] [153] [154] 2) The state dental boards have adopted this language, and some state boards have added to it. The effect is that in many states, **dentists are not allowed to tell their patients that mercury is toxic**. If their patients bring up the matter, they can respond, but only in a very guarded way. For a dentist to go against these edicts is akin to asking to have his or her license revoked.[155] So, our dentists are put in the unenviable position of weathering the storm that neither our public health authorities nor their professional association will address. The only ones put in a worse position are their patients.

Because of these obstructions to forthrightness, two ridiculous (if not harmful) conversations take place every day in most dental offices across the country. They go like this:
Conversation #1, about filling material: "Silver or white?" "Which would you use?" "Well, the white looks better." "Which costs more?" "The white." "I'll go with the silver."
Conversation #2: Your dentist tells you, "Those old fillings really should be replaced." "Why, aren't they doing the job?" "Yes, but they're old."

When Deborah showed the dentist the protocol her naturopathic physician had come up with to keep mercury exposure to a minimum, he just about flipped. Apparently it was unworkable. He explained the protocol he used, and the two came to an agreement on procedure.[156] He also gave us a cost range for the job.

Now the ball was in our court. I went to work and researched the Septocaine and Citanest and two of the other anesthesias that were possible candidates. With the background of Deborah's sensitivities, it made for very scary reading. I organized my research results and presented it to her, and we prayed about it. We then determined to let it rest to see how we felt about it in the coming days.

A week or so later we discussed it again, and both of us were peaceful to proceed exactly as the dentist had suggested. It was an amazing time—we felt like we were young children again, and in effect we were. Facing what we knew could severely cripple her for life, our sense was that of perfect peace and rest. We were resting in the hands of the same faithful and loving God who had seen us through the difficult birth of our son and who had seen us through so many other crises since that time.

Deborah had five amalgam fillings, a gold crown, and three gold overlays. In order to not subject the body to more toxic material than it could handle at one time (which is never a good idea), she and the dentist agreed to have the fillings removed in three office visits spaced about a month apart, with a heavy detoxification protocol in between visits.[157] Depending upon what the mercury level and liver enzyme test[158] results were, we would determine what to do with the crowns and overlays.

Preparation for Removal, and Detoxification from Removal
We were fortunate to understand before Deborah had the dental work done that there are many factors involved in the safe removal of mercury amalgam. We understood that regardless of how carefully the removal work was done, there would still be exposure, and it was imperative that the released mercury be fully discharged from the body. Specifically, the liver and kidneys need to be functioning properly, the lymph needs to be flowing without obstruction, and the intestinal tract—especially the bowel—must be working properly. **In other words, amalgam removal is a whole-body matter that cannot be managed adequately without the patient's clear understanding and involvement.** In our opinion, any dentist who does not emphasize the importance of these things to their patients is not qualified to do the removal work. Nevertheless, for reasons stated earlier, **it is the patient's responsibility** to educate themselves and bring up all the issues to

the dentist so that he or she *can* address them. By having this discussion, instigated and led by the patient, the patient can find out how serious a dentist is about the subject of dental mercury. **The removal of amalgam will expose the patient to mercury, and it is only prudent that the patient do everything he or she can to prevent the released mercury from lodging in the body.**

The protocol that Deborah's dentist followed for the amalgam removal was quite complex, so I have summarized that in a note.[159] Appendix V, at the back of the book, is a more complete list of recommendations put out by The International Academy of Oral Medicine and Toxicology, or IAOMT. It would be wise for anyone considering amalgam removal to be familiar with it *before* agreeing to have any work done. I am not endorsing any protocol or recommendations. I am simply letting the reader know that some people have taken the removal of dental amalgam seriously and have attempted to find a safer way to do the job.

[I should point out at this juncture that dentists have been trained to think in term of mechanics first, of life second. So they plug holes in our teeth and reconstruct them when necessary, but for the most part do not think in terms of the biocompatibility of the materials placed in our mouths.[160] But a tooth is a living member of the body, and sometimes—quite frequently, actually—the body is not happy with the intruders placed in it.[161] Though dentists are trained to understand the dangers of infection, and stress this frequently, they are usually mum on the subject of health problems related to the materials used in their trade.]

Deborah's follow-up detoxification after each dental appointment was also quite complex, so I have also put that in a note.[162] If all these precautions seem a little "over the top," they are. Mercury poisoning is "over the top." Deborah had known enough of it, and it was obvious from our research that her life was on the line. By "life," I mean any quality of life. The research we did spelled out many potential health issues in graphic detail.

Unfortunately, many people have not understood the potential dangers involved in having mercury fillings removed and have greatly poisoned themselves. No doubt, much of this is due to inadequate precautions by dentists; but the process is dangerous, difficult, and inexact. There are many factors involved, and everyone's body will react in its unique way. **We should not think we have no responsibility in the matter and expect miracles from our dentist. The patient should be proactive to help his or her body discharge the metals released!** A high percentage of the cases of amalgam removal poisoning are likely due to inadequate participation by the patient. The patient must take the lead to help the body eliminate the poisons that are stirred up in the process.[163]

Of course, we do not know if all the precautions Deborah took were necessary, but our attitude has always been that we will approach things the best we possibly can, and after that leave it in the Lord's hands. As you can tell if you have read this far, neither of us are comfortable being sloppy, and neither of us believe in luck.

The result of the removal of the five fillings was that there was decay under every one. In other words, mercury from the mercury/ amalgam fillings had been leaching into Deborah's bloodstream at a steady rate for who knows how long![164] She had no clue that there was any problem with any of the teeth, and it was only then that we learned what dentists never tell you—that they cannot see decay under a filling on those X-rays that they insist that you have. That had never occurred to us.[165]

After the removal of the amalgams, Deborah needed to go on a soft food diet for a few months to give the subject teeth the best chance of surviving. Most of the fillings were large (at least some of them had been replaced once before) and the teeth needed to be re-constructed. During this time, she dropped more than twenty pounds—and she was not overweight to begin with.

After all the amalgams were removed, repeated testing over several months revealed that there was still mercury in Deborah's blood. The count was reduced considerably but was still high, probably indicating that there was still exposure. Because of the decay under the amalgam fillings and the high blood count, we knew we had to replace the crown and overlays because it was possible that there was some amalgam or decay under some, or all, of them. When that work was done, we found that one tooth was okay, the other three were infected. There was also some amalgam under the filling material on three of the teeth.

Deborah lost one tooth shortly after the work was done, and another that had been worked on was lost three or four years later.[166] Also, as with many people who have had tooth decay, Deborah's jawbone was compromised.

Amalgam Conclusion
1. Multiple "unexplained" health problems can be a signal of amalgam illness. How many people are made sick by amalgam fillings no one knows. Somewhere between the dental industry's stance that nobody is and the claims by others that amalgam makes everyone sick lies the truth of the matter. There are a large number of factors involved, and meaningful statistics may be impossible to produce. However, two things are certain: Mercury is a neurotoxin of the worst sort, and putting it in the mouth has caused considerable harm to a very substantial number of people.
2. Amalgam illness is usually, but not always, from low-dose exposure over a long period of time. Often decades.
3. Sometimes people get sick right after dental work in which mercury was used or disturbed. In that case, we think it is wise to aggressively detoxify, and after the crisis is over to continue to detoxify at a lower rate.
4. Removal of amalgam fillings may or may not be a wise thing to do. If the patient is in great health, to carefully remove a small amalgam filling is one thing. If the patient is not healthy, *or* if the patient has a mouth full of amalgams, that is another. Also, some people are far more sensitive than others. Most people who are stung by a bee have a little discomfort for a day or so, and that's the end of it. For about one in 1,100, however, the sting can be life-threatening. Likewise, some people are far more sensitive to heavy metals than others. Like the bee sting— but with more frequency—new exposure to mercury when it is released in the process of amalgam removal can be very dangerous. Therefore, we think that to slow down, learn, and make an informed decision is the only wise course of action. **It is not merely a matter of getting a knowledgeable and careful dentist to do the work!** The patient can—and we think

must—do a lot to protect himself or herself by preparing for the treatment and by following up after treatment with adequate detoxification. We believe that the stakes are too high to do otherwise. Having said that much, in many cases it probably is a good idea to get amalgam removed. If you have mercury poisoning, there may not be a good alternative. Without removing the source of the poisoning, the effectiveness of any treatment is quite limited and can in fact be harmful. If you have amalgam fillings—especially if you have several—and you do not have any health issues, consider yourself lucky. But also realize that you are carrying around a potential time bomb and you do not know if, or when, it may go off. **I am not advising the reader to do anything; I am merely stating some points for consideration.**

5. Some people can recover from amalgam illness simply by having the amalgam removed. Many cannot. Many actually get sicker after amalgams are removed. Percentages are impossible to state, but all three responses are common. Remember that the effect may not be realized for months or even years. A significant number of people who have had longstanding serious health issues (like Deborah) are likely to need further medical treatment after amalgams are removed. And after removal, many people will require more extensive dental work.

6. If you tell your doctor that you suspect you have amalgam illness, he will probably think you are nuts. That is what his medical training taught him to think, and any other evidence notwithstanding, that will likely be what he will think of you.

7. **Dental gold** typically contains 50-90% gold, 1-30% silver, 0-20% palladium, and 0-12% platinum.[167] I found no evidence of mercury being used in dental gold, but anything is possible. The question in some cases may not be one of mercury but of reaction to *any* metal.

8. Porcelain crowns are often mostly nickel covered with a thin coating of porcelain. That nickel makes many people sick.[168]

9. Many people have adverse reactions to the nickel in stainless steel that is used in **dental braces**. If you have both amalgam and metal braces in your mouth, electrolysis is taking place and it is possible, if not likely, that the amalgam is corroding.

10. It is needful to say here that **tooth decay, though looked at as easily remedied in our society, is in fact a serious matter.**

First, infection can seriously compromise the immune system, and like Deborah, you may not know that a filled tooth is infected. Second, once a tooth is compromised, it may need to be attended to many times over a person's life, each time requiring more elaborate treatment and expense. And who knows what the potential harmful effects of the new filling materials may be or how our body chemistry may change?[169]

11. In my opinion, anyone considering amalgam removal should read Part II of this book carefully and also read Huggins' books. (See Resources) **The removal of amalgam fillings often turns into a significantly larger project than the patient anticipated**, so it is prudent to understand what the variables are. It is also worthwhile to see the downsides of various dental procedures that your dentist cannot or will not discuss with you unless you bring up all the talking points. Huggins has made it quite easy for us by stating what those talking points are.[170]

Read Directions Before Use

WARNING *Ingestion:* May cause Neurotoxic Nephrotoxic effects.
Inhalation: May cause Bronchiolitis, Pneumonitis Pulmonary Edema
Eyes & Skin: May cause redness and irritation to eyes and skin.
Acute Exposure: May cause sensitization dermatitis and possible visual disturbances.
California Prop 65 Warning: This product contains mercury, a chemical known to the State of California to cause birth defects or other reproductive harm.

Store at temperature no higher than 25°C.

Mercury Complies to ISO 1560: 1985

Keep Out Of Reach Of Children

Caution: Federal law restricts this device to sale by or on the order of a dentist.

Approximate Alloy Content:	Silver	41.5%
	Tin	30.5%
	Copper	28.0%

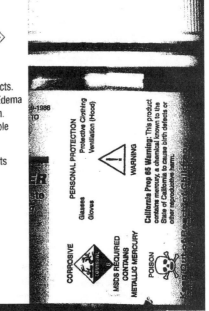

Above and next page: Dental mercury container label and warnings.

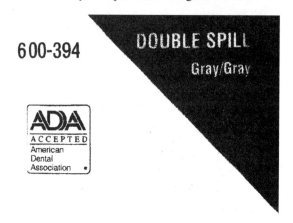

600-394

DOUBLE SPILL
Gray/Gray

ADA
ACCEPTED
American
Dental
Association •

EACH CAPSULE CONTAINS:
600 mg. ALLOY/600 mg. MERCURY

WARNING: This dental amalgam product contains mercury. The placement of a dental amalgam in a patient will increase the level of mercury in the body of the patient. The use of a rubber dam may decrease the amount of mercury absorbed by a patient during the removal or placement of an amalgam.

The health authorities of the various countries including Canada, Germany, France, the United Kingdom, Norway and Austria have recommended against the placement or removal of an amalgam in certain individuals such as pregnant and nursing women and persons with impaired kidney function. You should check with the authorities in your country that govern the practice of dentistry and dental materials to determine what recommendations or restrictions apply to the use of dental amalgams. The United States Food and Drug Administration and the World Health Organization have stated that there is no basis for any restrictions on the use of amalgams.

In rare cases, a patient may suffer a localized hypersensitivity reaction to dental amalgam.

Proper care should be taken when handling this product. Protective measures such as the wearing of gloves, using the product in a well ventilated area, using an enclosed amalgamator when mixing the product, proper disposal of spent capsules and any excess unused amalgam, and the use of HGX, or similar-type mercury absorbing compounds in the event of spillage, should be employed. These precautionary procedures should always be used in addition to procedures recommended by your local regulatory agency and dental association.

The following information is contained in the Health Hazard Data section of the Material Safety Data Sheet for this product.

Effects and Hazards of Eye Contact: Irritant. Acute Exposure: Contact may cause irritation. Mercury is corrosive and may cause corneal injury or burns. Chronic Exposure: Mercury may be deposited in the lens of the eye, causing visual disturbances.

Effects and Hazards of Skin Contact: Irritant/Sensitizer/Neurotoxin/ Nephrotoxin. Acute Exposure: May cause redness and irritation. Chronic Exposure: Possible sensitization, dermatitis and swelling. Mercury may be absorbed through the skin causing urinary problems.

Effects and Hazards of Inhalation: Irritant/Sensitizer/Neurotoxin. Acute Exposure: Inhalation of mercury vapor can cause cough, fever, nausea and vomiting. Chronic Exposure: Inhalation of high concentrations of mercury vapor over a long period may cause mercurialism. Findings are extremely variable and include tremors, salivation, stomatitis, loosening of teeth, blue lines on gums, pain and numbness in extremities.

Effects and Hazards of Ingestion: Neurotoxic/Nephrotoxic. Acute Exposure: May cause nausea, vomiting, kidney damage and nerve effects. Chronic Exposure: Symptoms include central nervous system (CNS) disorders.

California Prop 65 Warning:
This product contains mercury, a chemical known to the State of California to cause birth defects or other reproductive harm.

CAUTION: FEDERAL LAW RESTRICTS THIS DEVICE TO SALE BY OR ON THE ORDER OF A DENTIST.

"Clinical studies in adults and children ages 6 and above have found no link between dental amalgam and health problems."
FDA website 4-30-13, "About Dental Amalgam Fillings"

Chapter 11
Three Other Mercury Poisoning Cases

In this chapter, I want to tell you about three other mercury toxicity cases. Discussing these cases here will give a better overall picture of typical mercury poisoning in the US today. Again, this book is only about our experiences or the experiences of people we know. These are real people, and thanks to mercury, we have become close to them.

Jane

Jane was a florist for about twenty-five years and had spent a great deal of time making arrangements with cut flowers. Many cut flowers come from South America. They need to be protected from fungus, so guess what is sprayed on them before they are shipped? You guessed it, mercury. Of course they don't call the product mercury, but that is the active ingredient in some of the fungicides of choice.[171]

Over the years, Jane started becoming fatigued. She eventually had to quit work and then became nearly incapacitated. She started losing her memory. At first she thought it was just part of getting a little older, but then the condition progressed to the point that she did not dare leave the room if she turned on the stove or started the bath water. There was no possibility that she would remember that she had done so.

The mercury in Jane had settled in her brain. And it is not so easy to get it out.

Bill

Bill is a medical doctor and researcher from the Seattle area whom I met while writing this book. He worked his way through his undergraduate schooling by painting houses and apartments in the summertime. Most of the work was indoors in vacant homes, and if the job was far from where he lived, he would stay in the home he was painting overnight. Sometimes the evenings got uncomfortably cool, and when they did he would shut most of the windows. He got used to the paint fumes, and after a while they did not bother him. Later, after he got his medical practice established, he acquired a great fondness for sushi and would eat it a few or even several times a week.

When he was in his fifties, he became quite ill. He was tired all the time and could not remember anything. He went on a leave of absence, but the condition only got worse. About that time, the fish scare came out, and Bill decided to get his blood checked for mercury. He did, and the test results came back very high. He had a few DMPS treatments (I'll tell you about that later) and afterwards felt much better. His memory and energy came back, though he still struggles at times.

As we swapped mercury stories, Bill told me that he thought that his exposure was from the fish and the phenyl mercury in the paint, and then added, "But of course, I'll never really know."

Bill asked me what Deborah's glutathione count was. I told him I didn't know. He expected it would be (or had been) quite low, and he went on to tell me that people with mercury poisoning typically have a low, or even a very low, count. His had been very low. When I got home, I checked Deborah's blood tests and all indicated that she had maintained a high count. When I told Bill that, he then asked me if she had been taking heavy doses of vitamin C. I told him that as long as I could remember she had been taking between 1,000 and 2,000 mg a day. "Well, that explains it," he said. "Vitamin C stimulates glutathione production. That's why she didn't get worse."[172]

Jean

Jean is a business colleague whom Deborah went to see from time to time. She has a son, Sammy, who has **autism**.[173] If you know anything about autism, you know that it is far from rare. Now. It was virtually unknown thirty years ago. You probably also know that the severity of the cases varies considerably.

The spike in the number of autism cases coincides precisely with the increased number of vaccines on the CDC immunization schedule beginning in 1988, and consequently given to infants born after that time.[174] Almost all of these vaccines were preserved with—you guessed it—mercury. Of course, they don't call it mercury, they call it thimerosal.[175]

Jean's son, like countless other autistic children born in the US between 1988 and 2003, was injected with between 12.5 and 25 micrograms of mercury before he left the hospital as a newborn.[176] According to the CDC schedule, he, like the millions of other babies of that era, received another 175 mcg total at his "well baby" examinations at two months and at six months. For a baby, 1.5 mcg in a single day *was* considered "safe."[177]

At about eighteen months, Jean went to the doctor to get another 87.5 mcg of mercury injected into Sammy. Of course, she didn't know that.

A few days after the injection, she lost Sammy. Oh, he didn't die; she just hasn't seen the same child since. The once lively, smart, and affectionate Sammy stopped talking. He would no longer make eye contact with his mother or father. He started having diarrhea. At times he began screaming while holding his stomach. As the days went on, it got worse. He began flapping his arms wildly. He did not seem to be aware of anyone else. Sometimes, at the slightest noise he would cover his ears and scream uncontrollably. At other times, he became silent and seemed to be in a state of bewilderment. It got worse. And worse.

The same scenario was played out in tens of thousands of American homes during that era. It went like this: 1) Parents have a healthy, happy baby. 2) Parents take the baby to the doctor for "well-baby" immunizations when he is between one and two years old. 3) A few days or weeks after the immunizations, the baby falls into the abyss of autism.

In many more cases, the onset of problems was earlier or later, or less or more severe. Of course, most of the children immunized at that time did not develop full-blown autism. But more than 100,000 did, and a much larger number of others developed less severe neurological disorders such as ADD and ADHD.[178]

Is it a wonder that Sammy has a high level of neurotoxic mercury in his body? That he is autistic?

Several class-action lawsuits over thimerosal went to trial, and the parents of the autistic children lost them all in the federal vaccine court.[179] There was simply not enough "scientific" proof that the mercury in thimerosal caused autism.[180] [181] The parameters given by the court for the cases are perhaps a perfect example of how you can make your "science" say anything you want. The plaintiffs had to show that at least fifty percent of the cause of their children's autism was thimerosal.[182] According to the judges, they could not, so thimerosal was exonerated and judged as not harmful.

Somehow, lost in the fervor of the early part of the litigation was the fact that the CDC had not conducted any further examination into the cause of autism, or more specifically, why suddenly one in 166 instead of one in 10,000 American children developed the disease.[183] [184]

I think it is easy to understand the ramifications if one of the judges' decisions had gone in favor of the parents. Settlement payouts could have been reminiscent of the tobacco suits, and there is no way that those in authority were going to allow that to happen. [185] Whether or not mercury (or the vaccines for that matter) likely played a major role in these kids developing autism was immaterial; those who had the most to lose did everything conceivable to cover their backsides.[186]

I will mention just a few high points (or is it low points?) of the history of what led to the litigation. First, some parents of autistic children born in the late 1980s or early 1990s discovered that their children's symptoms were very similar to some of the classic symptoms of mercury poisoning in adults. They investigated and eventually found out that mercury was in the vaccines given to their children. From the time the mercury/vaccine/autism hypothesis was presented by the parents to health officials, the parents had a tough time of it. When they brought this information to the authorities, what they received were the typical placating, condescending responses that those with politically incorrect diseases are accustomed to.[187] There would be no cooperation.

The parents were first told that there was no epidemic of autism, but rather the increased number of cases was due to better diagnosis and reporting. The number of autism cases was the same as it had always been.[188] So, a search was made for the hundreds of thousands of adults with classic autism who had preceded this group of children and should have existed, but obviously they were not found.[189]

Later, as the human genome project heated up, and it became popular in "scientific" circles to say that everything was genetically caused, the authorities placed the blame on genetics. Sadly, it was not until 2004 that the CDC would admit that there was an epidemic of autism cases in American children. Epidemics are caused by environmental factors, not genetics. So much for the genetic theory.[190]

At one point, the naysayers went so far as to say that the ethyl mercury used was not toxic because it was always excreted out of the body.[191] However, those who made that claim turned down a proposal for a scientific study that would have shed significant light on the issue. The proposal was this: Since the health authorities, vaccine makers, and certain pediatricians and researchers were so confident that ethyl mercury was not a cause for alarm, would they not be willing to be injected with a corresponding amount of ethyl mercury that the children were injected with? There was certainly a large enough candidate pool for the proposed study, but unfortunately there were no volunteers, and a great opportunity for science was lost... Or maybe it wasn't lost.

Thankfully, some highly respected, well-placed people, such as Boyd Haley of the University of Kentucky, and Neal Halsey of Johns Hopkins, went against the tide of the medical community to one degree or another concerning the supposed safety of the use of mercury in the trade. But those who did were few and far between.

Many "scientific" studies came out after the litigation began. The odds of any of them being objective are nearly nil.[192] Regardless, no amount of "scientific" studies will change the fact that mercury is a neurotoxin like no other and that these kids were injected with doses of it that were far above what the EPA considers safe. That thought being unpalatable to the public health authorities, the fishing industry instead has taken a good hammering, and the mothers of autistic children were blamed for eating too much fish and passing the mercury on to their children.

The problem is not that there was not enough evidence presented against thimerosal in the trials. The records of the initial clinical trial and FDA approval of the product, back in 1930, were found to be spotty, destroyed, or sealed from public view. Thimerosal was simply given the status of being "grandfathered in." Through the decades of use, there were also plenty of warnings given to health authorities about the mercury in thimerosal from reputable sources that were uncovered during the litigation that could not be denied.[193]

Also exposed in the trials were enormous conflicts of interest between the public health agencies and the medical and pharmaceutical industries. Many CDC and FDA officials were paid "consultants" for the drug companies, and as is commonly the case in government agencies, top personnel cycle between industry and top government positions. Due to this revolving door, in many cases there is, for all practical purposes, no difference between the two. The government agencies simply do the will of industry.[194]

For this reason, when it came to dealing with the parents, decency was thrown out the window, and those who were harmed the most by the failure of our "public health" system and our "health care" system received the full fury of their combined forces. It did not matter that these children and their parents had suffered irreparable harm from gross negligence, or that their homes and lives were shattered. Court cases are war, and they would be slapped in the face and crushed. [195] [196]

Unfortunately, many internal government records on thimerosal have been sealed by court order.[197]

To this day, the CDC maintains that "there is no convincing evidence of harm caused by low doses of thimerosal in vaccines except for minor reactions like redness and swelling at the injection site."[198] [199] [200]

In other words, by looking at the CDC website, we are to believe that mercury released from coal-fired industrial plants came down in rain and poisoned the fish that these mothers ate, but their babies were not poisoned by having mercury injected into them at concentrations 40 to 100 times higher than that which the EPA calls dangerous.[201]

Autism is not so simple. There are almost certainly other factors that are responsible for its rise as well.[202] But, that high concentrations of the earth's most toxic non-radioactive element and a known neurotoxin contributed significantly to the epidemic cannot reasonably be denied.

So, on one hand, we are left with the CDC telling us that "there is no convincing evidence of harm caused by low doses of thimerosal in vaccines." On the other hand, when the amount of mercury being injected into infants was revealed, the director of The Institute for Vaccine Safety told a reporter, "My first reaction was simply disbelief, which was the reaction of almost everybody involved in vaccines. In most vaccine containers, thimerosal is listed as a mercury derivative, a hundredth of a percent. And what I believed, and what everybody else believed, was that it was truly a trace, a biologically insignificant amount. My honest belief is that if the labels had had the mercury content in micrograms, this would have been uncovered years ago. But the fact is, no one did the calculation."[203] [204]

I have purposely kept the thimerosal discussion brief. For a better understanding of the topic, please read all the notes in this section and see Resources.

I will close this section by stating that chelation for some of these autistic children produced excellent results.[205] With others, the results were minimal, if it had any effect at all. Treatment as soon as possible after exposure is the biggest factor, but certainly not the only factor for successful chelation.[206]

Conclusion of the Thimerosal/Autism Issue
Compare the 1983 and 2010 immunization charts on the next pages.

"Studies have shown that there is no known harm from thimerosal preservative-containing vaccines."

FDA website, February 22, 2013 [207]

CDC Mandatory Vaccine Schedule 1983 vs. 2010

For children, from birth to 6 years (recommended month)
(Most of the increase was in 1988)

US 1983	US 2010
DTP (2)	Influenza (prenatal)
OPV (2)	Hep B (birth)
DTP (4)	Hep B (1)
OPV (4)	DTap (2)
DTP (6)	Hib (2)
MMR (15)	IPV (2)
DTP (18)	PCV (2)
OPV (18)	Rotovirus (2)
DTP (48)	DTap (4)
OPV (48)	Hib (4)
	IPV (4)
	PCV (4)
	Rotovirus (4)
	Hep B (6)
	DTap (6)
	Hib (6)
	IPV (6)
	PCV (6)
	Influenza (6)
	Rotovirus (6)
	Hib (12)
	MMR (12)
	Varicella (12)
	PCV (12)
	Hep A (12)
	D Tap (15)
	Hep A (18)
	Influenza (18)
	PPS (24) (if high risk)
	MCV (24) (if high risk)
	Influenza (30)
	Influenza (42)
	MMR (48)
	DTap (48)
	Varicella (48)
	IPV (48)
	Influenza (54)
	Influenza (66)

CDC Immunization Schedule, 1983

TABLE 1. Recommended schedule for active immunization of normal infants and children (See individual ACIP recommendations for details.)

Recommended age*	Vaccine(s)[†]	Comments
2 mo.	DTP-1,[§] OPV-1[¶]	Can be given earlier in areas of high endemicity
4 mo.	DTP-2, OPV-2	6-wks-2-mo. interval desired between OPV doses to avoid interference
6 mo.	DTP-3	An additional dose of OPV at this time is optional for use in areas with a high risk of polio exposure
15 mo.**	MMR[††]	
18 mo.**	DTP-4, OPV-3	Completion of primary series
4-6 yr.[§§]	DTP-5, OPV-4	Preferably at or before school entry
14-16. yr	Td[¶¶]	Repeat every 10 years throughout life

*These recommended ages should not be construed as absolute, i.e. 2 mos. can be 6-10 weeks, etc.

[†]For all products used, consult manufacturer's package enclosure for instructions for storage, handling, and administration. Immunobiologics prepared by different manufacturers may vary, and those of the same manufacturer may change from time to time. The package insert should be followed for a specific product.

[§]DTP—Diphtheria and tetanus toxoids and pertussis vaccine.

[¶]OPV—Oral, attenuated poliovirus vaccine contains poliovirus types 1, 2, and 3.

**Simultaneous administration of MMR, DTP, and OPV is appropriate for patients whose compliance with medical care recommendations cannot be assured.

[††]MMR—Live measles, mumps, and rubella viruses in a combined vaccine (see text for discussion of single vaccines versus combination).

[§§]Up to the seventh birthday.

[¶¶]Td—Adult tetanus toxoid and diphtheria toxoid in combination, which contains the same dose of tetanus toxoid as DTP or DT and a reduced dose of diphtheria toxoid.

1983 childhood immunization schedule

Industry Guidelines; Gnats and Camels

As far as we can tell, none of the stories of mercury poisoning that I have related to you in this chapter came from large industrial exposures such as what happened in Minamata, Japan. Nor, as far as I know, were any of these people exposed industrial workers. But the stories given of the people in this chapter are no less real. And they are far more common. A more subtle disaster has taken place here in the US that, after the dust settles, may in fact dwarf the disaster in Minamata. Though our health authorities as of yet have not significantly changed their rhetoric, the amalgam and thimerosal issues are not going to go away. There is no denying that mercury commonly accumulates in the body and that these are two known sources of exposure. The only argument is over what sources of exposure we are going to call harmful.

I commend our federal health agencies for learning a lot about mercury poisoning from what happened in Japan and later in Iraq. And I commend them for what they have learned from the exposures of people who worked in, or lived near, industrial plants where mercury is used. But I do not believe that those kinds of exposures represent the majority of mercury poisoning cases in the US. Nor do I believe that basing studies and industrial guidelines upon exposures such as those in Japan, in Iraq, and in industrial sites is advantageous to the cause of public health.[208] Further, the current medical practice that excludes looking for mercury unless there has been a known "industrial" exposure is tantamount to closing your eyes. By focusing attention only in politically correct places, and refusing to look in other places, our public health agencies have brought us into a state of affairs where stories like the one I will tell you next are commonplace.

On August 10, 2012, liquid mercury from a wall-mounted blood pressure meter leaked out of the device and onto the floor in a doctor's office in South Miami. As required by law, the incident was reported, and soon the Miami-Dade Fire and Rescue people were on the scene. The large, multistory building was evacuated, the area was cordoned off, and a Haz-Mat team came in to deal with the highly toxic substance. It was found to be a very small spill (probably a few ounces) and was cleaned up by people wearing special protective clothing. Eventually the building was reopened, but not before news of the dangerous spill was flashed across the nation.

On that very same day, that same shiny, silver-colored metal was placed in the mouths of 100,000 people in dental offices all over the US.[209]

Sounds to me like straining out the gnat and swallowing the camel.

A Short Story of Lead

The dangers of lead poisoning were well known long before we started adding tetraethyl lead to gasoline in 1923. Even the key figure in the development of the compound, Thomas Midgley Jr., suffered greatly from his own invention. But that did not deter him from swearing that it was perfectly safe. Likewise, many people died in the production of the product, and many more went insane or were otherwise left in sorry shape, but that did not deter the companies that produced it.

Not surprisingly, when in the 1950s, a researcher by the name of Clair Patterson determined to understand why we had such a huge increase of lead in the atmosphere, he invariably came up with either wrong or misleading information. It turns out that the "studies" done on lead safety had been funded by the manufacturers of lead additives.

Patterson found out that the great majority of lead in the atmosphere came from automobile tailpipes, and after a long fight, lead was finally removed from US gasoline in 1986. Shortly thereafter, lead arsenate was finally removed from pesticides, and later lead was removed from most paints.

But that lead is still with us—once extracted, we can't put it back into the rocks from which it came—and Americans now have hundreds of times more lead in their tissues and bones than they did before it was discovered that engine knock could be eliminated by tetraethyl lead and that bugs could be killed by spraying lead on them.

Chapter 12
Detoxification and Chelation

During the time that the first round of Deborah's dental work was going on, she and I researched what to do next. What we needed to do was find a way to get the havoc causer, the mercury, out of her tissues.

Now that she knew the likely underlying cause for three decades of ill health and the further health threats she faced, Deborah was on a mission. She wanted to get the mercury out yesterday, if not sooner. The train was moving, and I felt like I was running full speed in my research to try to keep up with her so that a check could be made on her decisions. There was no good alternative. She had suffered enough and was intent on trying to minimize the chances of developing Alzheimer's, Parkinson's, or one of the other diseases commonly associated with mercury toxicity. At the same time, I was becoming aware of the possible consequences if we made a mistake. I am very thankful that Deborah and I had good coordination. She was ahead of me in understanding on several points, and I checked her findings, which of course brought up more questions, which I also researched. I was a student again, in effect taking a tough biochemistry course for which I did not have the prerequisite courses. I went over some of my findings with Deborah and shielded her from others because I felt they were too scary and would not be beneficial to her.[210]

While the mainstream medical system is dancing around the subject of mercury poisoning, there are many people who are suffering greatly and do not have time for the politics of the matter to play out. Thankfully, there are professionals on the periphery of the medical system or outside of it altogether who are writing about the subject. However, their opinions on what constitutes dangerous exposure and what treatments are beneficial vary considerably.

Our job was to find out what was most credible from the better sources and develop an appropriate course of action.

Detoxification Sequence
As we saw it, and still see it, detoxification of mercury has to be taken in steps. The first step is to get a good understanding of what

you are dealing with and eliminate all known sources of exposure. **Eliminating** fish from the diet is pretty easy. **Removing** amalgams is not. For that, there is some preparation and cooperation needed, as I discussed in the chapter on amalgam removal. The **filtering** organs may need to be strengthened or fortified so that they can do their jobs adequately, and collectors, or **binding** agents, need to be taken to help in the **removing** of the metal from the body that is released during the dental work.

To rid the body of **loose** mercury, that is, mercury from new exposures, is one thing. To mobilize mercury that has been **embedded** in the tissues is entirely another matter. That is declaring war. With war, careful preparation is required, and some ugly things are likely to happen. Next, after the mercury has been removed from the tissues (as much as can be determined), then it is time to go after that which is lodged in the brain.[211] Last, after these steps are accomplished, there is by necessity a repair and maintenance period. A war-ravaged country is not healed as soon as the shooting stops.

During and after the dental work, Deborah took massive doses of chlorella[212] (fresh-water algae) and NAC (N-acetyl cysteine) to try to "bind" the loose mercury[213] and move it out of her system **through the bowel**. She drank plenty of water to **flush the kidneys**. She took heavy doses of vitamin C to **boost her immune system**. [Important information on the use of glutathione, cilantro, and chlorella is in this note.[214]] She also had massage treatments that varied from deep tissue massage to lymphatic massage in order to maximize **the flushing action of the lymph**.[215] She brushed her skin daily with a skin brush and took clay baths to **release toxins through the skin**. However, Deborah was convinced through everything she had read that these methods alone—though very effective for loose mercury—would not get the mercury out of the tissues. She believed that she needed to extract the embedded mercury with something more effective; that is, with chemical chelators.

To remove mercury from the *tissues*, a process called chelation may be needed. **Chelation** is the process of pulling heavy metals out of the body tissues by having them bind to another substance so that they can be released into the bloodstream, filtered out by the kidneys and liver (primarily), and then removed from the body through the urine and feces.[216] Though there are some "natural" chelators for mercury (such as vitamin C), by themselves they appear to be limited in their effectiveness. Also, if used incorrectly they can in fact be dangerous. Alpha lipoic acid and cilantro are two good examples. The severe warnings on these two are that they enable mercury to cross the blood-brain barrier. If mercury is suddenly released, as it is during amalgam removal, or if it is released from other tissues during chelation with other chemicals, it can go into the brain instead of out of it. Hence the importance of proper protocol. According to some experts, these products should not be used for some time before or after dental work.

In common usage, the line is somewhat blurred between what is called a chelator and what is called a detoxifier. Since the most effective means of chelation are pharmaceuticals, the term "chelation" often refers to using these products. The drugs used to chelate mercury were developed initially for industrial workers who had heavy metal poisoning. In the US, the drugs are recommended for acute poisoning shortly after exposure, because that is when they are most effective. However, there are many more people who have chronic metals poisoning, and from what I can tell, our mainstream medical system has for all practical purposes denied the condition and turned its back on them.

Chemical Chelators
All the medical people we saw (who would talk about metals poisoning) and Deborah's naturopath were of the same opinion, that the mercury could not be extracted from her tissues without the use of a powerful pharmaceutical. The drug most suited for chelating mercury is dimercapto-1-propanesulfonic acid, or DMPS.[217] It is not surprising that the dangers of the drug are considerable.[218] [219] That is virtually always the case with pharmaceuticals, and not only for ultrasensitive people like Deborah. Mary, whose case is worse than Deborah's, had a course of DMPS and it weakened her for years.[220] Due to her sensitivities, DMPS looked far too dangerous for Deborah. If we could, we would avoid it.

We consulted with health professionals of different persuasions who were at least somewhat knowledgeable about mercury toxicity.

Some offered chelation treatments, some did not. Our interview with one physician was most interesting. Concerning mercury, he said, "That is wicked stuff." "Wicked" is not a common word in a physician's vocabulary now days, but this man (who did not provide chelation treatment), explained to us that seemingly untraceable amounts of mercury can cause great havoc in the body. He told us that a minute amount of mercury can cause severe damage to the nervous system and to the glands. But neither he nor the others we saw had a viable alternative for DMPS when it came to chelating mercury. Most of these professionals told us that the two other chelators sometimes used for mercury poisoning, dimercaptosuccinic acid, or DMSA, and ethylendiaminetetraacetic acid (EDTA) are very effective for chelating lead but are not nearly as effective as DMPS for chelating mercury.

Interestingly, DMSA and EDTA are FDA approved[221]; DMPS is not fully approved. Some writers on the subject say that DMPS needs more testing and they are hopeful that one day it will be fully approved. Others say it is a bad drug and should not be used. Since DMPS has been around for more than fifty years and has proven very effective for the chelation of acute mercury poisoning, I don't think that a lack of testing is the reason it has not been fully approved. The reason may be this: When a drug is fully approved by the FDA—say a drug developed for a heart condition—a physician can prescribe it for toenail fungus or any other condition if he wants to. In many cases, taking that kind of liberty with a drug is a very bad thing to do.[222] It certainly is with DMPS. For this reason, DMPS must be under the supervision of a physician specifically licensed to prescribe and use the product.

The lack of more recent testing in order for DMPS to gain FDA approval is easy to explain. It is an old drug and is very inexpensive. No one is going to spend the enormous amount of money required to test something for FDA approval if they can't make any money on it.

DMPS can be taken orally or intravenously, and state laws may affect the form in which it can be prescribed. When Deborah was considering chelation, none of the professionals we spoke with said anything about the oral option, and if I came across it elsewhere in my research, the information did not stick. As I said earlier, the train was moving on our decision, and I was playing catch-up to check Deborah's suppositions.

There are two ways to take DMPS intravenously: an injection of the substance, also called a "push," and an IV drip. The push takes a few minutes, the IV a couple of hours. The "push" assaults the system very quickly, and for that reason, Deborah and I are not in favor of it. We also strongly disagree with using DMPS in <u>any</u> form without taking appropriate detoxification precautions, which I discuss in more detail later. Many people have been harmed by what was in effect a redistribution of mercury provoked by DMPS because they did not take the necessary precautions. For this reason, the DMPS challenge test,[223] which is sometimes used to diagnose mercury poisoning, can in fact be harmful. (See DMPS Backfire in Resources.)

A "Touchy" Situation

I should mention here, in the main text of the book, that when I began my research on chelation, I had no idea that the entire subject of mercury was so hyper-sensitive in "public health" and medical circles. Also, I could not understand why, when it came to chelation or treatment, the public health websites I found were not helpful in the least. Several medical doctors wrote or said something about chelation on their websites, but the CDC was for all practical purposes mute. What I did pick up from the public health departments was the general attitude of mainstream medicine toward "non-industrial"[224] mercury exposure and toxicity. It goes something like this: "It's the fish; and don't let your children play with thermometers." At the same time, those sources I did find (on the web and at doctor visits) who were recommending chelation did not say *anything* about the fact that chelation is much more effective for acute cases than it is for chronic cases. That understanding was to come to me later.

From our reading, we *did* understand that if an internal mercury environment has been established in the body, it becomes increasingly worse unless drastic measures are taken to reverse the process. Therefore, we did not feel we had a good alternative,[225] and our next step in the game plan for dealing with mercury was to go to a doctor who provided DMPS chelation. As with the dental work, we had to find a skilled practitioner familiar with the procedure who would listen and not subject Deborah to unnecessary risk.

Strangely, we found out that few physicians provide or monitor chelation treatments. We were on the edge of "medical" practice and "alternative" practice. [226] This surprised us, and we would not really understand why until I was writing this book. The fact is that any medical doctor who even mentions mercury, let alone acknowledges that it is a problem, could be treading on thin ice with the medical establishment that holds power over his or her medical license. Like the restrictions placed on dentists referred to earlier, chelation for heavy metals toxicity—especially mercury—is not something that can be advertised or even spoken of freely by those in the industry. If they would be so bold as to say that they treat metals poisoning, they would be fortunate if they were only shunned by the medical community.[227]

[While writing this book, I contacted a physician who I found out was knowledgeable on the subject of mercury poisoning. He was very interested in Deborah's case and was excited that I was writing the book. We talked for some time and agreed to meet in person and discuss our experience and findings in more detail. The next day I picked up a message from him telling me that he had just received what was in essence a threatening letter for his public comments about mercury toxicity. Another medical doctor, Jane Hightower, a practicing physician in San Francisco and the author of *Diagnosis Mercury: Money, Politics and Poison*, was advised by a colleague that if she continued looking into mercury poisoning, she "would have no friends."[228] [229]]

The first doctor Deborah saw who practiced chelation would not listen. In speaking with him, it became evident that he would treat her just as he would any other patient; that is, with his standard determined dosage of DMPS in intravenous form. He had no flexibility and did not see any reason to approach Deborah's case any differently. He did not understand that Deborah is far more sensitive to nearly everything than most people.

After more than three decades of suffering with her sensitivities—and dealing with doctors who did not believe her—we were convinced that the risk of putting ourselves in his hands was far too great. We had read about the dangers of DMPS and realized full well that he could easily administer treatment that would leave her in a very sorry state for the rest of her life. This doctor was not interested in Deborah's history, did not believe her concerning her sensitivities, and apparently did not consider the risk involved. What he wanted to do was his standard, aggressive, full dose protocol. He wanted to start the next day, and it would be $1,200 down.

Thanks, but no thanks.

In my opinion, he was a presumptuous man wielding a very dangerous drug who had little respect for the complexity of the human body. I wish he was an isolated case.

Anyway, we were once again in that position we had known so well—we knew of no way to get help. We always hit the same roadblock with medical doctors—they simply either do not believe or do not care that some people are far more sensitive than others. It was always, "I've never heard of that before." By that time, we had heard that song and dance for more than thirty years, and we weren't buying it.

It seems many of these folks have been trained very well not to listen to their patients but rather to tell them of their competence. The concept that not everyone will react the same—that is, like the "scientific" model—is either past their mindset or purposely put out of mind. **This common industry practice of treating people as if they had no more uniqueness than automobile transmissions is for Deborah and for many others very dangerous.**

Deborah's Chelation

Through her "mercury comrade," Jean, Deborah learned of the clinic that Jean took her son to for DMPS treatments.[230] Deborah saw a naturopath there who listened. She was also told about the limited success of vitamin C chelation for some heavy metals. It was safe, but by all reports was not very effective for chelating mercury. Nevertheless, Deborah wanted to try it, and her naturopath was okay to go along with that. Deborah had four or five sessions of intravenous vitamin C, but test results showed that very little progress was made. The rate of extraction was far too slow. I was not surprised and neither was she, and I'm sure the doctor thought, "I told you so." But we had to try.

The good thing was that the vitamin C was able to chelate a significant amount of cadmium. Her levels were still high, but had decreased.

Next, Deborah agreed to try an intravenous treatment of a reduced dosage of DMPS dispersed in a saline solution. It was about 30% of the normal dose. If she could tolerate that, she and her naturopath agreed that they would increase it in steps. The last thing we wanted was to loosen up lodged mercury and dump it into the system without getting it all the way out of the body.

Deborah did okay with the DMPS in lower doses, and, over four months, worked up to full-strength, or 250 mg, treatments.[231] We slowed down the rate of the intravenous drip so that the session would take about three hours. Typically the IVs go much faster, but we felt that slower may be better. During the sessions of full-strength DMPS, Deborah usually looked gaunt. Sometimes she would cry with no conscious thought as to why.[232] She knew what was going on. That stuff that was going into her veins was a poison, and it was loosening up other poisons. Until both were eliminated, it would not be good. She came home from each treatment depleted and went straight to bed.

[By the way, I took her to the clinic for the chelation sessions and during that time saw many autistic children (some of whom had high mercury levels) come in for DMSA or DMPS injections. Seeing the suffering of those kids and sometimes of their parents from the constant strain of living with autism could break your heart.]

After each chelation session, Deborah collected her urine for 24 hours and then sent it in for testing. When she came home from the chelation treatments and had recovered enough strength, she soaked in a clay bath. She also took heavy oral doses of chlorella, bentonite clay, and NAC (N-acetyl cysteine)[233]. She could not tolerate another suggested detoxification product, alpha lipoic acid, which is supposed to be effective in removing mercury from the brain, because it will drop the blood sugar substantially.[234] [235] Within two or three days after the treatments, she was functioning pretty well again.

According to the principles of detoxification (as discussed in Chapter 8), Deborah realized that if detoxification was to be effective, it would make her feel somewhat ill. That is normal. To become too ill, however, is a signal to back off. We need to be able to function.

All through chelation, she kept up the high doses of vitamin C—per Klinghardt, spacing it as far apart from the chlorella as possible. She continued the massage treatments as described earlier and kept up an exercise regimen to detoxify the muscle tissues as much as possible. She also had regular colonics in order to cleanse the bowel as thoroughly as possible.

Deborah set up her project so that every known pathway for excreting the metal was addressed: the bowel, the lymph, the urine, the skin, and the maximum function of the organs. [236] In other words, she gave it her best shot.

Deborah insisted that she wanted to get her mercury count down to zero. She was advised that that might not be a realistic goal and was also told that she could have future exposure. [237]

The DMPS-provoked urine tests after the chelation treatments showed a large amount of mercury being discharged.[238] The other metals were being chelated out too. After three sessions at a reduced dosage, Deborah had three full-strength chelation sessions of DMPS. After these sessions, and because the *blood* tests continued to show levels of mercury, she determined to get the other dental work done (previously described in the chapter titled Amalgam Removal). After the balance of the dental work was completed, she had four or five more sessions of DMPS.

The test after the second to last session showed that the amount of mercury being chelated had dropped considerably. Her last full-strength chelation session was different from all the others. She did

not feel bad at all—it was as if she was being infused with water—
she felt nothing. She even checked with the nurse to be certain that
she had been given DMPS. The last test result came back clear—no
mercury was detected.[239]

When we saw the test results, she cried, and we gave thanks.
Deborah even broke into a spontaneous "happy dance." But we
were also very sober. We knew full well, just as we did with the
dental work, that we were far from out of the woods. By means of
chelation, mercury had been loosened from the tissues, but if it was
not all discharged, any remaining in the body could resettle
elsewhere and cause problems. And we might not know the full
effects for months or even longer.

By the time Deborah was done with all the dental work and
chelation, three years had passed and she weighed just 98 pounds.
Her five foot six body clearly showed the effect of the poisons that
had been flowing through her.

**A Summary on Chelation and Detoxification of *Chronic*
Mercury Toxicity**:
I have told you what we did and why we did it. What I am going to
say in this summary—as in the rest of the book—is just my
unprofessional and unqualified opinion that is based upon our
experience. I am not telling the reader what to do, nor have I
suggested a protocol for anyone. What I have done, to the best of
my ability, is presented the considerations and factors involved in
mercury detoxification as far as I understand them. **The
information here is for the benefit of those who take full
responsibility for their actions.** As stated in the warning after the
preface, if that is not you, you should not be reading this book.
There are needfully many warnings in this summary. There is also a
lot of hope for those with chronic metals poisoning through
detoxification and chelation. I hope that while warning, I have
encouraged as well.

These are the conclusions we have come to:
1. Chelation is not something to take lightly. If you decide to do
   chelation, you need professional help. There will likely be times

of crisis, so *the patient* needs to know how to deal with them as well.

2. The biggest danger with chelation is probably the risk of redistributing mercury (and other metals) into other parts of the body. If imbedded mercury is loosened up, it needs to be thoroughly eliminated from the body or significant harm can be done. Therefore, the importance of proper and adequate protocol cannot be overemphasized. Do we know for certain that the clay baths, the chlorella, and all the other items of the protocol that Deborah followed were the right thing to do? ABSOLUTELY NOT! We simply researched as best we could, counseled with the best professionals we could find, and made the best judgment calls we could.

3. We think that any detoxification for a *chronic* heavy metals condition has to be gradual so that the body can safely discharge the poisons.[240] If we ingest a poison and have an *acute* poisoning case (such as what happens sometimes with amalgam removal), I think every effort should be made to get it out as quickly as possible before it settles in the body. Dealing with a chronic case of poisoning is very different. In that case, the poisons are already settled in the body, and to release them too quickly can result in an acute poisoning case.

4. We think that the second biggest danger in chelation is that it may deplete the body of needed minerals. In our opinion, if there is a shortage or imbalance of needed minerals, restoring a proper balance of those minerals needs to be a priority, because their deficiency can cause potentially serious problems. For one thing, mineral deficiency may attract toxic metals.[241] Minerals may be monitored by regular blood tests, however, what is in the blood and what is in the tissue can be very different. This is another reason to have qualified professional help.

5. One of the most important items in any detoxification regimen is to keep the bowel moving properly. **Close to 90% of the body's mercury burden is discharged through the bowel. If the bowel is not emptying completely, or if the transit time of waste is too slow, toxins such as heavy metals are staying in the system and re-poisoning you.** A 12-hour transit time, from the time food is eaten until the waste from that food is excreted, is healthy. Anything more than 24 hours is definitely unhealthy. For detoxification of metals, you want the bowel to

move completely at least twice a day. (For help on this, see Bernard Jensen's book in Resources.)

6. The same can be said for the kidneys. They also do their job of filtering out toxins such as mercury. Like the bowel, the kidneys are one of the prime storage places for mercury in the body. If we do not drink enough water, kidney damage can result. How much more so while chelating!

7. For any detoxification program, we need to be as healthy as we can be. Proper nutrition and exercise are all-important. In our opinion, any doctor who does not approach chelation from a holistic standpoint cannot be of much help. We think that to eat a high fiber, healthy diet and supplement it with basic vitamins is prudent. We also think we need adequate protein and healthy oils.[242] Klinghardt and others warn against using DMPS with a high carb, low protein diet.

8. I believe it is prudent to slow down and learn before embarking on any detoxification or (especially) chelation program. You may want to read Dr. Mercola's protocol, Cutler's book, and Dr. Klinghardt's paper first (see Resources) and then read the other protocols. There are several protocols on the web, but I did not find any others that came close to adequately addressing what we believe to be the necessary details. By looking at the others, you will see why I mention Mercola, Cutler, and Klinghardt. However, some of the other websites have additional information you may want to check out. (You can search the web for "mercury chelation protocol" and a number will come up.) I do not think it is wise to trust what anyone says until you have considered conflicting points of view and have a good understanding of the subject matter yourself. If you have a knowledgeable doctor you can work with, that's great. If not, in our opinion, you need to find one. In our opinion, the last thing you want to do is just go along with what _anyone_ says. The stakes can be too high.

9. It is very helpful to read about the experiences of others who have gone before. However, it is probably not wise to pattern your program after people who chelated two months ago and now say they are all better. Better to see what they say in two years. Because of redistribution, other problems—sometimes worse ones—can show up later.

10. Chelation is very individual-specific. I think it is wise to know the specifics of your case (which metals are involved, etc.) as well as you can before submitting to any chelation protocol.

11. I cannot see any benefit from chelation before amalgam dental fillings are removed. (What value is there in dissolving your mercury fillings?) Also, if you have any metal parts in your body, chelation may not be a good idea.[243]

12. Our experience, and that of others we know of, tells us that if we are going to chelate, we need help. Too many things can go wrong and we need someone *who understands our protocol* to look after us *both professionally and at home*. Brain fog is very common during chelation, so we need to have someone at home who can help us when help is needed. We cannot evaluate and make good decisions when we do not have the mental clarity to do so.

13. Detoxifying agents are target-specific. For example, Klinghardt says that chlorella is great for getting mercury out of the gut. Cutler says alpha lipoic acid gets it out of the brain. See Cutler and Klinghardt.[244]

14. When to stop chelation is a huge question. Mercola and some others say you keep going until the provoked urine test count goes down to single digits or until you feel better. It is good to keep in mind that the possibility of depleting necessary trace minerals, or causing an imbalance in them, are big factors.

15. There are several "nutricutical" therapies on the web that are purported to be effective for heavy metal detoxification. If any are, or if any are dangerous, I don't know. (And I don't believe in magic pills.)

16. If you are chelating, you may want to slow down. There is no sense in re-poisoning yourself!

17. If you are chelating, it might be a good idea to rest. You will need the strength.

18. Having the benefit of hindsight, if we were to do DMPS chelation again, we *might* do it differently. Very shortly after all amalgam was removed, using DMPS in the form of intravenous drips, *in Deborah's case*, I believe was a good decision. Beginning about a month and a half after all the dental work was completed (and that exposure dealt with by the IV DMPS), I would consider using oral DMPS, as Cutler suggests. The oral method is much slower, but is also considered safer by some

experts. After a thorough discussion *with different professionals*, and particularly with the one who would be monitoring the treatment, we would make a decision.[245]

19. Some people have better results with chelation than others. Some people get hurt. To offer statistics on this would be meaningless because there are too many factors. What we can say is that how well designed and carried out the treatment is has a lot to do with the degree of success. So does the extent of the condition, the number and kind of toxins involved, how long the condition existed, overall health, and many other factors. Few people who have had chronic metals poisoning for an extended time are completely resolved with chelation. It is seldom a magic bullet for anyone. Our intention was to arrest the deterioration of Deborah's health that was due largely to mercury toxicity. In this it appears that we succeeded.

20. Some medical doctors performed chelation for heart disease for a period of time, then dropped it because they found it not to be the panacea it was purported to be. Recently someone sent me a CBS News article titled, "Chelation Brings Slight Benefit In Heart Disease Study, But Experts Unconvinced." The article said that 100,000 Americans "use" chelation. I mention this article to make two points. First, if these doctors or patients are approaching chelation as a means of cure without addressing the factors that cause the disease, in my opinion they are deceiving themselves and/or their patients. Second, this article, and thousands of other half-baked "news" items like it, are good reason not to read or listen to the "news" from sources that are in fact entertainment-based.[246]

21. After all we went through with Deborah's mercury chelation and detoxification, we are convinced that if someone has a heavy metal problem, they need professional help **and that means not just one person's advice**. We think it is a good idea to research different—and conflicting—resources. We also think it is prudent to only deal with people and sources that have something to lose. Long established practitioners who deal with the problem on a regular basis are probably more trustworthy than what an inexperienced physician may say because he heard or read something somewhere.

Resources are at the back of the book.

Chapter 13
The Repair and Maintenance Phase;
Mercury Conclusion

The damage that mercury, lead and other neurotoxins do to the body is often quite extensive. Therefore, detoxification from chronic poisoning from these sources can be a very long and even incomplete process. I suppose we are all conditioned to think in terms of quick fixes, but in the case of mercury that has been settled in the body for decades, the process is not so simple.

Actually, a year after chelation, Deborah did not look as healthy as she did before we decided to go after the mercury. We knew something of what we were getting into when we decided to stir up the mud at the bottom of the pond, but considering her condition (see Chapter 6) and the high probability of a continuing decline in her health, we felt that in the long run it would be the best choice.

It was not until about a year after the last DMPS treatments that Deborah began regaining her weight. In another year, she was back to a normal weight. Thankfully, her liver enzymes are now at healthy levels. Over the years since she began treatments, her liver and gallbladder have discharged very well with the aid of a supplement regimen that includes an herbal remedy.[247] The results can be seen in the blood tests and in the colonic tube. In the colonic sessions, a lot of bile—green from the gallbladder, deep neon-yellow from the liver—was discharged. A DMPS-provoked urine test a year and a half after completion of chelation showed no mercury.[248] Her blood tests also have shown no mercury.

Deborah is now in a stage of repair. The process is slow because damaged cells and tissues need to be replaced, and a healthy body equilibrium needs to be established.

After the removal of her mercury fillings and during chelation, Deborah was able to expand her diet. After being limited to five foods for nearly two decades, she was up to about twenty-five foods that she could eat without getting a headache or otherwise feeling ill. As of this writing, many other things have also improved. Her reaction to electromagnetic fields (EMFs) has been reduced considerably. Smoke is not nearly the problem it once was. And we have taken trips to the mountains without her getting elevation sickness. But she is far from "all better now." (A little more on Deborah's status is in the epilogue.)

Many stories of other people who have had chronic mercury poisoning for a long time and have chelated heavy metals are similar. Mercury poisoning and chelation are war. From what we have read, it often takes a year or more to feel that much better, and there can be large fluctuations in how you feel during that time. There is also no guarantee that all the mercury is chelated out after the initial session even though the test results seem to indicate so. As the body adjusts, the effects of treatment or of remaining metals deep in the tissues can surface at a later time, hindering further healing or causing one to feel ill again. Also, how much irreparable damage was done by the metals we may not know for a long time.

Project Management
I almost don't need to say anything about this. You can see from Chapter 4 on that for Deborah, caring for her health has been a project. She has approached everything systematically. From educating herself, to formulating a course of action, to calculated experimentation, to execution of the plan, to adjustments to that plan—all has been done systematically, even scientifically, in the true sense of the word.

I was so pleased, while writing this book, to come across Andrew Cutler's book, *Amalgam Illness: Diagnosis and Treatment*. Mr. Cutler also had a severe case of metals toxicity, and he charted out his recovery in the same manner that Deborah did hers. He has a PhD in chemistry; we do not have that kind of background.

Regardless of whether we have a strong scientific background or not, we need a good, workable plan in place. Mercury poisoning is *war*. We need trusted, capable allies, adjustments will need to be made, and strength is needed throughout the fight. Having gone through this with my dear wife, I think that nothing like tackling mercury poisoning should ever be tried alone. Further, I think it is wise to be flexible and pay attention to our body more than to any protocol. The last thing we want to do is make ourselves so sick that we cannot function.

It is important to mention that, just as with many complex projects that are not fully defined, we had cost and time overruns.

I need to make one additional very important point as I conclude this section on Deborah's mercury removal: She worked through the whole thing. The days that Deborah had chelation she took off of work, and some other days she took off too if she was ill, but those other days were relatively few. (Thankfully she was able to work flexible hours.) Working helped Deborah not be overly focused on her body, and that was a wise decision.

The Most Common Question We Are Asked

The most common question we are asked is: "How do you get mercury poisoning?" I stated in the preface and at the beginning of Chapter 9 that any short answer to this question is not a good answer. I hope that point has been made abundantly clear.

The better question may be this: "If we are all so exposed to mercury, why do some people suffer from mercury poisoning and others do not?"

First, many people *do* have harmful levels of mercury in them that have caused or are contributing to health problems, but they are not aware of it. Frequently they are being treated for other illnesses or diseases (including mental illnesses) that may not be the root problem.

Second, the bodies of some people latch onto and absorb mercury at a much higher rate than others do. Since 90% of mercury excretion is through the bowel, the frequency and completeness of evacuations is crucial. The longer waste stays in the body, the more mercury is returned into the system.

Third, a mineral deficiency can attract unhealthful metals. If we don't have a proper balance of the healthy minerals, we can be inviting the unhealthy ones to stay.

Fourth, some people filter out mercury and other heavy metals much better than others do. In other words, the filtering system of some people gets overloaded or weakened and no longer works adequately. The liver, kidneys, bowel, and skin take the lead in the gathering and discharging of heavy metals, and our overall health will determine how well these and other organs work.[249] Likewise, how well these organs work will determine our overall health. The body is one and should be treated as such. **Therefore, the value of the remaining chapters in this book cannot be overstated.**

Mercury Conclusion:

Three of the most common sources of exposure to mercury are fish, dental fillings, and vaccines. The health threats of two of the three are denied by our public health departments and by mainstream American medical practice. This being the case, it is not surprising that we cannot find one bit of practical help on how to deal with chronic mercury poisoning from these sources other than to be told to eliminate fish from the diet. So, it appears that we are going to have to go elsewhere. That is one side of the issue.

The other side is composed of the claims of those who offer various detoxification products and/or treatments. All are very positive about their products and methods and nearly all boast of great results. But dealing with heavy metals is no simple matter, every case is different, and some of those protocols for treatment, while maybe helpful for some people, are potentially harmful for a significant number of others. The basic defect, we believe, in most protocols is that they are not broad enough; that is, they are not (truly) holistic in scope.

Thankfully, there is a third side from which to view the subject; that is, from the testimony of those who have had the condition and treated it. To be helpful, a large sampling needs to be looked at. Thankfully (or sadly), we have a significant number of cases available to us. (See Resources.)

That the public health authorities will eventually acknowledge the dangers of amalgam and thimerosal is inevitable. Too many scientists, medical practitioners, and patients know the truth of the matter and have given more than ample proof of it.

Forty-some years ago, after more than sixty years of balking, our health authorities and the medical establishment finally stated what any reasonable person already knew—that cigarette smoking is harmful to health. As the evidence mounts concerning mercury, it will be the same with dental amalgam and thimerosal. No amount of "scientific" studies helped tobacco, and no amount of "scientific" studies will help these two common vehicles of heavy metal poisoning. [250]

In a clandestine way, the acknowledging of the dangers of amalgam and thimerosal is already in progress. First, thankfully, thimerosal has been removed from most vaccines. Second, the US EPA and the US Agency for Toxic Substances and Disease Registry (ATSDR), who do not have to take the heat directly, tell us that amalgams and thimerosal may in fact be problematic. The EPA is especially concerned about dental mercury because it has been proven to be a major source of mercury pollution in our water. The ATSDR says, "Removal of dental amalgams in people who have no adverse effects is not recommended and can put the person at greater risk if performed improperly."[251] By saying "people who have no adverse effects," the ATSDR is admitting the fact that some people do. Even the FDA now admits that "removing sound amalgam fillings... exposes you to additional mercury vapor released during the process."[252] Eventually, new people will come into the public health departments and say something more responsible than their predecessors have on both thimerosal and dental amalgam. It is only a matter of time... and of finding a way to turn this liability into an asset.

In the meantime, for some of us, this is not an academic debate. The question for many people is, "What do I do if I have or think I have a metals problem?" After going through what we have, I think we are wise to educate ourselves as much as possible by gathering the best information we can from conflicting sources, then study it, ask questions, and if necessary chart out a plan and have it reviewed by trusted professionals. The utmost care should be taken regardless of what we do or don't do.

Some Closing Points:
1. Heavy metals poisoning is a common component of many diagnosed, undiagnosed, and misdiagnosed illnesses. This is especially true with autoimmune disorders such as allergies,

MS, arthritis, and chronic fatigue, with any problem involving the central nervous system, and with mental illness.

2. It is a huge mistake to think of mercury poisoning by itself or simply as heavy metals poisoning. Our bodies are not that simple, and there are always other factors involved. **The fact is, no one knows at what level heavy metals may be toxic to someone.** It largely depends upon the presence of other metals, other toxins, and overall health.

3. We should take abnormal liver, kidney, bowel, or immunity function seriously. Proper function of the filtering organs and good immunity are our best protection from having mercury exposure become mercury poisoning.

4. Many of the symptoms of hypoglycemia are duplicated or intensified by mercury poisoning.[253] If you suffer from hypoglycemia or any kind of glucose intolerance, and proper diet does not correct it, or if several allergies persist after correcting the diet, you may want to get your metals checked.

5. Though we may be very ill with heavy metal toxicity, *standard* laboratory tests that our doctor orders for us will very often come back "normal." In some cases, this may be because medications and/or dietary supplements influence the tests and mask a problem. Even if something is flagged as abnormal, the last thing the doctor will suspect is heavy metals poisoning. Probably the only case in which a medical doctor will consider metals toxicity at all is when he or she is confronted with lab tests that show high levels of metals.[254]

6. A physician is trained to not make a diagnosis for chronic mercury poisoning unless there has been an industrial exposure. Therefore, it is likely that he will think of his patients with metals toxicity symptoms as psychotic. After all, that is what he learned in medical school. This may (will?) especially be the case if the patient tells their physician that they suspect amalgam illness or any other kind mercury poisoning. Also, medical textbooks and journals have a tendency to assess cases where there are a number of undiagnosed symptoms as psychological problems, so most doctors go along with that thinking.[255] The fact is, metals toxicity *is* often a component of mental illness, and someone with mercury toxicity will likely have mental challenges of one sort or another. If we want drugs to control the *symptoms* of a mental illness, our medical system

has plenty of them to "help" us with. If we want to get to the *cause*, we are largely on our own. Many times the cause of mental illness is nothing more than improper diet or heavy metals toxicity.

7. About the cost of treatment: Because mainstream medicine does not acknowledge "non-industrial" metals poisoning, insurance probably will not cover a significant portion of the cost of treatment. Dental plans are not going to pay the extra amount required to have amalgams removed safely. (Or to fill teeth with other than mercury/amalgam either.) Medical plans are unlikely to pay for chelation except, *maybe*, in the very worst cases where you are almost dead from metals poisoning. (All this is explained in Chapter 15.) This means that a very substantial part of the cost of treatment is going to come out of your pocket, regardless of whether you have "good insurance" or not. We think the best way to make use of funds is to understand the condition and treatment as much as you can. That way you are more likely to know if you are being led down a pathway that is a waste of money. I hate to say this, but every practitioner would like to make as much off of you as possible, and if you have a serious problem you are prime picking. The only way to keep a lid on costs is to manage the project yourself. Last, when insurance is involved, many practitioners give a substantial discount if you pay by cash or check. In other words, if they do not have to go through your insurance company. The insurance companies beat them up pretty good, so it is well worth asking about. If you don't ask, it is unlikely they will offer the discount!

8. Either we will manage our body or someone else who may not know it as well or care about it as much will. The choice is ours.

How Deborah got mercury poisoning could perhaps be summed up in one word: sugar. Without the ingestion of sugar, there would likely have been no tooth decay. Without tooth decay, there would have been no mercury/amalgam fillings. Without the mercury/amalgam fillings, there would have been no leaching of mercury and other contaminants into the bloodstream, and no release of mercury vapor into the mouth. Without the grossly unnatural ingestion of sugar, Deborah would likely have been stronger. Had she been healthier, she perhaps could have filtered out the mercury that she was otherwise exposed to.[256] [257] Further, without the undermining of her health by these means, it is unlikely that her diet would have become so restricted, leaving her with few food items that she could tolerate other than tuna, which is a known source of mercury exposure.

Do we know what portion of Deborah's illness was caused by the decay under her filled teeth and what portion was caused by mercury and other metals? No. We only know that sugar played the major role in the initial tooth decay.

As stated in Chapter 9, there is no lack of sources of mercury exposure in our environment, so we will never know for certain where all, or even the major part, of Deborah's exposure came from. Nor can we know for certain why her body could not filter it out. It is not possible to obtain "scientific" proof for the preceding and we are not foolish enough to insist upon it. We can only understand what can be understood, and that is that the probability of what is stated here is very high.

Remember:
What is written in this book is what my wife and I did and the conclusions we came to. We have shared it with you with the hope that, if you have the need, you will find it helpful in your own research and in your discussion with your doctors or other health care professionals. What you do in your situation is entirely your responsibility.

Resources are at the back of the book.

Part III

"Let Your Food Be Your Medicine and Let Your Medicine Be Your Food."

Hippocrates[258]

Chapter 14
The Smokers' Circle and Sugar

In 1970, while in boot camp, I lived in a barracks with fifty-nine other men. When we first arrived, we were issued our uniforms and all of our personal effects were taken away from us. We did not even have our wallets or watches. And the smokers did not have their cigarettes.

At that time, there was a lot of debate in our country over whether or not cigarette smoking was addicting. This was before, one after another, the heads of the various tobacco companies, under oath, testified before a congressional panel that they did not believe that cigarette smoking was addicting.[259] Everywhere people were debating this issue. The sixty men in our barracks didn't need to debate it. We saw for ourselves.

On the third or fourth day of basic training, the drill sergeant gave permission to those who smoked to get into their personal effects and get their cigarettes if they wanted them. Fifteen men did. We then lined up, stood at attention, and were marched outside. The drill sergeant then pointed out the smoking area and barked at us: "If you've got 'em, smoke 'em. You've got three minutes."

What happened next was truly phenomenal. Most of the men who had the cigarettes ran to the designated area, which was about thirty feet from the rest of us. There they huddled in a circle, and with trembling hands began to light their cigarettes. Many were shaking severely. Two other men who had brought their cigarettes stopped short. They, like the rest of us, saw what was happening. We all watched as the thirteen struggled to draw as much of that drug into themselves as possible within the three minutes allowed. Those two men quit that day. They had not known the depth of what they had gotten themselves into. One of the two had actually joined the smokers' circle but turned around and walked back toward the rest of us. I will never forget the shocked look on his face. As he went by me, he said something to the effect of, "I will never do that again!"

As for the thirteen smokers, if they did not know they were addicted before that time, they surely knew it then. I remember the tenor of some of the comments that some of them made later—things like: "Well, I just have to," or "Whoa!" But mostly it was a shock beyond words. For all of us. These were young men; most were between nineteen and twenty-one years old.

The argument over whether cigarette smoking was harmful or habit-forming was silly. But it was not funny. Many people died from smoke-inflicted lung cancer and other diseases while the "experts" argued over the matter. There never needed to be an argument—the smoker's cough told everyone loudly and clearly that this habit was a very serious threat to health. But real people got caught up in this deception, and many lost their lives over it. When I was growing up, our next door neighbor lost her life to lung cancer when she was in her thirties. Another neighbor woman a few doors down followed her about four years later. Young kids were left without a mother. Why?

Those who smoke today show clearly that the root problem is quite deep.

Sugar Addiction
It is the same with sugar addiction. It is foolish to argue if there is such a thing—just try quitting. Try staying off of all sweeteners, including artificial sweeteners, for one month.

I know I am talking about an old family friend here. Refined sugar has been with us for five or six generations now. We grew up with her and we all learned to love her. But she has stolen our health. Her predecessors—honey and molasses—gave nourishment to the body; she takes our stored nutrients and leaves us depleted. [260]

Any grade school teacher can tell you of the ill effects of sugar on children—just ask them what **the worst day of the school year** is. Without fail, they will tell you, "the day after Halloween." After they have finished rolling their eyes, they will describe to you in detail how the kids turn into monsters from eating all that sugar.

But this too is not funny.

The current crisis we have with so many children unable to sit still long enough to learn in school could be turned around very quickly simply by a change in diet. In the last few decades, too many people have proven this with their own children for there to be any argument over the benefits of kicking the sugar habit.

If we want to keep the kids from bouncing off the walls, if we want them to have an attention span that is longer than that of a gnat, the solution in most cases is very simple: Cut out the sugar.

One of the greatest scourges in our society today is what is called **attention deficit disorder**, or ADD. I have read several "scientific" articles about this condition, all of which tell how complex the condition is, and all of which go around and around the issue but miss the obvious. Regardless of the complexity—and lack of scientific proof—a little common sense is in order. If the nervous system has not been damaged by mercury poisoning, the most common root of the problem is simply overstimulation. Get yourself and the kids off of junk food and get away from the over-stimulation of the brain that comes from the quick flashing images on the television. Sugared-up, fast-burning junk food stimulates the brain too much. Likewise, the hyper pace of the images on the television gives no time for the child's developing brain to process the information. All that information becomes a blob. And this is during the years that those little brains are being formed! Under these conditions, it is a marvel that any kid can learn anything.[261] If we have dull children, children who are hyperactive, or children who simply cannot concentrate or solve problems, we should not think it strange considering what they are fed and what they are exposed to. What has become commonplace is NOT normal.[262]

Of course, we can ignore this and go along with some distinguished medical school professors who have come out with gems like these: "There is no valid evidence that sugar affects behavior." "Studies have failed to link hyperactivity in children and sugar consumption." "There is no scientific proof [demonstrating behavioral effects and sugar.]" "Most claims identifying [sugar] as a harmful substance have been refuted by scientific evidence."[263]

I disagree with these esteemed professors. I also disagree with the system that has allowed the lobbying of pharmaceutical companies to succeed in getting approximately 10% of ten-year-old boys in the US on Ritalin or similar drugs for the treatment of ADHD and similar conditions.[264]

We cannot flirt with sugar if we want to beat addiction to it. We will not win. **The need is to re-educate our palate** and the palates of our children so that we and our families eat natural foods that burn at a slower and more even rate. From what we have seen, more than ninety percent of the cases of hyperactive children can be solved that simply.

The behavioral problems caused by excessive sugar consumption are not only with children. **Why are so many young people who are new in the workplace functionally illiterate?** Oh, they can read. As long as it is a short sentence. But many cannot read well enough to follow simple instructions that would require reading three or four sentences. This kind of illiteracy is very different than the illiteracy we knew forty years ago. The new illiteracy is not because people failed to learn to read, but because their attention span is too short to make anything but the simplest reading impractical. Such people are in fact disabled, and the condition is far too common. Why? The same two reasons: 1) They have grown up hyped on sugar. 2) They have grown up with their senses greatly overstimulated by watching too much television and by spending an excessive amount of time playing computer games. Take away the first, replace it with a good diet, add in outdoor exercise, and the desire for the second will drop off by itself.

The pandemic of new health problems, nearly unheard of a generation or two ago—diseases of the bowel, autoimmune diseases, the great increase in cancers—where did they come from? I have heard and read many people who blame "the environment" for these diseases. My response is: "What environment?" We may not be able to do much about the outward environment we live in, but we can do a lot about the environment that we create by what we take into our mouths and into our minds and hearts.

We live in a society where most of us have a perverted appetite. Why has diabetes gone rampant? Why is this disease that was rare before 1880 now affecting a third of our population? [265] Why are people at a younger and younger age being diagnosed with it? **We need look no further than to a ruinous diet, the anchor of which is sugar consumption.**

It is important to understand what I am talking about when I say "sugar." I am including high fructose corn syrup and all other refined caloric sweeteners. The chemical sugar substitutes for caloric sweeteners may be even more unhealthful.

Sugar is added to everything. One cannot understand this until the food labels are looked at closely—that is the ingredients, not the claims made on the front of the packaging. Even the roast beef in the sandwich that we buy at a deli has a 20% dextrose and water solution added to it. Look at the ingredients of a common breakfast cereal. Many are composed of nearly 50% sugar, and the rest is simple carbohydrates, which turn to sugar almost immediately upon ingestion; and then most people add more sugar on top of that! Many of us grew up that way. And many of our parents did too.

Unfortunately, if we grew up consuming refined sugar, we likely passed some of the resulting weakness of our bodies on to our children.

There is a way out of this mess—break the sugar habit!

To break the sugar habit, the biggest need is to stop lying to ourselves.[266] To do so, it may be helpful to look at some basic statistics.

1. Sugar became available after its refining was perfected and made economical in the late 1870's. Before that time, the sweeteners used were mostly molasses and honey. Abuse of these natural sweeteners was limited, largely because few people wanted too much of either of them. As we well know, it is not that way with sugar.
2. By 1913, sugar consumption in the US had grown to about 40 pounds per person, per year. Most of that consumption was of the sugar added to canned fruit.[267]
3. In 1967, the figure was 114 pounds per person, per year.[268]
4. In 1997, the figure was 153 pounds per person, per year.[269] [270]

Please understand in reading this that I once liked apple pie as much as anyone, and my mother made the best of them. She also made pumpkin pies, apricot pies, and boysenberry pies, all of which the whole family enjoyed immensely. We thought we were eating fruit. And Mom used less sugar than the recipe called for, so we thought we were pretty healthy eaters compared to most people.

We didn't know better. The problem was that, like so many other families, we all got addicted to refined sugar. Sugar killed my grandfather. It killed my dad. The effects of sugar consumption helped my brother get a bypass. And those same effects have left their mark in me, though I turned away from this destroyer of health decades ago.

> **What I am proposing here—to break the sugar habit—is not some strange thing. It is only suggesting that we go back to the pre-1870s rate of sugar consumption. That is, to zero.**

Developing a Successful Withdrawal Plan

The earlier the sugar habit is broken the better. Granted, it may be too late for some, but in most cases it probably won't hurt to try.

Don't say you can't keep kids from sweets. Yes, the more they have been trained in the habit the harder it may be, but we know too many people who have succeeded. **Arm yourself with knowledge, develop a plan, involve the whole family, prepare well, and take it one day at a time.**

The plan should take into account the level of addiction. A young adult who has grown up largely on sweets and other junk food their whole life should probably transition slowly. A two-year plan may be needed to completely free someone with that kind of history from sugar. Hopefully they have that long before the result of such a diet causes serious health problems.

As I write this, I am thinking of so many young people I know who are in their twenties and thirties and who are now just beginning to reap the ill effects of a sugared-up diet. It is heartbreaking for me to see this among them—diabetes, obesity, bowel diseases, etc. How I hope some of you are helped by this book!

Thankfully, most cases are not as extreme as described in the preceding paragraphs, but the number of people descending into the pit of a grotesquely sugared-up diet has increased dramatically. The downward slide of our society toward this abyss, as shown in the sugar consumption statistics just mentioned, is very great.

In order to free ourselves and our family from sugar bondage, we need to devise a plan according to where we are in our overall sugar consumption. Those with a truly small habit can go "cold turkey."[271] Those with anything more than a truly small habit may do better if they take a more moderate approach. Many people have followed a plan similar to the one below. By going after the worst offenders first, many of them have succeeded.

First, cut out soft drinks and the like—they have the highest concentration of sugar. Don't substitute with fruit juice; substitute with the whole fruit. The fiber in the whole fruit will help the sugar burn slower. That is the goal—to eat foods that burn slower.

Second, cut out candy. A reasonable substitute is fresh fruit in plain yogurt. Never buy the sugared-up yogurts!

Third, cut in half the number and size of cake, pie and cookie servings, and eventually phase them out altogether. A reasonable substitute may be whole grain bread with a little honey and cinnamon on it.

Whatever we do, as we are cutting down one classification of offenders, don't increase another offender to take its place. Be methodical. This habit can be beaten!

Start switching over from pre-prepared foods to foods you prepare yourself. This helps tremendously, because in doing this we have much more control of what we are actually eating.

Replace any remaining refined sugars with natural ones, and white flour products with whole grains.

Write the plan out, assign dates for milestones of progress, and don't be afraid to adjust as you go along. Just keep moving in a positive direction.

Remember the tortoise and the hare.

Cravings should start to diminish after three to four weeks and will completely go away after a couple of months of complete abstinence. If the habit is larger, more time may be required.

After we have been weaned from sugar, in social situations we can smell all we want. Smell is the greater part of taste. In time, we will find that we do not need to taste and in fact have no desire to.

Hidden Enemies to Success
There are many people in the medical field who are milder in their approach than the medical school professors quoted previously but who nevertheless argue that sugar is not a problem. That may be true for some people. At the present time. But for the majority of the population, sugar is, or will become, a significant health problem.

I once told a medical doctor that I could not eat certain kinds of foods because of their high (natural) sugar content. He asked if I was diabetic. I told him I was not, and he fired back, "Then what's the problem!" He had obviously been primed by someone or something else concerning this subject before my appointment, because he was lit and rebuked me sharply for being so stupid. He exclaimed, "Our bodies can't burn anything but sugar anyway! All foods are converted to sugar! What's the problem?"

All of this doctor's medical training had led him to the conclusion that I was one of the stupidest people he had ever met, not that fuels burn at different rates and that it might be wise to pay attention to the kinds of fuels we burn.

Although this gentleman's treatment of his patient was unusual, his concept of sugar was not. That is the stance of the medical mainstream. For this reason, we have ample reason to state that, in our opinion, it is unlikely that we can get much help on diet from someone who is in that system.

I need to say something about **"natural" sugars and fruit juices**. Since a large portion of the population has now come to understand that refined sugar is not good for you, many people have been influenced by slick marketing to think that "natural" sugars are healthy.

Unrefined sugars are in fact much better—when taken in moderation. *If* you do not have a blood sugar problem. And *if* you do not have a yeast/fungal/candida problem.[272] Don't let the discussion of the different kinds of sugar (fructose, maltose, sucrose, lactose, etc.) distract from the point. As a society, we are way "over the top" in *any* kind of sugar consumption, "natural" or otherwise.

The problem with the "natural" "health bars," "sports drinks" (great marketing names, eh?), and similar products should be obvious— they eventually damage the body and raise blood sugar levels.

Why not call these kinds of products what they are? I applaud Jolt for taking an honest name. But I am afraid that many people are being jolted one time too many.

Look What Happened to the Food Pyramid!
The Food Pyramid was developed in Sweden in the early 1970's. The intent was to show the basic food groupings and to make dietary recommendations based upon those groupings.

The Pyramid has gone through many changes since it was first published, and the USDA came out with its own version in 1992. The US version was considerably different from the Scandinavian one and had "sweets" added to it.

In the USDA version, sweets, oils and fats are at the top of the pyramid, indicating that they should make up the smallest portion of our diet. These, it is suggested, are to be eaten sparingly. Next are the proteins: dairy products, meats, eggs, beans, and nuts. The next level contains vegetables and fruits, and at the base of the pyramid are breads, cereal, rice and pasta, which it indicates should make up the largest part of our diet.

But get this! The USDA model made no mention that these foods should be whole, natural foods. So, with this left out, the pyramid was misleading from the beginning. If the grains and starches are highly processed, they convert to sugars VERY rapidly. Because these are the kinds of foods most commonly purchased, almost all of those foods at the base of the pyramid should actually go to the top! **In effect, the Food Pyramid got turned upside down!**

The Food Pyramid has been a source of controversy since it came out. Whether or not you agree with it is not the point. My point is that it got turned upside down.

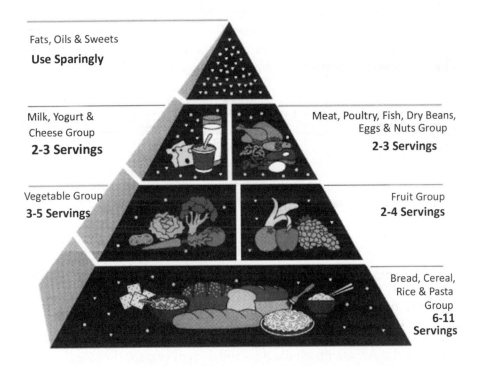

USDA Food Pyramid, 1992-2005

The newer USDA version, *My Pyramid*, which came out in 2005, was lobbied successfully by various interest groups so that what came out is so confusing that no one knows what it means. It was replaced in 2011 with *My Plate*. Both of these state the need to use whole grains, which represents a big step because it finally addresses the processed food problem, though in a very limited way. That the USDA will eventually take a stand against the use of refined sugar is inevitable, though in the meantime countless health problems are being produced in part due to this inaction.

Diabetes—All Too Common, but Not Normal

Diabetes is a condition in which the pancreas and liver can no longer control the rate at which we metabolize carbohydrates (including sugars). The result is that excess glucose is dumped into the bloodstream.

The first thing to understand about diabetes is that **the disease usually takes a few decades to develop.** Today's children who are given candy are tomorrow's diabetics.

The second thing to understand about diabetes is that **those decades could have been lived by our recent ancestors,** and we could have been born with a propensity to develop the disease much earlier.

The third thing to understand about diabetes is that **by the time the disease is diagnosed, a significant amount of damage to the body has already been done.**

"Do you have a sweet tooth? With a little planning, you can go ahead and enjoy your favorite desserts." So says the American Diabetes Association.[273]

This thought, expressed in a thousand different ways, is the position taken by the American medical establishment toward diabetes.

Let's check the objectivity of that statement. It is easy to do; just look at their own statistics.

Ugly Statistics

The same American Diabetes Association tells us that Americans spent $116 billion on diabetes in 2007.[274] To give this number some meaning, General Motors Corporation had a *worldwide* gross income of $156 billion for the same period.[275] The worldwide revenue of the diabetes industry is greater than that of GM and Ford combined.[276] Further, the upside for the diabetes industry is tremendous because the industrialized nations have exported their way of death to the developing world.[277]

Now, if you think any business is going to turn away from that kind of revenue stream, think again. If GM was "too big to fail," as we were told in 2008 before our tax dollars bailed the company out, I suppose we are to save the diabetes industry as well—regardless of what it does to our health.

It is not a strange thing then that the *prevention* of diabetes is not taken seriously by the medical establishment in the US. This stance is underscored by the fact that the US Center for Disease Control *and Prevention* puts diabetes way down in the list of causes of death in the US.[278] Diabetes is down the list because the statistics are skewed according to what is listed on a death certificate. The immediate cause of death is entered, not what brought about the cause of death.[279] Therefore we are told that the #1 killer is heart disease, #2 is cancer, #3 is stroke, and #7 is diabetes. If we look at the underlying cause of a large portion of cardiovascular disease,[280] what do we find? Bingo! Diabetes. About 65% of diabetics die from heart disease or stroke.[281]

According to the American Diabetes Association:
   8.3 % of Americans are diabetic
25.2% of Americans are "pre-diabetic" (see definition). Therefore,
33.5 % of Americans are diabetic as defined by Mr. Webster. That is, these folks typically have excessive amounts of glucose in their blood.

In other words, a third of the US population *is* in fact diabetic. Since most of these people are older, we can understand that **there are only two classifications of people in the US:**
   1. Diabetics (including "pre-diabetics")
   2. People who are likely to become diabetic

> **The discovery of insulin was truly wonderful because it saved the lives of thousands of diabetics. Unfortunately, the misuse of insulin has produced nations full of diabetics.**

When we first found out that Deborah had a blood sugar problem, I went down to the local university medical library and did a lot of reading. That was in the mid-1970s, before the Internet. One of the books I looked at was published in 1938 and was an account of an old doctor who had run a clinic in the South for decades. He described in great detail how he and the other doctors at the clinic rarely saw a case of diabetes until after Coca-a-Cola hit the market (1888). Within a short time, they began to see diabetes cases, and the number of cases multiplied exponentially over the following decades. The author even had a chart showing the number of diabetes cases at his clinic over the years and another chart showing the increase of Coca-a-Cola consumption in the US over the same period of time. The doctor who wrote the book stated that he was very concerned because he had no doubt that the dramatic increase of Coke (and sugar) was responsible for the epidemic of diabetes. He warned as stringently as he could, in vivid detail, that disaster was looming if the current trend continued.

What happened to that doctor's findings and to the findings of many others like him is not difficult to understand. Just follow the money.

If healthy living was practiced, diabetes would eventually once again become the non-issue it was in our society 130 years ago. But compare the above physician's findings with the tenor of the American Diabetes Association website, which is representative of the AMA stance. Simply stated, it goes something like this: "Oh you poor darling, you have a problem. We will help you, and you only need to change some things a little bit. Here are the drugs you need. We are here to help, and we will take care of all your needs."

Dangerous Self-Deceptions
In the information presented by the American medical establishment, there is much **emphasis on the genetic nature of diabetes**. This plays well into the hands of people who prefer to be irresponsible. How often we have heard something like, "Well, it's in my genes. There's nothing I can do about it!"[282]

In its discussion of diabetes, the Centers for Disease Control *and Prevention* website emphasizes exercise, which is absolutely correct. No improvement or correction of the condition can be expected without adequate exercise. **But the CDC will not touch the sugar issue**. It talks about weight control and eating "right," but hypocritically will not address the ill effects of **heavily processed**

foods and sugar directly. The processed foods industry is just too powerful. "Eating right," according to the CDC, is to eat smaller portions; eat less fat; limit candies, cakes, cookies, crackers, and pies; eat breakfast cereals made with 100% whole grains; eat plenty of vegetables; and drink fewer sodas.[283]

The problem with this approach is that we tend to compare ourselves with those who eat a worse diet than we do, and then think we are doing okay if we improve a little. Without stating clearly and emphatically the danger of *any* sugar in the diet, this kind of behavior is justified in the addict's mind. My, how we have seen this again and again! It is self-deception at its worst. From what I have seen, the compromise approach to sugar far too frequently leads to diabetes medication dependency.

We have ample reason to have a no-compromise stance with sugar. **We have seen the ugly side of diabetes**—the loss of hearing, the amputated limbs, the heart attacks, the loved ones who suffered for decades, and the friends who died far too young. So, I will not do you the disservice of sugarcoating the matter.

Diabetes, as a disease, has been known for thousands of years. Likewise, the connection between sugar consumption and diabetes has been known for generations. The discoverer of insulin, Frederick Banting, knew precisely what was responsible for the explosion of diabetes cases—refined sugar! [284] It seems it is only the current "scientific" community—the CDC, the AMA, and the American Diabetes Association—that will not admit the obvious.

If you have a problem with fleas in your house, don't spend your time chasing the fleas. Get the elephant out of the living room, and most of the fleas will go out with it.

Are we going to listen to all the "scientific" hoopla that distracts us from the obvious, or will we use good common sense and get sugar and other highly processed foods out of the diet?

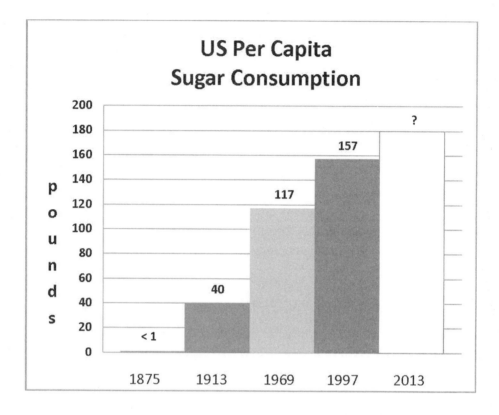

US Per Capita Sugar Consumption

Shortly after his discovery of insulin in 1922, Frederick Banting, along with several other top medical men of his day, was invited by the United Fruit Company to visit its hospitals in the Caribbean and in Central and South America. The company invited him because of the explosion of diabetes cases among its workers. While strolling through the docks in Havana, Banting saw many shiploads of sugarcane bound for the US. But he also saw something he did not expect—incoming cargos of refined sugar from refineries in the US. Seeing the volume being unloaded, he immediately understood. Diabetes, which had previously only been among the wealthy, by cheap imported sugar had become the disease of the poor as well.

Everywhere he went in his tour, he found the same thing. Refined sugar was now inexpensive everywhere. The raw substance—sugar cane—had almost never caused the disease; the refined product was quite another matter.

Rabbit Trails
Other than to say that both Type 1 and Type 2 diabetes stem from the same destructive diet (whether by the eater or by his or her forebears or both), I will not discuss the types of diabetes. The definitions of the types of diabetes have been expanded and changed in recent years, and are still changing. This has made the matter unnecessarily confusing, so I will not go down that rabbit trail. There is plenty of information available on the types of diabetes if you want it. There is not, however, much available that tells us a reasonable way of **preventing** the disease or of controlling it without medications. That is the intent here.

Therefore, I do not care one bit about "the latest findings on diabetes." Virtually all of that noise is a distraction from the main point. When dealing with diabetes or the threat of diabetes, the main point should be simply to return to a natural diet free of processed foods, the leading component of which is sugar.

Also, I do not see the least bit of value in counting calories in order to lose weight. From what I have observed, if sugar and other unnatural foods are eliminated from the diet, the "sweet tooth" will no longer control us, and the excess weight will fall off by itself. There may be exceptions to this, but I have not seen one yet.

Last, I find no value whatsoever in compromising the stance stated here against refined sugar and processed foods. According to everything we have experienced and observed, **a change to a more natural way of life is the only hope for a non-drug approach to prevention and control of the disease.**

For a longtime insulin user, it may or may not be too late. Many who have taken the "natural" way do not think it is too late, but the scope of this book is to share our direct experience only, and we have none in this regard. Therefore, I will refrain from commenting further other than to say that I do not think that a balanced, natural foods diet, free of sugar and simple carbohydrates, will hurt you. That diet, taken under the supervision of a health practitioner who can monitor your medications and whom you have taken on board to help you find a way out of dependency upon medications, may help you reach or at least come close to your goal.

Honest and Dishonest Terms

Fifty years ago, a term often used for diabetes was "sugar diabetes." That is an honest term. In recent years the term **"pre-diabetes"** has been introduced. Pre-diabetes is not an honest term. It is like saying you are half pregnant. Either you are, or you are not. You either have excessive sugar in your blood or you do not. Pre-diabetes is diabetes. When the term first came out, many doctors strongly objected to it because people with this condition *are* in fact diabetic. **They do have abnormally high and potentially dangerous levels of blood sugar.** Nevertheless, the new term won out and now many medical professionals and patients alike have gone so far as to refer to a diabetic as someone who is on diabetic medications. According to them, a pre-diabetic is someone not yet on medications.

Why the change in terminology? Perhaps because too many people have become diabetic and to say the truth would be too alarming. **Changing the definition has in effect cooked the books.**

Blood Sugar Dynamics and Normal Blood Sugar Levels

If we ingest too much in the way of sugars, simple carbohydrates or starches, the liver cannot convert these into storable forms of energy fast enough. The excess glucose that is produced then stays in the bloodstream, and the only way to neutralize it is to add insulin to the mix. This tires out the pancreas, and as described in Chapter 4, it also damages other glands and organs. **That is the ugly truth of the matter.**

Normal blood sugar levels, as stated by those in the health industry in recent years, have become more confusing. For about ten years now, a newer test, called Hemoglobin A1c, has been relied upon more than the testing that was prevalent in prior years. The A1c, instead of reading the current blood sugar level, is supposed to give an average count over a three-month period.[285] The value is an average and does not show the all-important highs and lows. There are also several factors that can affect the accuracy of this test. The result is that the patient is now more dependent upon his or her physician for interpretation of blood sugar level.

Historically, a blood sugar level of 80-110 mg/dl was considered normal. There is an inherent shortcoming in giving this number, however, because the level of sugar in the blood goes up after a meal and comes back down a few hours later.[286] Therefore, to get any accurate understanding of blood sugar level swings, it is necessary to test before eating in the morning, an hour after the meal, two hours after the meal, and about four hours after the meal. This, repeated **under normal conditions and under abnormal conditions**,[287] on different days and at different times, will give a reasonably accurate assessment of a person's actual blood sugar level.

Now days, it is very difficult to get meaningful numbers for "normal" blood sugar levels from the traditional sources. What used to be quoted no longer is, probably because without a full explanation any number can be misleading. But I did find a medical clinic website that stated what I think is pretty reasonable.[288] The numbers they gave are:

Fasting, before breakfast: 70-90 mg/ dl
One hour after a meal: 90-125
Two hours after a meal: 90-110
Five hours after a meal: 70-90

Whether these numbers are optimal or not, I don't know. I am not qualified to say. But the principle, I believe, is correct, and I don't think the numbers are too far off. I have seen more conservative numbers where the high is 115.

You may find it helpful to do what Deborah and I did when we needed to get an idea of what was going on with our blood sugar. We got a test kit, collected the data, compared it with sources we trusted, and discussed the results with a health practitioner.

Having a history of these tests has proven invaluable. As our bodies changed, we needed to make adjustments.

In the diabetes industry, there are different blood sugar ranges with higher numbers given for a "pre-diabetic" than for a "diabetic." Why, I don't know; and I won't go there.

Diabetes-Related Heart Disease
In the US, thirty percent of **open-heart surgeries** are on patients who are currently classified as diabetics.[289] However, there are three times as many "pre-diabetics" as there are diabetics. The actual percentage of open heart surgeries performed on people with high blood sugar levels, therefore, is obscured by not counting the newly-called "pre-diabetic" diabetics.

The number of bypasses performed in the US has fallen by about a third in the last eight years.[290] The surgeries were once touted as being necessary, but a heated battle over the effectiveness of the procedure erupted within the medical community. Those who were pushing the surgeries lost the battle. Whether the data shows that the operation is not nearly as successful as previously thought, as is now stated by some, or if the decrease is for cost savings purposes is still being debated. Regardless, the outlook does not look good for the consumers of those services.

Economics 101
If the flow of diabetes patients was cut off, that would be bad for the economy—at least as far as the drug companies and those who produce other related "health care" paraphernalia are concerned. Those businesses that make their living off of encouraging the disease would have to find something else to do.

Don't misunderstand me. I am thankful that there are medications for diabetes. And I am sure there are some people who need them. **What I object to is the focus on the treatment of the disease with medications instead of focusing on the prevention of the disease, and if necessary, the treatment of it by means of a diet that is free of sugar and simple (processed) carbohydrates.** This improper focus has unquestionably led to the epidemic abuse of diabetic drugs.

To understand the mess we are in with diabetes medications, let's talk about the Opium Wars in China.

For centuries, the British wanted to trade with China. The problem was that though China had many goods that the British wanted, the Chinese did not want anything that the British had. The British tried everything, but the Chinese were not interested. They wanted to be left alone. Finally someone figured out how to get that lucrative trade. There were poppies in Afghanistan (then British-controlled territory) that when processed and smoked produced a state of euphoria. Voila! Traders began to give some of the stuff away in China and quickly developed an extremely lucrative market. Now, at last, there was something that the Chinese wanted! A lot of people made fortunes, and China was finally opening up. Many big businesses got into the act. Did the British people involved in the trade with China know what was really behind that trade? Of course they knew *something*. Undoubtedly many said, "That's not my problem if those people want to smoke the stuff."[291]

We Americans have become the most lucrative part of the worldwide diabetes trade. This has happened right under our noses, and we are in such a stupor we don't even realize it.

I am not talking about "corporate greed." There is no such thing. People are greedy, not institutions. And people can be just as greedy in their desire for more and more sweets as they can be in their desire for more and more money.

Here is what I mean:
We know a woman, a diabetic, who tested her blood sugar for the sole purpose of seeing if she could justify (in her own mind) a piece of cheesecake. We know another diabetic who would eat a stack of cookies and then give herself a shot of insulin. She was pretty good at figuring out how to trick her body until her feet went numb and had to be amputated. Neither of these people cared for anything but satisfying their craving, and it was all paid for by Medicare and "good insurance." Unfortunately, these are not uncommon cases and are typical examples of "health care" that, in fact, isn't.[292]

Destructive lifestyle habits have one thing in common: a lack of discipline. And I have never known any worthwhile mode of living that did not require discipline.

A word of warning is needful here: If you are on blood sugar medications, don't think it is so easy to get off of them. Without professional help you could harm yourself. The medications given for diabetes are strong—once you take them, they tell your body what to do. Your body is no longer in control—that medication is.

Making a Turn From Sugar Addiction

I am well aware that many people seem to get away with eating sugar. But that does not mean that they will always be able to, or that someone else in their household or family does not need their help or cooperation.

Where do we get the strength to turn away from sugar addiction? From being honest with ourselves. In turning away from the sugar habit, I found out a lot about myself, and frankly, some of the things were not pleasant. But the truth has a way of setting us free.

If you want to be freed from the sugar habit, you can prove the same thing. Being honest with ourselves undermines the power of unhealthy slavers, and they will fall.

Smoking and sugar addictions *are* difficult to overcome. You will be nervous just like any addict is during withdrawal. With tobacco, cold turkey has worked for many people. With sugar, it may be prudent to go slowly but surely, and eventually abstain completely. After a short period of abstinence, a switch will be thrown in your metabolism and you will be free from that slaver. Just don't go back. Many have proven that going back to eating a "little" sugar throws the metabolic switch back.

If we suffer greatly for ingesting sugar, the process of quitting is easy. If we do not, it may be considerably more difficult. But why wait until the body has been damaged further?

Yes, kicking the habit may be difficult, but where there is a vision of a better life ahead and an understanding of how to approach this as a project, it is not *so* difficult. It is only where there is no vision that people cast off restraint. **The good news is that there is a way out, and many people have gone before and taken it.**

The reward? Besides increased energy, a clear head, and generally feeling better, I have heard people say, **"I can taste my food!"** How many times I have heard that from someone who just gave up drinking, smoking, or the sugar habit! People who give up sugar find that celery, cottage cheese, and a Granny Smith apple are indeed sweet. Frequently they don't want anything sweeter.

Conclusion

My premise is entirely this: Diabetes was rare before refined sugar came on the scene; therefore, removal of sugar from the diet is *the* key to elimination and control of the disease.

> **What is offered here is only what I consider to be a more reasonable approach to the plague of diabetes than that which is offered by our public health agencies and the medical industry. I have no professional training and am completely unqualified to give the reader any medical advice. Therefore, what is stated here is not advising you to do anything. What you do with this information is entirely your responsibility. I am only a reporter, reporting what we have experienced and observed, and the conclusions we have drawn from that experience and observation.**

Resources

The Case Against the Little White Slaver, by Henry Ford, 1914 see http://medicolegal.tripod.com/ford1914.htm
This is Mr. Ford's observations on tobacco use. T. A. Edison, who observed the same, wrote the forward. It makes for interesting reading in light of the fact that our medical system did not condemn the practice until fifty years after this book was written. You can read it on Google Books.

See Chapter 22, Diet Treatments, for more on diabetes

Reversing Diabetes, by Julian Whitaker, MD, 2001

Chapter 15
Why Our Medical System So Frequently Cannot Help Us

The history of diabetes presented in the last chapter is a classic example of the points made in this chapter. But it is only one of many such examples. If we have an acute medical emergency such as a broken leg or a ruptured appendix, our medical system may be as good as any to help us. But if we want to prevent or treat chronic illness, that same system has failed us miserably.

In this chapter, I want to look at the principles that govern our "health care" system in order to show how it works and how it leads us away from caring for our health. *Please understand that I am writing about a system here, not about individuals.* We have doctors and nurses in the family and not a few friends who are in the field. Many of these people, and many others like them, got into a medical career largely because they wanted to help others.

That notwithstanding, any "health" *system* is destructive that does not emphasize—above all else—the nourishing of life and the avoidance of that which is contrary to life. Hand in hand with that statement, and in equal weight with it, if we do not practice a healthy lifestyle, but instead expect our "health care" system to bail us out, the very best we can hope for is supervised neglect. Having said that, I believe these are the leading reasons why our medical system so frequently cannot help us:

A. Follow the Money.
The reporters who cracked the Watergate scandal that ended the Nixon presidency had an informant who told them that the case was not hard to solve. All they needed to do was follow the money, and they would find what was behind the events that took place. We should do the same when it comes to the $2 trillion industry that is referred to as "health care."

Our medical system is compromised from the beginning. Who funds the medical schools? The pharmaceutical industry makes very significant contributions to many, if not all, centers for medical education. Many of these are "charitable contributions." Pharmaceutical companies *as a matter of course* also fund endowed professorships and research positions in medical schools.[293] They have legions of these people sitting on various kinds of "advisory boards," working for them as "consultants," and giving lectures funded by them.[294] They give thousands of grants to these institutions for "research."[295] They often pay for the required "continuing education" of medical doctors. Do you think they do not expect a return on their investment? Do you think the administrators of these schools and medical centers, and these professors and researchers, can be objective when their living, or a significant portion of their living, is funded by these companies?[296] Will they not favor the products of those who are paying their bills?[297] Behind the white lab coats are people just like you and me.

How does a physician decide to prescribe a particular drug? Is he or she influenced by the all-expenses-paid seminars at five star resorts in exotic places paid for by pharmaceutical companies? The elegant dinners, the sporting events, and the celebrity performances that he or she is invited to—all paid for by sales representatives of the drug companies—do these affect their judgment?[298] Will they continue to be invited if they don't prescribe the host's goods?[299] These practices are denounced from time to time in one of the major medical journals (usually after a major scandal that goes to Washington), but has the practice stopped?[300]

A recent article in the *New England Journal of Medicine* described the results of a *voluntary* survey of 3,167 American medical doctors. 35% of them *admitted* receiving reimbursement from the pharmaceutical industry for costs associated with professional meetings or continuing education. 28% *reported* receiving payments from drug companies for consulting, giving lectures, or enrolling patients in drug trial programs. 83% reported receiving food; 78% reported receiving drug samples.[301] [302]

As a patient, is this in your best interest? Do we not need to arm ourselves with the truth and with a sober mind, and protect ourselves and our families from this onslaught?

When we see the magazine advertisements and the television commercials for new medications, it is good to bear in mind that the companies that offer those goods also heavily support political campaigns. Do you think there could be a connection between these "donations" and the laws that are passed? Are most of our laws really written by our legislators, or are they in fact written by corporate attorneys and our legislators simply sign them?[303]

If something gets into the medical textbooks—look out! Physicians are covered by law if they follow the accepted protocol. If they break ranks, they open themselves to greatly increased liability. They are tied into a system where the only safe thing for them to do is to push the new pharmaceuticals, have you hooked up to the latest gadget, or suggest the latest industry-blessed procedure.[304]

When a new drug reaches the market, the pharmaceutical companies have thirteen to twenty years to make their money on it before it goes generic.[305] After that, we are told, "We have something better now."[306]

Does what is described here have anything to do with caring for your health?

B. Its Commitment to Spreading Chemical Dependency

I have three questions. I believe to ask them is to prove the validity of this subtitle.
1. How often does the average patient leave a medical doctor's office without at least one pharmaceutical prescription in hand?
2. How many of these drugs are easy to get off of once you start them?
3. After investing a billion dollars on a drug in order to get it approved *and marketed*, how do you suppose the pharmaceutical companies are going to get a return on their investment?[307]

I also have a few comments:
1. Pharmaceutical medications routinely suppress the immune system, yet it is only a strong immune system that stands between us and degenerative disease. The concept of using drugs to inhibit or highly stimulate bodily mechanisms greatly underestimates the complexity of living organisms.
2. Leaf through any modern medical textbook and see what the emphasis is. It is easy to come to the conclusion that these manuals for "health care" are really cookbooks, the purpose of which is to dispense the latest goods of the pharmaceutical industry.[308]

3. From a business point of view, there are two disasters that can take place in the pharmaceutical industry. One is to accidently kill people with your product. The other is to cure them. The goal is NOT to cure; it is to treat. In other words, to make it so the patient repeatedly, or better yet, continually, needs your product(s). **Put more bluntly, users of medications become an annuity for the pharmaceutical companies.**

4. In 1997, the FDA started allowing drug companies to run ads on television. That has drastically changed the medical profession, as now people go to the doctor and tell him or her exactly what to prescribe them. And the doctors (if they want to keep their customers) comply. Even children are enticed by pharmaceutical industry advertising by use of their favorite TV characters.[309] Another result of this FDA decision has been an easily recognizable boom in new neighborhood pharmacies which make it convenient for people to get their drugs of choice 24 hours a day.

Do we really want to be part of this system?

C. Gag Orders

In Chapter 10, I gave the example of the gag order that our dentists are under concerning the dangers of mercury in dental amalgam. The same, in principle, applies to a physician speaking out against any industry-blessed protocol. Can a medical doctor say that he does not agree with giving children so many vaccines? Can he say that he believes that sugar consumption causes diabetes? Can he warn his patients that CT scans are dangerous because they expose them to far too much radiation? Can he say that _____ (You fill in the blank.)

I understand that professional associations and government agencies do not want "loose cannons" to make reckless statements that are likely to cause harm to patients. But disagreeing on the points mentioned above is far from reckless. *In practice*, the concern does not seem to be to protect the patients' interests, but rather the interests of business. Because of what are *in effect* gag orders, responsible medical professionals who disagree with the industry mainstream are, for the most part, silenced, and open debate (within the medical industry) on too many basic matters concerning our health is virtually nonexistent.

Countless people go to medical doctors every day to get help and instead run into the herd of sacred cows that blocks the streets of doctor/patient communication. If your doctor does not want to lose his license, he does not dare to bump into them. So, frank doctor/patient communication on many subjects has ceased. Is it any wonder that people are leaving this system in hordes?

D. Pseudoscience

When you pay for your science to say something you want to say, that is not science. As a matter of course, many abstracts of "scientific studies" that are published in well-respected journals are not scientific at all but are in fact marketing pieces. This is not me saying this. See "Sounding Board: Buying Editorials" in *The New England Journal of Medicine*, Sept. 8, 1994.

When medical "science" chooses only the results of experiments that suit its object and carefully sets aside everything that may disagree with those results, that is a falsifying of both the facts and science.

Some typical examples of pseudoscience:

1. Phony "studies." A much quoted "study" on the autism/ethyl mercury connection traced the medical history of 33 children who received vaccinations containing thimerosal. That is hardly an adequate number.[310] Ditto with the "study" of the effects of mercury on dentists in which 267 dentists filled out questionnaires, and of those 62 were selected to "study."

2. Phony citations of "studies." The FDA tells us that "clinical studies in adults and children ages six and above have also found no link between dental amalgam fillings and health problems."[311] Five paragraphs down from that statement is this one: "...[the] FDA does not recommend that you have your amalgam fillings removed or replaced. Removing... exposes you to additional mercury vapor released during the removal process." OK, which is it? Is there in fact "no link to health problems," or is there an exposure here that we should avoid?

3. Phony new medical conditions or diseases. These latest inventions of the pill pushers are aimed at enticing people to

buy their latest model. There are too many examples to name. Just turn on the radio or TV for 15 minutes, or glance through any magazine.

> **The person who phrases a research question can get precisely the "scientific findings" they want to get. Never regard any "scientific" study without *carefully* reading the parameters given for that study. Your teeth will just about fall out if you read the parameters given for many of the "scientific" studies that are quoted in what are considered to be reputable sources.**

E. Treating Symptoms, Not the Cause

The accuracy of this statement should be obvious enough. If you go to the doctor and tell her that you have a headache, she gives you something to take the pain away. If you complain of a stomach ache, she tells you to take an antacid. If you can't sleep, she prescribes a sleeping pill. If your skin breaks out, she gives you some cream to put on it. What is this!

The problem with medications is that they mask the underlying cause of our symptoms. Then we don't know what is really going on in our body. For example, pain is a message our body gives us to tell us that something is wrong.

> **When we take medications for pain, high blood pressure, high blood sugar, or just about anything else, we are in effect killing the messenger and ignoring the message.**
>
> **Is that good medicine?**

The same goes for many surgeries. I am thankful that certain surgeries are available. I am very thankful for the surgeon who operated on our neighbor after his appendix burst and for the surgery performed to sew back the severed finger of another neighbor. Likewise, I am thankful for the surgeon who operated on Grandma when she broke her hip. But many surgeries are not so obviously needful. Should we not ask before submitting to a surgery if surgery is in fact the only way to rectify the problem? Above all, should we not look for the *cause* of the condition and treat it first and foremost before treating the effect?

The typical coronary bypass operation is a good example. Now that it is acceptable to do so, an increasing number of physicians are speaking out against bypasses as being overprescribed. But patients with insurance like them. They have been conditioned to believe that they will be just fine afterwards. The statistics show that many of them will not be.

F. Sold Out to an Unhealthy Way of Life

In the thirty-five years we have dealt with hypoglycemia, we have always heard or read medical doctors say or write that if your blood sugar goes low you should "eat a candy bar" or "have some sugar." Not once have we heard or read a medical doctor say or write "eat an apple" or "have a bite of fruit."

G. Seeing Parts, Not the Whole

Two blind men grab hold of an elephant. One has hold of the tail; the other has hold of the trunk. Both describe what their understanding of an elephant is, and they are very certain of their assessment. But in fact neither has seen the elephant.

Actually, the men aren't blind; they are medical specialists.

When a general practitioner does not know what to do, he sends us to a specialist. We better hope he chooses the right specialty, because a carpenter will always try to fix things with a hammer, an electrician with a screwdriver, and a sheetmetal worker with a pair of tin-snips. That is natural enough; that is what they know. And medical specialists have bills to pay too.

H. Built-in Financial Disincentive

1. The sicker we are, the more we spend on medical "care." (Or the more other people pay for our medical "care"—whatever the case may be.)

2. Medical professionals do not get paid primarily for taking care of their patients' best interests. They get paid for performing procedures and prescribing medications.[312] And they protect their living by performing the procedures and prescribing medications that have received the blessing of political lobbying.

I. Tied Hands

Medical professionals take a tremendous risk seeing patients at all. This is reflected in the exorbitant malpractice insurance rates they pay. Since our legal system has made it easy for a physician to get sued, they need to limit their liability as much as possible. Whether a case is won or not, it is costly because the loser typically does not have to pay court costs. Every day your doctor must go to the office with a defensive mindset. He or she must focus on self-defense in order to survive. Therefore, your doctor will do nothing but the standard procedures that have been approved by their medical association (or Medicare for older patients) in order to protect themselves. Typically, it is only after covering all of the bases with all the standard procedures and tests that a medical doctor will dare go out of the small box he or she is put in. And that hesitatingly. By that time you are out of money, are much sicker, or both.

Actually, your doctor may have other tools in his "bag." But in too many cases his hands are tied and he will not use those tools before using all the "scientific" ones—provided of course that you have the insurance to pay for them. "Scientific" means that there is an expensive treatment. "Non-scientific" means it is a remedy that simply works—like giving yourself an enema, cutting refined sugar out of the diet, or taking vitamins, for example.

As stated earlier, if physicians follow industry-blessed protocols they are covered; if they deviate, they're not. Sad to say, they have largely become box-checkers, often using no more intelligence when we see them than a postal clerk does when he or she handles our packages for us. There are codes for all the diagnoses and procedures just as there are zip codes and street addresses. If you use the right zip code and street address, your package arrives just fine. If your doctor checks the right box, he gets paid and probably won't get sued. It is as simple as that. [313] [314]

And our doctors' actions are tied into databases.

To a significant extent, a profession that once attracted the best and the brightest students has now become a resting place for those who are willing to follow orders and leave their own thinking out of the equation.

I told you at the beginning of this chapter that we know many people in the medical profession. We also know some who were in it and got out. One former nurse told us, "What I was doing was not helping my patients." A retiring medical doctor told me, "I know that the direction [the medical system] has gone is not in the best interest of the patients." Another told me, "I was just checking boxes and passing out drugs." A high percentage of those who remain in the business struggle with these things on a daily basis. Many have borrowed deeply for their education, and now the only way they can pay the bills is to...

J. A Service That is Self-Serving is Not a Service
"Union! Union! Union!" shouted the longshoremen as they marched down the Embarcadero pumping their picket signs up and down. The medical establishment usually does not take to the streets like that, but their tactics can be similar. Anything to preserve the brotherhood.

Don't think so? Turn to the back of the book and read Appendix IV. There is a long history of the AMA refusing to cooperate with any health practitioner who is not in their ranks. This practice has been diffused somewhat in recent years, nevertheless, the history is telling.

K. Advocating Improper Dependence
The best way to illustrate this point is with a story.
A friend of ours, James, was put on medications to lower his cholesterol. This was a real blow to him because he has a family history of high cholesterol and heart disease, and he thought he had done enough differently in order to be able to avoid the medications. His blood tests showed otherwise, so James went on the medications.

But he did not feel any better, and because he had seen his father suffer not only from the condition but also from the medications,

James was determined to get off the meds if he could. He read up on high cholesterol, realized he could do a lot better, wrote up a plan for himself, and presented it to his doctor to see if he thought it would work. His doctor was caught off guard and was quite uncomfortable about James doing this. He admitted that in fact James' plan might work, but he cautioned him not to go off the medications while trying the diet. James agreed and said he would continue to have the lab tests every three months to see if the medication could be reduced or not. After more discussion, the doctor reluctantly agreed. James was determined to do his best to not need the medication, but he said his doctor acted like he had been caught with his hand in the cookie jar.

My point in telling the story is that **if a health practitioner really has his patients' best interest in mind, he will try to work himself out of a job.** That is, he will help his patients not need him other than for routine checkups. Many practitioners (of all disciplines) do not practice in this way but rather help people live in an unhealthy manner and then try to make up the difference by treating them in one way or another. If a practitioner's focus is on having you dependent on him, it is unlikely that he can truly help you.

By the way, James' tests are now in the normal range, he is off the medications, and he is feeling better, but he quickly adds that it is a work in progress.

L. Unhealthy Secrets and Outright Deception
There are many tightly held secrets in the medical industry that are to our detriment. I'll name just a few.

1. The rate of hospital-contracted infections. That is, what is the chance that you will pick up an infection just by checking into a hospital? Though no hospital will divulge records of infections contracted in their facility, no honest, knowledgeable hospital professional will deny that hospital-acquired infections have reached a far from acceptable rate.

Deborah has a friend whose middle-aged husband checked into a hospital for a "routine" procedure. Two weeks later he died, not from the procedure, but from a staph infection. Such cases are common. We know of a similar death with a thirty-year-old.

2. The risk factors of a colonoscopy are also a very heavily guarded medical industry secret. If you ask your doctor, he or she will *always* tell you: "The risks are very low." This must be what they are required to say by the governing powers that hold their medical licenses. (How else could they all say the same thing and never divulge any practical information whatsoever?) [315] **This assessment of the actual risk is far from the truth**.

Hospital studies or other reports get posted on the web from time to time. You will have to use Google Scholar or PubMed to find them, as most will not show up readily in a typical web search. From the studies that I have seen, the incidence of serious complications is about one in 200. The perforation rate is estimated in different studies as being between one in 500 and one in 2,000. About 90 % of the other complications are when a biopsy or polypectomy (polyp removal) is performed. If the bowel wall is punctured, major surgery is required, which many times results in complications the likes of which are not pleasant.[316 317 318]

We are told that it is a good idea to get a "routine" colonoscopy, but are not told of the severity of the risks involved or of the high statistics on complications. Would you submit to a "routine" colonoscopy if you knew the risk of serious complications was one in 200?[319] So they lie about the risks and they lie about the pain involved[320]—what else are they lying about?

3. When my neighbor's Uncle George died a couple of weeks after open heart surgery, the surgeon told the family that "the surgery was successful." How inappropriate it was for Uncle George to die afterwards! The worst part is that in the statistics kept on surgeries, Uncle George's surgery *was* a success. That is the box that gets checked because he lived for two weeks after the surgery was performed. So the "scientific" statistics are skewed. And consequently we often do not know what we need to know to make an informed decision.

What else are we not being told?

M. Genuine Lack of Interest in Politically Incorrect Conditions

---

"I've never heard of that before."

If we had a nickel for every time we have heard that from a medical doctor we would have quite a pile of nickels. Whether it was concerning my wife's difficulty with low blood sugar, her reactions to anesthesia, her reactions to EMFs, or her reactions to a number of other symptoms of mercury poisoning, the response was the same. We eventually realized that when a medical doctor says "I've never heard of that before," he is probably really saying, "I was not taught that in medical school, so I refuse to think about it." The closed-mindedness was, and is, astounding. Deborah told me once, "I hope I am done trying to make them understand."

By the way, all of her conditions are quite common.

N. The Common Use of Unnecessary Dangerous Drugs

A century ago laudanum, an opiate, was a popular drug that was used to treat just about anything. Mercurial salts were also very popular, again used to treat just about anything. Medicines with lead in them were also common. These were not the medicines of the medical fringe, but were the "science" of the day and were prescribed by the medical mainstream. Now we know that those drugs were not a good idea.

We also now know that the more recent "science" behind Rezulin, Vioxx, Avandia, and Zoloft (to name a few) was not so good.[321] But our physicians, who get a large part of their education from the pharmaceutical industry, apparently don't know any other way.

O. Arrogance

Due to many early successes in disease control during the late 1800s and early 1900s, there developed a kind of arrogance in the medical industry. Routinely, claims were made—and are still being made—that proclaim, in effect: "We are so smart, nothing can stop us now."

Such an attitude ignores the obvious. We are in fact very frail and do not even have power over our next breath. That breath can be taken from us at any moment. Then where is our boasting?

In the 1950s, our medical experts decided that tonsils were unnecessary, so they began taking them out whenever they had a chance. It was the same with the appendix. Who needs these parts that are so prone to inflammation and infection! The next generation of medical experts has told us that neither of those practices was such a good idea and that their predecessors were not as knowledgeable as they are. Oh? Has anything really changed? If so, why is it that now one in three American babies are delivered by C-section? [322]

I remember when the baby formula, Similac, became popular. That was right about the time our son was born. The manufacturer claimed that Similac was "better than mother's milk," and many doctors at the time were parroting that claim. Where is the wisdom in that? "Shall the thing formed say of Him who formed it, 'He has no understanding?' " [323]

P. The New Chameleons
A chameleon is a kind of lizard that changes color to adapt to its environment. It is still a lizard. It may change color, but it still thinks like a lizard, behaves like a lizard, and eats flies like a lizard.

Many, if not most, physicians have realized that the tide of public opinion is not with them as it once was. They are no longer looked upon with the respect, even reverence, they once were. Too many people are now turning to "alternative" means of health care, and the medical industry is suffering a credibility crisis. As a result, many medical doctors are now claiming to use "natural" methods.

At the beginning of a recent doctor's appointment, the doctor told me, "I don't like drugs." During the exam and consultation, he did suggest some natural means of care, but he kept coming back to medications. Just as surely as my knee reflex worked, he kept coming back to his roots. What he suggested in the way of "natural" treatments were sugared-up, additive-laced products. This physician claims to be "natural" and he treats diabetes as a specialty. But he has no clue as to the dangers of sugar consumption, and he always comes back to meds.

The problem is that all the training of a medical doctor is in another vein. If a physician has truly switched over to treating people naturally, medications will be the last thing on his mind. He will not offer them to you unless *after trying everything else* he knows no other means of treatment.

In other words, if your doctor eats flies, you may want to seek the professional opinion of someone who does not.

Q. About Insurance. What is Paid For; What is Not
From what I have heard from many people who have an HMO, when they go see the doctor they are likely to simply have generic drugs thrown at them and be shown the door. They tell me the business formula seems to be: "Stall unless the patient is dying," and at that point say, "There's not much we can do."

If you have "good insurance," those procedures and medications that make you dependent upon the medical establishment are paid for. Those things that help you help yourself are not paid for. [324] Ditto when it comes to what expenses may be tax deductible. That's the way it is. Get over it.

About twenty years ago, I went to Las Vegas for a business convention. While driving to the convention center, I passed a casino that was on the corner where I needed to make a turn. There on the marquee were the words, "Free T-Shirt With Minimum $20 Bet." As I sat in traffic waiting for the light to change, several people came out of the door under that marquee with big smiles on their faces and a T-shirt draped over their arms. I couldn't believe it. Those people were paying twenty bucks for a T-shirt! I even phoned my wife just to tell her about it.

Does that sound like a good deal? How about getting "free" medical treatment because you have "good" insurance? How many times have you heard someone say concerning an unnecessary or questionable medical procedure, "Well, my insurance paid for it?"

A compromised "health care" system that leads people away from the basic principles of health is not a good choice, even if you don't have to pay for it.

Actually, you may be paying a lot more than you think you are.

How to Talk to Your Doctor

I will let you in on a well-guarded secret in the medical community, and what I am going to say here is in itself worth the price of this book.

Because the consequences of our doctors going against their trade association (as previously discussed) are so great, when it comes to prevention of disease and chronic problems, the patient must take the lead in everything, beginning with educating themselves. We cannot go to them as dumb lambs and expect to be truly helped.

For example, many doctors are in fact in favor of their patients kicking the processed food and medication habits and living in a much healthier way. But they don't press these points, first of all because they don't think their patients want to hear it, and secondly because they are quite limited as to what they can say without jeopardizing their license or otherwise destroying their business.

So, if you want to kick the sugar habit, for example, and you feel you need some help, you may want to start by making a plan and taking some specific steps with which you can quantify that you are getting your diet under control. If you don't do this, no doctor will believe you are serious. Then, after some initial success, tell your doctor what you are doing. The doctor will only give you so much time, so you probably don't want to spend that time asking her what to do. That sets the wrong tone and often gets off on a rabbit trail. You might find it more profitable to *tell* her that you are determined to get off sugar and see how she responds.

If she will help you, great; if not, you may want to find a doctor who will. Just understand that you need to take the lead in everything. What you are looking for is not advice as to whether or not you should abandon the sugar habit. That is already cast in concrete. What you are looking for is a double check on your method and progress of attaining the goal that you have already set for yourself.

You must be fully convinced in your own mind of what you want to accomplish and have a plan *clearly and fully* thought out. You must have already taken some steps and had some success in order to convince your doctor that you are serious. The exception (in this case) is the diabetic who is on medications. If you are a diabetic on meds, you need your physician on board from the start.

Next, you must ask the right questions. For example, do not ask, "should I do this" or "how do I do this," but rather, "do you see any danger in me doing this?" Do not expect your doctor to help you more than that. She cannot. What I have said here is not theory. It took us a long time to figure this one out, and we and others we know have plenty of experience in what is a helpful approach and what is not.

Many physicians know that the direction that the medical establishment has gone is unhealthy. We have had some, in confidence, tell us so. If your doctor is genuinely interested in what you are doing, you may also want to give him or her a copy of this book. You would be amazed at how many people in the mainstream medical profession are very interested in what those of us "going natural" are doing. Not a few know that we are on the right track.

Once again, I must remind the reader that this information is only intended for those who take full responsibility for their actions. See the warning after the preface. Thank you.

Resources

Our Daily Meds by Melody Petersen, 2008

A well-researched and documented book. Petersen exposes a large part of medical "science" for the science fiction it is. A MUST READ for anyone who takes medications of any kind or is thinking about taking them.

Pro Publica publishes a list of payouts that fifteen pharmaceutical companies have made to doctors and health institutions. You may want to look to see if physicians you use have significant relationships with one of these drug companies. The data is very limited. Most of the industry money, gifts, etc. exchanged will not be listed. These are only amounts and relationships that are disclosed, but what is disclosed gives an indication of the practice. See http://projects.propublica.org/docdollars/   For information on the data, see http://www.propublica.org/article/about-our-pharma-data

To understand the government/medical industry relationship, see Jean's story in Chapter 11.

Chapter 16
An Unhealthy Spell

I don't like the title of this chapter, but I know of no other term that so accurately describes the unhealthy influence our society is under when it comes to taking care of our bodies. What is commonly called "health care" is not, and the resistance to common sense is often supernatural.

In ancient Greek, the word for sorcery is *pharmakia*. This is the word we get our English word "pharmacy" from. The word also has the meanings of medicine, drugs, spells, and poisoning. In ancient Greece, the use of drugs—whether simple or potent—was a part of the sorcerer's ritual. The ritual was designed to impress the applicant with the mysterious resources and powers of the sorcerer.[325]

Some things haven't changed.

I knew a man who was on twenty-eight prescription medications. His wife told me that his doctor was "a really nice guy."

I knew a young boy who was covered with eczema from head to foot for years. He was very uncomfortable and itching all the time, often to the point of bleeding. His mother had taken him to the doctor repeatedly and received no help whatsoever, yet when we told her what we knew, she would not change the boy's diet. Others had told her the same before we did. Her doctor had told her that the boy's diet was not a problem.

I knew a man who had some very serious health issues, including recurrent blockages of the bowel. He would not have a colon irrigation but did submit to a colonoscopy knowing full well that he stood a chance of serious complications.[326] Even after the colonoscopy—which showed no problems—he still would not have a colon irrigation but instead submitted to various medications that did not improve his condition but rather worsened it. It did not matter that a close friend of his had recently begun having colon hydrotherapy, had not felt better in years, looked much healthier, and kept recommending the treatment to him. It did not matter that the cost of the treatments was covered. It did not matter how bad he felt most of the time. Nothing else mattered because his doctor said it wouldn't help.

I knew a man who has diabetes and had a coronary bypass when in his late fifties. His father, his uncle, and his grandfather also had diabetes and all had major heart attacks in their late fifties or early sixties. Yet he still told me that the food he ate (a typical sugared-up American diet) was not sweet and his doctor had been taking good care of him.

This kind of thinking is commonplace. The American "health care" system is sick, and I dare say that those who are suckered into it are very likely to be also.

The problem is not merely physical. It is of spirit, soul, and body.[327] Many people are so strongly bound up in an unhealthy lifestyle that they will subject themselves to just about anything as long as they don't have to make a change. Other than that, all they seem to care about is that someone else makes all the decisions for them and they don't have to pay for whatever is prescribed.

Too many other people make decisions regarding their health or that of their families based upon what they hear on the "news."

A common link in all the cases given here is that these folks do not realize that they have been become merchandise. As puppets on a string, they are pulled this way and that while an unscrupulous system preys upon them.

Every society has benefited from their medicine men. I use the term in the purest sense, in the sense that there are some people in every society who understand health matters better than others. But when the medicine men become too powerful, they become tyrants over the rest of the people. Among some of the Native American tribes as well as among the ancient Greeks, there are stories of this phenomenon. Our society is supposedly more sophisticated, but the principle of improper dominance is the same.

How can we be freed from this improper and supernatural dominance? The first line of defense is the truth. Arm yourself with it!

Chapter 17
The Germ Theory of Disease and Dead Food

The Germ Theory of Disease
This phrase may seem odd to some readers. Some will probably think, "What do you mean, 'The Germ *Theory* of Disease,' everyone knows that germs cause disease! That's been scientifically proven long ago! What are you, some kind of nut case?"

Well, true science is more complex than that. The problem is in the word "cause." Yes, where many diseases are, harmful germs are present. But looking a little closer, those same germs are present anyway—in perfectly healthy bodies! The difference between a diseased state and a healthy one is not the presence of germs but rather which germs are running the show.

It could be said that germs cause disease to the same degree that flies cause garbage. Yes, where garbage is, flies are present. But if you take out the garbage, where are the flies?

Good science, what is truly science, takes into account all factors. It does not state a hypothesis, then go about proving it by throwing out every finding that does not support that hypothesis.

So we come to Louis Pasteur.

Mr. Pasteur is typically given the credit for linking germs with disease. Actually, there were many scientists before him who did so, but he had a famous case, the press got on it, and the rest is history.

Pasteur hypothesized, as did some other scientists of the day, that germs were in fact the cause of disease. Many other leading scientists of the day disagreed with him. They were no less intelligent, nor were their methods less scientific. The two groups simply drew different conclusions.

Another Frenchman, by the name of Claude Bernard, was a leading physiologist of the day. Bernard worked with Pasteur to develop the process that later became known as pasteurization. The two used the same kind of microscopes and lab equipment, worked on the same problems, and identified the same microorganisms. But as stated earlier, they came to very different conclusions. Bernard thought Pasteur went too far—that it was not germs that caused disease, but rather the terrain in which those germs existed that allowed the germs to thrive that was responsible for disease. Bernard believed that the relatively stable state of equilibrium within an organism was what was vital.[328] In other words, he understood the importance of what is today called an ecosystem, and he favored the practice of nurturing a healthy one.

Pasteur was set on destroying the offending germs. In his mind, and in the minds of some other scientists, germs were the enemy. Many other top scientists of the day, however, sided with Bernard. Perhaps this group had more respect for the complexity and perfection of the creation and therefore did not buy into the concept of eradication as a preferred means to treat disease.

But Pasteur's methods were shown to be immediately effective, there were serious health threats at the time, and government money (first in France, then elsewhere) was funneled to the scientists who were going to kill the germs. From that time until now, "killing the germs" has been the dominant "scientific" mindset. Scientists who disagreed were—and still are—ridiculed as being "non-scientific." Since that time, the government money has gone to schools that teach methods based upon the principle of eradication. And we have been taught that anyone who does not agree is a quack.

Unfortunately, the principles of eradication and nurturing don't mix well. It should be obvious, when speaking of matters of life and health, that nurturing should be at the forefront and eradication used only when absolutely necessary, but the problem is that money is involved. Lots of money.

There are hundreds of cases that illustrate how and where "public health" policy has gotten away from common sense and health-full-ness. The example I'll use will bring the matter into more modern times, will bring it closer to home, and will tie in perfectly with what has already been discussed in this chapter. It will also serve as the transition to the second subject of this chapter. The example is a more recent one—it is the story of unpasteurized milk and the Alta

Dena Dairy. I have chosen to tell the Alta Dena story because I am familiar with it, but there were also other dairies across the US whose stories are virtually identical.

The Alta Dena Story [329]
The Alta Dena Dairy has been in the Los Angeles area of California since 1945. The dairy has a long, honorable, and controversial history. It is the story of the politics of milk.

The Alta Dena Dairy became a "Certified Dairy" in 1953 and began producing raw milk[330] and raw milk products. Contrary to what we have all been told, raw milk is not unsafe. What can be unsafe in unpasteurized *or pasteurized* milk is how that milk is processed and handled. Actually, that should be obvious. Humans have been nourished by unpasteurized milk for thousands of years.[331] But when we've heard something—such as "unpasteurized milk is not safe"—over and over again, we often believe it. Repetitive advertising is very effective. The truth has not changed. The facts are still the same. But our response to the truth and to those facts can easily be changed.

The pasteurization of milk is a process in which milk is heated to about 160 degrees Fahrenheit. The heating does a good job of killing bacteria. But it kills nearly all the bacteria—the beneficial along with the harmful. Not only so, heating the milk changes the chemical structure of the proteins, destroys many of the natural vitamins, and destroys or alters many of the enzymes. Enzymes are the little-understood amino acid chains that enable us to digest our food. After pasteurization, what we are left with is dead milk. The beneficial bacteria are gone and so are the enzymes, vitamins, and who knows what else. What we are left with is a white liquid that is mostly some hard-to-digest protein and some fat, sugar, and calcium.

I know we were all taught that pasteurization is a good thing. But as one who drank milk directly from the cow when visiting my grandmother on her farm as a child, let me tell you this: If you leave raw milk on the kitchen counter all morning on a summer day, you will have sour milk by noon. That sour milk is actually better for you than "sweet" milk. But don't try doing that with pasteurized milk or you will have spoiled milk. The difference is the presence or absence of healthy bacteria.

To take this point a step further, milk allergies were rare before pasteurization; now they are common. Why? Because most of the common allergies to milk are in fact not to milk, but to pasteurized milk. Since our bodies cannot digest it well, the lactose in pasteurized milk can accumulate and become toxic, causing an allergic-like reaction. Enough of this and we develop an allergy.

The original owners of the Alta Dena Dairy, the Stueve family, knew the health benefits of non-pasteurized, non-homogenized milk. They were convinced, as are many others, that the solution to unhealthful dairy products is cleanliness, not cooking the life out of the food.

The Alta Dena Dairy produced safe raw (unpasteurized and unhomogenized) milk for decades. It is not difficult to produce safe raw milk—you just have to keep high health standards and use common sense. But in what can be a filthy industry, what Alta Dena was doing made a lot of other dairymen look bad. Besides, as people became more health conscious, the Alta Dena Dairy grew and the other dairies were losing customers. Alta Dena's cleanliness standards far exceeded those of other dairies, and those other dairies could not, or did not want to, follow in Alta Dena's steps. So they lobbied the government.

The government then, through the California Department of Food and Agriculture, began a campaign to pull raw milk off the market in California.

Beginning in 1965, a long battle was played out in the California courts. It began with the San Diego County Director of Public Health, who individually issued an order that banned all raw milk in San Diego County. The ban was based upon his claim to have found *Staphylococcus aureus* in Alta Dena milk. (*S. aureus* bacteria are very common in humans, it is only when they get the upper hand that they have been a problem.) It did not matter that there had not been any cases of illness due to the consumption of raw milk; the health official was on a campaign. Alta Dena sued. After three years in the courts, the 4th District Court of Appeals ruled that the health officer had exceeded his authority, and Alta Dena's raw milk products went back into food stores in San Diego.

But that was only the first of what would be many times that Alta Dena's raw milk products would be pulled from store shelves. The ball was rolling. In 1967, while the San Diego case was pending, the California Medical Society got into the act and passed a resolution calling for the pasteurization of all milk sold in California. Responding to this, some other counties began to follow San Diego County's lead.

In 1969, the Los Angeles Health Department chimed in and claimed that raw milk could lead to Q fever, which is spread by the *Coxiella burnetti* parasite that can be carried in ticks on cows. There were no reported cases of Q fever, but a ban was put on raw milk in Los Angeles County anyway.

At that same time, the *Los Angeles Times* began what was to be a long propaganda war against raw milk. The Stueve brothers, knowing the hoax, responded to the ban and all the bad press by putting a label on their raw milk that said it was "for pet food, not for human consumption." For this, Harold Stueve was arrested for contempt of court. The charges against Mr. Stueve were not dropped until it was shown clearly to the court that Q fever was in fact not caused by drinking raw milk but by inhalation of the airborne parasite, usually from being around dirty animals. In fact, six of seven cases of Q fever in the US were of people who lived near, or worked in, dairies.

Foiled again but not deterred, in 1974 the California State Health Department issued a statewide ban on all of Alta Dena's raw milk. The reason stated was the threat of brucellosis fever, which is spread by *brucella* bacteria. The claim did not state any physical evidence but only a threat. Alta Dena had its entire herd tested. No trace of *brucella* was found, Alta Dena went back to court, and the ban was lifted. But only after tremendous financial loss.[332]

Since the *S. aureus, Q fever,* and *brucellosis* scares didn't work, the next attempt in the attack was made with *salmonella*. Again, the State Health Department led the attack, and it was against all the raw milk dairies in the state. In the mid-1970s, a state lab claimed to have found *salmonella* in Alta Dena milk. Again, no one got sick, but the department declared that a *salmonella* outbreak was imminent. The outbreak was limited to the press.

No *salmonella* contamination was found in any raw milk in the state, and the records of the claim somehow disappeared. But all of Alta Dena's raw milk products had been pulled off the shelves again—and most of it was forcibly destroyed.

That's expensive.

As if that were not bad enough, with all the hysteria, when the milk was allowed to go back on the market, Alta Dena and the other raw milk dairies were forced to put very scary warning labels on their products. No doubt, that fear tactic was successful on a lot of consumers, but many people (ourselves included) did not believe any of it. Fifty thousand letters were written by Alta Dena supporters and sent to the governor, but the damage had been done. We all watched as the Alta Dena Dairy slowly deteriorated. It was pitiful. You could see the decline in the upkeep of their delivery trucks, in the drooped shoulders of the delivery men, and in the ever shrinking space Alta Dena products had on the grocery store shelves. Availability of their raw milk products became spotty, then disappeared altogether. Another victim of *Corruptus governmentus*.

Raw milk was not pulled from the marketplace as a result of any illnesses. In fact, the heated public battle over raw milk in California took nearly twenty-five years to resolve, because during that time **there was not one case of illness that was proven to be due to raw milk**. But Alta Dena's opponents had deep pockets. They were funded by taxpayer dollars.[333]

The Stueves sold the Alta Dena Dairy in 1992. It no longer produces unpasteurized milk. [334][335]

Dead Food
Take the Alta Dena story, multiply it times 1,000, and you have a significant part of our current "public health" policy pertaining to food "safety." This policy of death is a tragedy and it is costing us our health. [336]

Today, we spray our crops with chemicals, then heat or radiate our food to kill the germs, then preserve it by killing the enzymes, then add other chemicals for various reasons, and then call it "safe." Our food supply is "safe" and dead. "Safe" and void of nutritional value. "Safe" and lacking the life-essence of food. "Safe" and stripped down to compounds of unhealthful, chemical-laced pseudo-nutrients.

Most of us are generations removed from having raw milk and other raw dairy products. We are exactly the same number of generations away from having a healthy intestinal tract.[337]

To understand the current epidemic of colon diseases, look no further than to the heavily processed foods we consume. Many health professionals now understand that we cannot digest them properly, that they putrefy in the bowel, and that they cause disease. Unfortunately, those who understand this and will speak out about it are in the minority.

Raw foods are not unsafe. They simply need to be handled with the respect we would give to any other living thing.

So now, to try to make up the difference for the dead things we ingest, we take probiotics—a term not even in the dictionary twenty years ago. Today, you see this term plastered on a lot of food labels, and even many medical doctors have started recommending their use. We used to just call them "acidophilus," or "cultured foods."[338] Now also, many of us realize the need to take enzyme supplementation. And of course vitamins. All these were once in the diet of our ancestors but now, unless we grow our own food, they have to be added back in—an adding which in no way comes close to the healthfulness of food that is not stripped of these things in the first place.

One of the preferred ways to make food "safe" is to add preservatives. What are preservatives? They are enzyme killers. Preservatives stop the decaying process. That is, they stop the digestion process.

About twenty years ago, there was an article about urban garbage in *National Geographic* magazine. A professor decided to dig down into a landfill in order to observe the recent history of our way of life. As he dug down into the pile of garbage, at a certain point he found newspapers that were twenty years old, so he knew how old the garbage was at that level. Alongside the newspapers were some hot dogs. That surprised him. They were not decomposed at all. Those hot dogs looked just the same as they had twenty years prior to that time! His conclusion was the obvious: Whatever was used to preserve those hot dogs sure was effective!

How do you suppose your digestive system deals with those hot dogs? Can it break them down? Sorry to say, we get the flavor on our palate, absorb the sugar and the fat, but do not get much else in a positive way. We do get a lot, however, in a negative way.

The first commissioner of the US Food and Drug Administration (FDA), Harvey Wiley, was particularly concerned about preservatives being added to foods. In a Committee on Interstate and Foreign Commerce, in February of 1906, Wiley was in the midst of a heated debate over benzoic acid, a common food preservative. The proponents of the use of benzoic acid pointed out that it was found in some foods such as cranberries, and therefore was harmless. Wiley responded with this:

> "The human body is required to do a certain amount of normal work. That amount of work is a beneficial exercise of the organs. If you diminish the normal work of an organ, you produce atrophy—a lack of functional activity. If you increase it hypertrophy ensues, and increase of functional activity. Nearly all of the organs that wear out do so from one of those causes, not from normal exercise of their functions. Therefore, assuming that the food of man, as prepared by the Creator and modified by the cook, is the normal food of man, any change in the food which adds a burden to any of the organs, or any change which diminishes their normal functional activity, must be hurtful."

Well said.

I read where one health advocate stated: **"Don't eat anything that won't rot; just eat it before it does."** That is a highly intelligent statement, and we would do well to follow it.

I'll tell you what we're getting if we move away from this maxim. We get:

    * "Natural" flavoring (derived from _any_ biological source [339]),
    * Artificial flavoring (derived from _any_ source [340]), and
    * "Enriched" food products

It is important that we know what the term "enriched" means in the food industry, so I'll tell you the story of bread in a very brief and to-the-point way.

For thousands of years, man has taken grains, ground them into flour, and made bread of them. So nutritious were these foods that they became known as "the staff of life."

Then in the 1890s, as a result of finer milling and separation processes, white flour came into being. White flour has the germ and bran removed from it. Those parts of the grain are the parts that are susceptible to spoilage. (Lifeless things don't spoil.) So if you remove them, the flour can be stored for a much longer time. Furthermore, dough made from white flour rises much more, so within a short time after the advent of white flour we had fluffy breads and "melt-in-your-mouth" pastries. The downside that was eventually discovered is that there was a great increase in disease among people who ate white bread. This eventually was proven, and "enriched" flour—that is, white flour with vitamins added to it—came out in 1941.

Since that time, we have been told by the food marketing folks that though they strip the flour of every nutritional element, they put those elements back in. Their wonderful, tasty products are "enriched" and "have all the vitamins and minerals you need."

Sorry gentlemen, but calling white flour "enriched" is like leaving the chicken on the barbeque for a week, scooping up the ashes that are left onto a plate, throwing a piece of wilted parsley on it, and calling it a chicken dinner. That is _not_ a chicken dinner, and your flour is _not_ enriched. It is a stripped and horribly unhealthful product that should never be placed in a human mouth.

In recent years, whole grains have made a comeback, but usually with plenty of chemicals thrown in to retard spoilage. I find it amazing that for thousands of years people handled grains in a way to keep them from spoiling (most of the time), but in our modern age we have trouble doing that without adding harmful chemicals.

Unfortunately, on your grocery store shelf there may not be one loaf of bread that in any way resembles what bread was 125 years ago. The "staff of life" has become a "rod of death." And many of us are being beaten to death by it.

I need to point out here that all this food alteration has been done in the name of "science." When it comes to food—and health in general—**one of the big problems we face is that, by following our palate instead of our head, we have been duped into not knowing the difference between science and marketing.**

You can make your "science" state anything you want.[341] That should be abundantly clear from many of the mindless "health studies" that our tax dollars are paying for and that are reported on the "news." We should not listen to such things. Unfortunately, they appeal to the tabloid mentality of a segment of the society, so we are deluged with this trash just as we are with raunchy magazine covers when we come to the checkout counter at the grocery store.

Where will all the madness of dead food stop? Ten years from now will our cottage cheese need to be "safe" after we have left it in the back seat of the car for a week?[342] As our society is dumbed down more and more, will the next generation have any idea that food should be something of life? Or will we live out Huxley's *Brave New World*, where the only sane person is considered a savage!

How's Your Bank Account?
Our health is a bank account. The problem is we want to withdraw and not deposit, to take and not give. We want to eat junk that depletes our body's vitality and think we can make up the difference by eating an occasional carrot stick and taking some vitamins. Though some people (almost always younger) *seem* to get away with it, for most of us that kind of behavior will not work, and eventually bankruptcy is at the door.

It is senseless to think in terms of which straw it is that "breaks the camel's back" of health. It is equally senseless to take a pill to counteract each straw. The problem is not with any individual straw or straws. The "camel" simply needs to be unloaded by eliminating those things that undermine our health.

Claude Bernard was not unscientific. Cancers and other diseases find a welcome host in a compromised immune system just as flies easily find garbage.

Much of our problem with dead food stems from the deception that "life is more fun if you just do as you please." Is it? Is the alcoholic having more fun? Are diabetics having more fun? Are drug addicts having more fun? Are the children who eat candy and are constantly restless and unable to learn having more fun? Is the man who eats a bowl of chocolate ice cream every evening having more fun when he lives a life of sleep deprivation because of that habit? I don't think so. For a fleeting pleasure, hordes of people have been suckered into a life that is far from optimal.

It does not have to be so. We can turn this ship around!

Some people say that it takes too much time to eat healthy. Oh? In a very real sense, time is not what the clock shows, but the strength we have to perform. If we are dragged down by a bad diet, all we have strength for after work is to sit in front of the TV where we are enticed to eat worse yet. What is the value of that kind of time?

If we eat properly, we probably will not spend our time that way. We will find that we not only have strength for preparing a decent meal, but will also have the strength to exercise both physically and mentally as well.

Some folks also say that it costs more money to eat healthy. Not so! If we use the money that is thrown away on the stuff that is bad for us, we will have plenty. Healthfulness is a long-term, day-by-day investment; and it all comes back to taking individual responsibility.

Resources:
For sources of raw milk, go to www.realmilk.com. Laws are constantly changing, but as of now (June, 2013), raw milk is once again available, though in a limited way, in 39 states.[343]

Chapter 18
Soil and Digestion; Nutrients and Adulterated Food

Soil

There is a natural wonder that is greater than Yosemite Valley, greater than the Grand Canyon, and greater than the Old Faithful Geyser at Yellowstone National Park. It is greater than the Giant Sequoias, greater than the migration of all the songbirds, and greater than all the animals in the Serengeti. It is the wonder that can be found in a handful of dirt—the wonder of healthy soil.

Healthy soil is the foundation of all life on land. Other than what we obtain from the oceans, almost all food comes out of soil that is at least somewhat healthy.

There are millions of microorganisms in one cubic inch of healthy soil that are working tirelessly in concert with larger organisms to break down spent leaves and other decaying organic matter and transform them into nutrients that can then be assimilated by growing plants that in turn feed the whole earth.

For thousands of years, mankind has worked the soil and been sustained by it. For the most part, we have done a pretty good job of it. If this were not so, we would not be here. But there are plenty of cases where the soil has become unhealthy at the hands of those who have been charged to till it. We can read of several civilizations that once thrived in what are now all but barren deserts. The life had gone out of the soil—and sometimes at their hands.

This being the case, it seems strange indeed that in many places modern tillers of the soil habitually kill the life in the soil that nourishes us. We spray herbicides to kill unwanted plants, apply fungicides to kill the various life forms that work so hard to break down dead vegetation, and often go so far as to purposely sterilize the soil that gives us life.

The problem with poisoning the soil is that its effects are accumulative. Apply herbicides in an orchard one year, and that's one thing. Do it for ten years, and that's another. Do it for thirty, and you may have not only lost your orchard, you may not even be able to plant another one. You have killed the soil. Actually, in the first application enough damage could have been done to create an almost irreversible problem. We have made some farm soil so dead that it can no longer break down the leftover vegetation from the previous crop when it is plowed under.

Of course, we can put our trust in the folks who sell us those poisons, who without fail tell us that what they are offering us is safe. But what happens when they are wrong—like they were with DDT, and have been, and continue to be, with hundreds of other products? Can we afford to continue to pay the price of being left with dead or deadly soil?

I am not suggesting that some of these products are not safe, nor that some may not be beneficial. But with more than 10,000 agricultural poisons registered in California alone,[344] and new ones coming out every day—nearly all of which are very complex chemical formulas—how can we possibly know which ones are in fact safe and which ones are not? And what about the combinations of, and residues of, those poisons that are used year after year and remain in the soil? Should we have that much faith in "science?"[345] In our government officials?

As in medicine, the chemical mindset, I believe, is problematic. Life is delicate, and if we think we know more than the One who brought it into being and sustains it, we are setting ourselves up to be humbled. And unfortunately we can take others down with us.

Remember the Titanic.

Digestion

Most of our food is now grown in depleted soil.[346] The food may look the same as highly vital food, but it is not the same. So we have to eat more food—a lot more food—to get the same amount of nourishment. This requires our digestive system to work harder, which in turn requires us to take in more nourishment.[347]

Our bodies are made from the dust of the earth and perform in precisely the same way as the soil does. The digestion and assimilation of our food follows exactly the same principles. We need an army of various microorganisms in our digestive tract to help us break down and assimilate the food we eat.

What happens if we sterilize the intestinal tract? What happens if we eat the natural glue in wheat instead of the whole grain? Are these smart things to do? How many millions of people are highly susceptible to disease because their immune system has been effectively put out of commission by antibiotics and dead food! And how many millions of people in the US eat far too much and are obese, yet are malnourished!

From digestion we assimilate that which makes up our body. And what we assimilate also affects our clarity of mind.

What Nutrition Is and What it Is Not
True nutrition is not difficult to understand. What is nutritious and what is not is clearly evident by how we respond to what we have eaten. Foods that are nutritious satisfy our hunger.[348] Foods that are not nutritious make us want to eat too much.

If we have been weaned from junk food, a meal of an apple, or of sunflower seeds, or of a vegetable with a little lightly seasoned chicken with it will leave us satisfied. We only want to eat so much, and then we stop eating. A meal of Oreos, or of popcorn, or of pizza produces quite a different response—we always want to eat more.

That is the principle of junk food—it is a teaser. It always leaves us unsatisfied. We eat, but do not have enough. Why, after the hamburger with fries and a coke do we always want to eat the last of the french fries even though we are already full? And why, after we eat such a meal, do we feel lethargic and generally not well? We do not feel so well because of the assault we have just made on our digestive system. Our digestive system is now working far too hard and wants the body to rest.

Why do the weight loss diets based on counting calories eventually fail? Because they ignore the basic principle of what nutrition is. Willpower to control overeating is not much of an issue if we eat the proper foods in the proper combinations.

I will discuss food combinations in Chapter 21, but here I want to tell you two stories in order to further explain what nutrition is.

When I was a young boy in school, I read about the Indians who had lived in the deserts of Southern California. I read how they had traveled hundreds of miles nourished almost entirely by a small quantity of seeds. I marveled at this and wondered how it could possibly be so. Many years later, I visited Joshua Tree National Monument and saw a display at the visitor center there that explained the same thing. They even had some of the seeds and a very small animal-skin bag that the Indians had carried to keep them in. For more than three decades, from the time I first read about this, I could not understand how it could be so. How could a human being derive so much energy from such a small quantity of food? Then I was forced to change my diet, and I had to explore new ways to get energy. By that time, I had been hypoglycemic for a few years and was accustomed to eating something every two to three hours in order to keep my blood sugar up. One day, I decided to try whole sesame seeds and purchased some. At my usual 11 a.m. meal, I was quite pressed for time, so I put some of those seeds in a teacup and took it with me back to my desk. About five that afternoon, it dawned on me that I had eaten nothing that afternoon other than about three tablespoons of those seeds. The mystery of the Indians in Southern California was solved.[349]

I have an uncle and aunt who came to visit us on their way back from a month-long trip to Thailand where they had gone to help build a school. I picked them up from the airport, brought them home, and my wife served us a nice meal. They were quite excited about their trip and we were equally interested in hearing about it. While my aunt taught the schoolchildren, my uncle worked with some other volunteers putting in the foundation of the new school building. The foundation and floor of the building was built of concrete that was all mixed by hand. That is brutally hard labor. Their porters for carrying the bags of cement to the mixer were Burmese women. The Burmese provide much of the heavy labor in Thailand, just as people from Mexico do here in the United States. My uncle was astounded at the strength and stamina of those women. He explained that they were very small in stature and weighed no more than 90 pounds. The sacks of cement weigh 94 pounds. And those women carried them all day.

Later, my uncle got into his luggage and brought out some photographs from their trip. He showed us a photo of the men pouring the concrete slab floor and many other photos. When he got to the bottom of the stack of photos there was a photo of him and my aunt sitting in a restaurant in Thailand where they ate dinner just before catching their flight home. In front of them on the table was a bowl of fruit. In the bowl was cut cantaloupe, some grapes, a pineapple and other fruits that we are accustomed to. This surprised me, and I asked him if they did not have local fruits. "Oh yes, but they're not very good. They're mostly skin and seeds. Only the poor people eat them." I don't know if anyone else at the table heard what I heard. But I just heard how those Burmese women got their great strength and stamina.[350]

THAT, dear reader, is nutrition.

You may rightly ask, "But why don't we get that kind of nutrition from our food?"

The answer is simple: We eat adulterated food and food that is commonly grown in nutrient deficient soil.

Nourishing Food vs. Adulterated Food
From the very beginning, tillers of the soil began picking out the larger seeds from their harvests to plant the next year. Cross pollination to develop new varieties of plants has also been going on for a long, long time, and many ancient peoples developed more favorable crops. At the same time, ancient peoples learned how to breed livestock animals for the traits they wanted. This being the case, there are very few foods that we eat today that have not been tweaked by human hands. Wild foods, such as blackberries, elderberries, mustard greens, black walnuts, and wild caught fish are exceptions, but such foods are in very limited supply.

Most of the foods we eat have little resemblance to the plants or animals they were originally derived from. The fruits we buy from the store today are a good example. Undesirable qualities, such as a thick skin, large or abundant seeds, and tart flavor were eliminated from these fruits long ago. What we have instead is fruit that is sweet, easy to eat, and delicious, but not nearly as rich in nutrients.

The process of crop and animal manipulation continues. A good example of this is the tremendous change that has taken place in the apples grown today in the US in comparison with those grown here forty or fifty years ago. We used to buy Pippins, Romes, and Spartans. These are hard to find now. Instead we have Gala, Braeburn, and Fuji, etc. What is the difference? Sugar content. The consumer has demanded a sweeter and sweeter apple.

Don't think the only harmful sugars are the refined ones. The problem is the balance of sugars with other nutrients—or the lack of it.

The grains that we eat today also have little resemblance to the grains eaten in former generations. The ratio of gluten to bran, germ, and other components is much different than it was 150 years ago. The kernels are much larger, the yield per acre is several times what it was, but the healthfulness of the food has been compromised. Of course, if we throw out the bran and germ and just eat the gluten, our bodies will pay the price for that. The new, widespread problem of negative reaction to gluten is no mystery.

In the last 150 years there has been an explosion in food crop manipulation, and a lot of it is detrimental to our health. Unfortunately, in agribusiness crops are thought of as commodities, not as food, and all that counts is tons per acre. Tons of what?

Is it any wonder that where we are "helping" the peoples of poorer countries by giving them "better" seed, so that they can get larger harvests, they are now coming down with diseases they never had before? [351]

Today, the greatest food tweaking ever is taking place—genetically modified organisms. GMOs, as they are called, are when someone decides what genes we want in a plant and what genes we don't want. No doubt their training has taught them what is beneficial for us and what is not. Or maybe not. But the practice has taken over the food industry, and because these new organisms are stronger than the others, it won't be long before it will be very difficult to get seed that is not genetically modified. We are probably there already with some crops. What is behind the frantic rush to develop all these GMOs? Is it really to "help feed the world" as we are told by the proponents? Don't believe it! The goal is to secure patents on food and reap the royalties from those patents.[352] [353] [354] [355]

The marketing people behind the development of the GMOs tell us that their products need to be developed so that we can get away from using chemicals on our crops, or at least use less of them. They state the obvious, that the method we have used for generations of poisoning our crops is not working no matter how greatly we increase our efforts. They tell us that their scientists who are engineering life are smart enough to develop plants that will not need insecticides, because the plants will be toxic to insects but not to people, and that their products will be good for us. Do you believe that? Do you believe they are smarter than the One who created all life? Will not their pride be shown as folly just as that of their predecessors has been?

By all accounts, the use of insecticides has not been working out nearly as well as we thought it would. Seems the bugs can adapt to whatever we throw at them. And the GMOs are being developed only to *resist* herbicides. So now we can have both herbicides and GMOs for breakfast.

All that is written here is not to cast a dark cloud, but rather to bring to light what has happened to our food supply. What we need is nutritious food, as close to the way God made it as possible.

The FDA
You may well ask, "Where is the Food and Drug Administration in all of this?" Answer: The FDA, like the CDC, AMA, or any other organization for that matter, has never made a decision. People make decisions; and the decisions we all make are founded upon our understanding and even more upon our character. Unfortunately, money is a great corruptor of character. We all need money, but if we use it, or if it uses us, is the question. This is the case whether we run a business or agency, or we merely work in one. A brief history of the FDA bears this point out very well.

What is now the FDA started out in the Department of Agriculture which was established in 1862 by President Lincoln. The Department began as an aid to agriculture, mostly for the purpose of collecting agricultural statistics in the different farming regions and making their findings public. The chief focus was on seeds—specifically which ones were most beneficial for different regions.

It did not take long for advocacy groups to form and begin lobbying for various business interests. In 1887, the Hatch Act provided for federal funding of agricultural experiment stations in the various states, and political lobbying increased exponentially.

A large part of the US food industry had become industrialized by that time, and there had been countless cases of abusive and even downright dangerous practices. As now, there were then many questions about the safety of the chemicals used in the growing, processing, and preserving of foods. Also, misbranding and false claims were as common then as they are now. For this reason, Congress eventually passed the Pure Food and Drug Act of 1906. A preface to the Act begins like this:

> "The sentiment back of the Food and Drugs Act is well understood. Everyone will agree that, so far as it can be done by legislation, the laws should protect the public from being deceived in the foods which nourish them or in the medicines which are relied on to cure their ills. But to formulate a law which will effectively protect the public without depriving it of freedom to eat what it may choose to eat and to take such remedies as it may wish to take, *and without serious disturbance of business conditions...*is a matter of great difficulty." [356]   (Italics mine)

A noted chemist and medical doctor, Harvey W. Wiley (referred to in the last chapter), took a leadership role in the passage of the legislation. He was an advocate for federal regulation of both food and drugs. Because of his respected work in the industry, Wiley became the first commissioner of the USFDA. As the above quote implies, that was, and is, a tough job.

In 1907, not long after taking responsibility for the FDA, Wiley published a book titled ***Foods and Their Adulteration***. He began to feel the heat immediately after it came out because now his opinions were not just his opinions; they also greatly affected many businesses.

Wiley was staunchly against most food adulteration. Of bleached (white) flour, he wrote, "At the present time flour is extensively bleached for the purpose of making an inferior article resemble a superior one." Strangely, at the same time, Wiley thought sugar (probably "raw" sugar) was a valuable food. He wrote that "next to oil and fat [sugar is] the most complete food for heat and energy that can be consumed...The value of sugar as a food is not appreciated as it should be, since it is valued mostly for its condimental and preservative properties." These statements and many more like them, such as his comments against benzoic acid described in the last chapter, ruffled some feathers. In 1911, he was dismissed from the bureau on a technicality. The details of the story are pretty ugly, as Wiley's name was dragged through the mud in the press and he was even brought up on charges. The outcome? Wiley was exonerated, benzoic acid is still used as a preservative, sugar has done marvelously beyond anything Wiley could have imagined, and for several decades most people didn't know anything but bleached flour.[357]

In 1929, at the end of his life, Wiley wrote a "tell-all" book titled, *The History of the Crime Against the Food Law: The Amazing Story of the National Food and Drugs Law Intended to Protect the Health of the People Perverted to Protect Adulteration of Foods and Drugs.*

The title says it all.

But I don't think Dr. Wiley could have imagined of the day in 1960 when the FDA ordered the confiscation of honey, apple cider vinegar, and books touting their use from the shelves of a health food store because the honey and apple cider vinegar were placed within five feet of the books, and that, according to the FDA, constituted mislabeling.[358] Nor do I think Wiley could have thought that the agency he once headed would determine that black currant oil was a "food additive" and have a supplier's stock confiscated in 1988 for not labeling it as such.[359] Nor do I think he could have foreseen the drug-bust style raid on a health co-op in 2010 where

US Marshals brandishing automatic weapons stormed the shop and confiscated the unpasteurized milk that the co-op was selling illegally.[360]

Another story: Do you know where "**USDA Choice**" came from? Probably not. I didn't either until I started doing the research for this book. During the Depression, certain agricultural businesses were stuck with a lot of grain that they could not sell at anything resembling a decent price. So what did they do? The same thing that most large businesses do when they are facing a crisis—they lobbied the government. They suggested that the grain be used to fatten cattle. Oh, and it would be nice if that was mandated.[361] [362]

There were many unhealthful practices used for fattening cattle before this time that were endorsed by the USDA, such as feeding the cattle sawdust,[363] but the action taken on grain-fed beef ratcheted things up and transformed the entire cattle industry.

Prior to the mid-1930s, the majority of beef cattle sold in the US came straight from the pasture to the slaughterhouse. In other words, it was grass-fed beef. Grain-fed beef is very different than grass-fed beef. Stockyard, grain-fed beef is marbleized with fat; grass-fed beef is not. The fat in a grain-fed animal is also very different chemically than the fat in a grass-fed animal.

One other thing: Cows were not designed to eat grain, at least not more than the tiny amount they would normally eat in the form of grass seeds. So what happened? The cattle in feed lots have their livers severely overworked. They cannot live for more than about four to six months on a grain diet, so they were (and are) fattened up until their livers are blown out, and then they are slaughtered and the meat of these greatly distressed animals is sold to you and me as—you guessed it—USDA Choice!

It's worse than that. What are you going to do with all those sick cows in the feed lots? Put them back on their God-given diet of grass? Oh no; they won't fatten up nearly as fast.[364] We'll feed them a constant diet of antibiotics and shoot them up with more antibiotics so they can live just long enough to get them good and fat. And so it was. And is.

This decision to fatten cattle with grain, a decision blessed by the USDA, was not just bad for the cows, because the cows were not the only ones who were dropping dead because of a grossly unnatural diet. People began dropping dead too. Heart disease, high blood pressure, high cholesterol, and a host of other human health problems that had been rarities now became prevalent.[365]

Beef is not bad for you; marbleized beef is. Wheat is not bad for you; stripped wheat that is too high in gluten is. Dairy foods are not bad for you; pasteurized dairy foods can be.

Within a generation after the success of the grain lobbying that gave us marbleized beef, we had the FDA allowing Camel cigarettes to advertise that their product helped improve digestion. Later, in the early 1980s, after people began to realize the evils of processed sugar, the FDA stood by as the refined sugar industry ran an ad campaign saying that sugar "is good food." And until recently, what was labeled as "whole wheat" bread could in fact be 10% whole wheat and 90% caramel colored bleached flour.

P. T. Barnum never pulled off a hoax as great as any one of these!

Resources
Silent Spring, by Rachael Carson, 1962
Though this book is often mentioned, apparently it is seldom read. If it was, we probably would have made a lot more progress in the fifty years since it came out.

"Power Steer," by Michael Pollan, published in the *New York Times Magazine*, March 31, 2002
An inside look at the beef industry. The story follows the life of a typical steer.

Chapter 19
"Organic" Food: What it is; What it is Not

"Organic" means grown without pesticides, right? Well... no, not exactly. The same US Department of Agriculture we talked about in previous chapters sets the standards for what can be labeled "organic" in the US and what cannot. So, what we have today is a situation where "organic" crops can be grown on top of a ground cover of plastic sheathing, can be rooted in a mulch of newspapers and styrofoam, can be sprayed with viruses[366] and certain soap-based insecticides, and can be irrigated with chemically enriched water. Similarly, beef cattle that are not fed plastic pellets[367], only get shot up with antibiotics when a vet says it's okay, and meet a few other restrictions can be labeled "organic." That's not exactly what we thought "organic" was, is it?

But then we knew something not so good was up when "organic" made its way to the large grocery chains, and a lot of the "organic" produce started looking more like table decorations than food; didn't we?

I am sure that beef cattle that are administered antibiotics on an as-needed basis are healthier, on the whole, than those that have a constant diet of antibiotics as described in the last chapter. But to call cattle "organic" that are fed grain—a food that is unnatural to them and causes them great harm—is at least somewhat misleading.

The controls placed on "organically grown" crops for the most part may produce healthier foods than "conventionally grown" crops, which are commonly grown with nearly a no-holds-barred attitude toward health. However, many of the allowed practices in "organic farming" are contrary to life itself and therefore undermine the health benefit that people desire (and think they are getting) when they purchase "organic" foods.

You can look up the regulations for "organic" foods on the web. The URLs are too long to bother typing them in, so just do a web search for the National Organic Program, Part 205 and that should get you to the Electronic Code of Federal Regulations and to all the information that you would rather not know about what "organic" can be according to the USDA.

In the early days of "organic" foods (the 1970s and 1980s) mainstream agribusiness did not care what the "organic" farmers were doing. If anything, they ridiculed the idea or said it was phony. But the idea of "organic" caught on, and too many small farmers and small food companies started doing very well. It soon became obvious to big business interests that the idea of more natural foods was not going to go away and that there was an enormously profitable opportunity in capitalizing on it. So, since they couldn't beat 'em, they joined 'em.

Certainly there were abuses before 1990 when the USDA got into the "organic" act. We are all cut from the same cloth. Nevertheless, whatever gets lobbied successfully by large agribusiness is now labeled "organic." For this reason, what was "organic" twenty years ago is not what it is today, nor what it will be ten years from now.

Obviously, the federal regulations for organic farming greatly favor the large producer. The small farmers (what few are left) get buried in paperwork and have to quit. Economy of scale has forced out many of the small farmers and retailers in the country, but not all have fallen by that means. Many have fallen to unfair regulations that favor the mega-corporations.[368] When it comes to producing healthful food, that is probably not a good thing.

Besides USDA certification, there are also local private farm product certification associations throughout the country. Oregon Tilth is one of the largest, and its certification is well respected. Organic Consumers Association was formed in response to the USDA's permissive regulations and serves as an excellent source of information. These associations, and others like them, promote what can be called "alternative food" in the same way that others promote "alternative medicine."

The Bottom Line in Food Purity
During both World Wars, what were known as "Victory Gardens" were encouraged both in the US and in Britain. That is, these

governments encouraged their people to grow as much of their own food as possible in order to reduce pressure on the food supply, and just as importantly, to give the people a sense of involvement in the war. We are in a different kind of war today—a war against our health that is waged by a more subtle adversary. Any progress against this assault starts at home and begins with a practical understanding of what food is. And we have at least as good a reason to have a garden for growing our food (if we can) as there was during those earlier wars.

[An added bonus for having a garden is that it is great for family bonding. Children who have grown up keeping a garden are less likely to want to hang out at the mall when they are teenagers.]

It would be nice if we could all grow our own food, but obviously that is not practicable for most of us. The next best thing to do may be to buy from trusted small local farmers—even if they are not certified "organic." Small businesses with a good reputation may be more conscientious when it comes to growing healthy food than a large certified grower. They have more to lose.

There is no way to protect yourself except to know and watch your local grower. And you may not be able to do that. Please understand that if your small local farmer is spending all his time on public relations, as many small growers are now doing, he or she cannot run a viable food business for very long. So we can get stuck with more agri-tourism instead of sources of wholesome food.

The solution to the mess we have gotten into with our food supply is not simple, but it starts with gaining an understanding of what real food is, supporting our local farmers, and growing what we can ourselves.

In some areas, a good way to support your local farmer is to sign up to get whatever they have that is in season. Many make weekly home deliveries on a contract basis. There are also many local cooperatives and farmers' markets.

Having said all this, most of us cannot purchase much of our food from small, local farmers or grow it ourselves. That being the case, there are advantages to purchasing our food from a health-minded grocery store. A "health-minded grocery store" will be big on fresh produce and other healthy foods, and will be very limited when it comes to the kinds of products that no one should ever put in their mouth.

If the produce doesn't look phony, or like it never saw dirt, it may be wise to purchase "organic" from the best sources that are available. After all, if the "organic" standards are commonly contrary to true healthfulness, what are the "conventional" standards?!

By the way, the soap-based pesticides that can be applied to an organic crop may be less harmful than the commonly used oil-based products. Unlike oil-based pesticides, soap-based pesticides that are applied directly to the crop can usually be washed off at the kitchen sink, unless the product is waxed or oiled.[369] And yes, many organic foods can be oiled.

Oh, and be happy when you see some aphids in your lettuce or holes in your spinach leaves. At least the bugs thought they were worth eating.[370]

Resources
Organic Consumers Association
http://www.organicconsumers.org/btc/BuyingGuide.cfm

www.localharvest.com and www.cafarmersmarkets.com (if in CA) may be good places to start if you want farm-fresh local food.

Chapter 20
Vitamins, Minerals and Dietary Supplements

After the discussion of our food supply in Chapters 17 through 19, it is appropriate to follow with this chapter on dietary supplementation. If we obtain our foods from modern industry, dietary supplementation to one degree or another is probably essential.

I am aware that there are a lot of medical doctors who tell us that taking vitamins and other dietary supplements is a waste of money. Some go so far as to say that dietary supplementation is all a lot of quackery. This being the case, let me tell you a story.

In 1749 a Scottish surgeon named James Lind discovered that citrus foods could be used to prevent scurvy. This horrible wasting disease had killed many sailors for centuries, and Lind proved that it could be prevented. The British Royal Navy accepted Lind's findings and began putting lemons and limes on their vessels. That almost stopped the scurvy problem. I say "almost," because it was not long before, instead of taking fresh fruit, many ship captains began taking lemon and lime juice in barrels in order to save space onboard. The scurvy came back. The Royal Navy then suggested that scurvy could be prevented simply by good hygiene, regular exercise, and maintaining good morale among the crew, rather than by using citrus foods. As time went on, other people proved that scurvy could be prevented on long voyages without the use of citrus. This was especially true in some long arctic expeditions where the crews survived on fresh seal meat, had no citrus, and had no scurvy on board. So, citrus foods were an on-again, off-again protocol for the Royal Navy for more than 150 years. When canned foods came along in the mid-1840s, they were thought to be "scientific," and the Franklin expedition—sent to find the Northwest Passage—took them along as well as lemon and lime juice stored in barrels. That expedition was a disaster in many ways. All the men eventually died, some from scurvy, some from starvation, and some from who knows what. The Royal Navy did its investigation and concluded that at least part of the problem was the lead used to solder the food cans. The Scott expeditions of 1903 and 1911 in the Antarctic also had trouble with scurvy. These men, as well as the other explorers, were top scientists of the day mind you. It was not until vitamin C was isolated, in 1932, that the cause of scurvy—vitamin C deficiency—was discovered.

Vitamin C can be found in many *fresh* foods. This explains why the barreled citrus juices were not effective deterrents.

The point I am making by telling you the story is that after Lind's discovery, 175 years passed while all this was being figured out. A lot of people died from scurvy during that time. You and I may not have that long to live while "science" figures out what too many people know from experience. That is, if we eat industrialized food, we will likely need dietary supplementation.

I won't attempt to tell you any of the science behind the vitamins here. I am not qualified to do that, and I will refrain from regurgitating what others have said. What I want to tell you is what we and others we know have experienced and found to be helpful.

Supplement Principles
1. What is stated in this discussion assumes that you do not grow all of your own food. I am talking urban and suburban USA here, and the foods that we have readily available to us.

2. What is stated here also assumes a good diet as set forth in this book—eating foods as much as possible the way God made them, refusing heavily processed foods, and greatly limiting the intake of natural sugars. If these things are not taken care of first, the effectiveness of taking vitamins and other dietary supplements will be compromised... perhaps greatly. A poor diet can make the hole in the bucket of health too big to be overcome by dietary supplementation. Sugar, especially, robs the body of vitamins, enzymes, and nearly every other healthful stored nutrient.

3. It would be nice to say that we just go down to our local health food store, buy a good multivitamin, and that's all we need to do. While that may be a good start—and probably everyone should do it—in fact it is usually not that easy. Especially as we get older.

4. It *may* be best to purchase vitamins and minerals that are extracted from food sources rather than those synthesized from non-

food sources such as petrochemicals. Food-source vitamins are more easily assimilated. What we cannot assimilate will, for the most part, pass through the urine.[371] Dosage needed of food-source vitamins and minerals will typically be very much lower than that of synthetically produced products. _However_, food-source vitamins and minerals are more frequently allergens and also commonly contain sugars and even yeasts. Furthermore, since the manufacturers of the more natural products like to put a large number of food products in their formulas, if you have allergies or a blood sugar condition, chances are that you will react to their products. For this reason we (Deborah and I) can rarely, if ever, use a product that has a long list of natural ingredients. Some vitamin manufacturers are obsessed with putting everything that anyone has ever heard is healthful into their products. In our opinion, they are selling celebrities, not healthfulness.

So, vitamin selection is not that simple. What is the point of getting an "all natural" product if you react negatively to it?

I realize that I have gone full circle, first telling you that food-source vitamins are best, and then explaining why perhaps they are not. This is purposeful because the marketing of these items ignores what I have stated here.

Selecting the products that are right for us takes some trial and error, but over time our bodies will tell us what is best for them and what is not. The benefit gained can be huge.

5. Cost. We often hear, "Vitamins and supplements are expensive, **I don't have the money for that!**" Yes, they can be expensive, but you can get the money from eliminating the things that rob you of your health. Just cut the alcohol, coffee, soft drinks, and over-the-counter medications off of your shopping list. (By the way, over-the-counter cold remedies, aspirin, stomach meds, etc., are virtually unknown in our household and in the households of some other people we know.)

6. **Always read the label**. We avoid products with sugar in them. We also avoid products with other unnecessary ingredients. In other words, if we need some vitamin C or B, it is not necessary to be ingesting fifteen other chemicals the names of which are difficult to

pronounce. There are some fillers that we cannot avoid. For example: Capsules are made of gelatin, magnesium stearate is used for flow of product into capsules, and silica and cellulose are used to make tablets.

7. We think it is wise to **purchase our supplement products at the healthiest food store we know of**. We avoid the cheap products sold at the large pharmacy chain stores. (Read the ingredients and you will see why.)

8. Don't know what brands to buy? The least reliable source of information is advertising. Besides reading the list of ingredients, I try to get my information from people who have no financial interest in what they tell me.

There is nothing as valuable as **comparing notes** with others who are on the path of healthy living. If you don't know anyone who fits that category, you may want to go to the healthiest *food* store you can and follow the shopping cart with all the green vegetables or other whole foods in it. The person pushing that cart respects their body. If you see a few vitamin or supplement bottles in the cart, talk to that person and ask them what they buy. Most likely they will be glad to help. (You may be better off not following the cart that is loaded with "power bars," "sports drinks," and frozen dinners.)

9. Supplement manufacturers are not static. Companies are bought and sold, and what was good yesterday may not be today. Many well-known brands are now owned by pharmaceutical companies, and the people in that industry see things differently. For example, a probiotic we took for years recently had titanium oxide added to it—for coloring. No thank you.

Some brands that we currently purchase are Jarrow, Twin Lab, Solgar, Solaray, Thorne, and Nature's Life. There are many other good brands.

10. **Not everyone will do well with the same supplement**. Deborah and I take different preparations of B12. What works for her does not work for me and vice versa. Our son takes a different B complex than Deborah and I do. He does very well with it; I tried it and it made me dizzy. Deborah, our son, and I all have glucose intolerance. For that condition, chromium picolinate is commonly

recommended. It works for Deborah and me, it does not work for our son. Deborah and I took a particular multimineral for years and seemed to do well with it. After a time, however, she found that it was not good for her. This kind of thing can happen with a lot of supplements. We adjust and keep moving forward.

11. Dosage, as stated on the package, may need to be cut down or increased. Deborah, being very sensitive, "sneaks up on it" to see if a new product will work for her or not. That is wise. If, after taking a supplement, your condition is made worse, the supplement itself may not be wrong; it could be that the dosage taken was too high. After getting "kicked in the shins" a few times in this way, we learn to use moderation.

12. Everyone purchases some products that do not work for them. Likewise, we all make mistakes. We learn and move on.

13. After starting a supplement regimen and getting it somewhat dialed-in, it may be wise to only add one product at a time. This gives the body time to adjust, and we will know what it is that we do well with, and what we don't do well with.

14. Deborah and I both keep a journal of what we are taking. The history is helpful and can save us a lot of time over the long run.

15. At first, I had trouble swallowing capsules. If the label does not say not to, we sometimes empty the capsule contents into a glass of water, stir, and drink our vitamins. I put some of mine—the ones that don't taste bad—into my bowl of ground sunflower seeds that I have for breakfast. Warning: Certain capsules are not to be opened.

16. We have found that it may be good to take some supplements for a while, but not for an extended time. Sometimes we can have a deficiency that needs to be addressed, and after it has been addressed, we reduce the dosage or discontinue use of the product..

17. Sometimes we will know right away if something is helpful or not. At other times it may take months to make that determination.

18. We don't get too complex. We listen to our bodies and they tell us what to do.

What We Take and Why

B vitamins

Almost everyone is short of the B vitamins. Why? Because they are easily depleted by a host of things in our modern society. Those depleters include, but are not limited to: refined foods, stimulants, medications (birth control pills included), stress, adrenaline rushes, tap water, and foods with poor vitamin content. (Yes, those foods can even be fresh foods; and no, you can't necessarily tell the difference.) We think a "B 50" complex is a good idea. That is, a complex of 50 mg of most of the B vitamins.

We don't take B vitamins after 2 p.m. if we want to go to bed at ten. They will keep you awake.

The vitamin C miracle

We take a minimum of 500 mg of vitamin C daily. We buy a product derived from citrus or with rose hips added. Note: People who have allergies commonly react to some natural source vitamin C preparations. Rose hips seem to be the least allergenic of the natural sources. If taking more than 2,000 mg daily, buffering is probably a good idea or a burning sensation will be experienced with bowel movements. You only need to make that mistake once.

Multiminerals

Since so much of our food is grown in mineral-deficient soil, we think taking a multimineral is a good idea also. There are several combinations, and some will agree with us better than others depending upon our particular mineral need. Looking at our blood tests with our health practitioner may be somewhat helpful.

Probiotics

Almost all beneficial bacteria have been removed from our food supply, and the dramatic increase of colon disease is telling us that that was not a good idea. We think it is wise to put some back. We can never do that as well as what God did in making whole foods, but we do what we can. We stay away from products that contain sugar (dextrose, fructose, sorbitol, etc.) and that cuts the number of products down considerably. It takes trial and error to see what is most effective for you. The goal is improved digestion.

Enzymes

Most of us do not digest our food very well, especially as we get older. There are a number of ways to determine this, the most glaring being to look in the toilet. Also, if we tend to eat too much, that is telling us we don't digest well. If our food is grown in nutrient deficient soil, it will be enzyme deficient, and our bodies will be too. Then we eat, but cannot assimilate. If we lack energy, don't feel well, or are hungry shortly after eating, it is probably because we cannot break that food down and we need some enzyme help to do so. Some people can get the enzymes they need through foods rich in enzymes such as papayas and apples. Others, like those of us who cannot handle the sugars in those fruits, may need to take enzyme supplements. Many enzyme products contain papaya. Other products contain ox bile, which has been helpful for me. With enzyme supplements, our bodies will tell us what to do.

A little bit about a few other vitamins and supplements

Vitamin D: In some cases, we may not be able to get enough from the sunshine. Vitamin D is essential for a healthy immune system.

Vitamin A: This one can be harmful if we do not know what we are doing. I would seek the guidance of a health professional before taking any.

Fish liver oils can be very beneficial if they do not have mercury in them. That's a big "if." If I think I need them, I will go with the most trusted source I can.

Herbs: Guidelines We Stick With

1. Many herbalists tell us to avoid using medicinal herbs with medications. The two camps don't mix very well. Some herbs are potent and can affect medications. We don't think it is wise to play with herbs. Some can be strong—maybe not for everyone, but for you. For example, many herbs will lower blood sugar, and taking them will throw diabetic medications off. If you want to get off medications and use medicinal herbs instead, it may not be such an easy transition. In our opinion professional guidance is needed.

2. We read the best herbal books we can, and get our information from multiple sources. We also talk to people who are experienced.

3. Many medicinal herbs should be taken as one would take a pharmaceutical drug; that is, for two or three weeks at the most. There are some herbs that we can continue to take, but we need to educate ourselves as much as we can first. If we take medicinal herbs, we need to learn how to listen to our body in order to know when to increase the dosage, cut it back, or stop it altogether. You may want to get professional guidance from a qualified herbalist before you embark on an herbal program.

4. Many medicinal herbs are greatly beneficial for some people but should be avoided by others. For example, ginseng is popular but for someone with blood sugar problems it can be detrimental. The same goes for licorice root and ginger root. Cayenne pepper is also very beneficial for many conditions, but it can be detrimental in some cases too.

5. Some fresh herbs are better than the same herb in dried form. Many herbals do not discuss this, but there can be a significant difference. A small herb garden is easy to maintain.

For a further discussion of herbs, see Chapter 8, Herbs. For a few specific herbal remedies, see Chapter 22, Herbal Remedies.

Use any information here at your own risk.

Summary of Vitamins, Minerals, and Herbs

1. We think it is wise to try to meet nutritional needs with foods. If we can't, then it's time to consider supplements.

2. Moderation is a virtue.

3. Remember, even the best baseball hitters only succeed a third of the time.

4. For a supplement regimen tailored to your specific need, you may want to consult the reference book, *Prescription for Nutritional Healing,* and a couple of good books on the use of herbs. After researching as thoroughly as you can, it may be a good idea to write out a plan and present it to a trusted health professional. Then you can make a decision how to proceed. Be prepared to make adjustments.

The Ongoing Battle Over Dietary Supplements

In the US, there has been a longstanding and ugly battle over dietary supplements between proponents of their use and the pharmaceutical and medical industries. The FDA is caught between the demands of the public and the heavy lobbying of the enormously powerful industries with which these products compete. This is a big subject and it affects us whether we realize it or not. I will only touch on the main points here.

1. In the late 1960s, prodded by the pharmaceutical and medical industries, the FDA went so far as to say that vitamins, as sold in health stores, could be toxic. In the ten year legal battle that ensued, evidence was provided showing that although a large number of deaths are attributable to aspirin every year, the FDA could not state one case of a death that was attributable to taking vitamin supplements.

That avenue being blocked, legislation was proposed that would have required vitamin preparations that exceed 150% of the USFDA Recommended Daily Allowance (RDA) to be sold by prescription only. That fight culminated in a 1976 law, <u>Public Law 94-278</u>[372] signed by President Gerald Ford, in which the FDA lost on every major point of contention.

Had it not been for vigorous petition signing and hundreds of thousands of letters written to our authorities and elected representatives at strategic times, the great majority of dietary supplements now available in health stores in the US would require a prescription from a medical doctor. That is the way it is in the European Union and in Canada, and it may yet happen in the US.

2. One of the key issues in the ongoing fight is what is classified as a dietary supplement, what is classified as a food additive, and what is classified as a pharmaceutical. Food does not require FDA approval. Non-food additives to food do, and of course, pharmaceuticals do. To have a formula of vitamins and minerals that greatly exceeds the US RDA is one thing. To add enzymes, amino acids, and a combination of herbs to that formula is another thing. To take it a step further and alter molecules and add those to the formula is quite another thing yet. All of these kinds of products are now sold under the classification of dietary supplements, and

the complexity of the formulas is becoming greater every day. This is stretching the envelope of what should be classified as a dietary supplement, and it is also stretching the FDA authorities.

3. At times, the battle has gotten completely out of hand. Federal Marshals have made numerous armed raids—drug bust style—on manufacturers of dietary supplements and on others involved in the business. Some of the cases would be laughable if they were not such an obvious abuse of power. It may be hard to imagine the confiscation of a shipment of primrose oil prepared by one of the finest supplement suppliers, but it happened.[373] Likewise it may be hard to imagine the drug bust style raid of the Life Extension Foundation and the eleven-year court fight in which the foundation was exonerated on all counts, but this also happened.[374] Certainly there have been warranted confiscations of products that clearly were not only in violation of law but were also from people who had no intention in conforming to the law. But why not just issue a warrant and settle the matter in court?

4. The Dietary Supplement Health and Education Act (DSHEA) was passed in 1994 and gave some reprieve, but its provisions are nibbled at daily by the lobbying efforts of those who oppose the supplement industry. Those of us for whom the medical industry has been a hindrance more than a help would merely like to take some of the most basic vitamins and herbs as we see fit. For many people, like Deborah, there is no good alternative. Thankfully, at this time we can freely purchase these products. But that right is threatened on one hand by the efforts of those who want us to get a prescription from a medical doctor for vitamin C sold in capsules greater than 100 mg., and on the other hand by those who manufacture and promote products that perhaps cross the line of what should be considered a food supplement.

5. Though there have been many serious threats of greatly regulating the supplement industry since DSHEA. So far the FDA has for the most part stayed out of it, other than to limit the claims that the manufacturers make. However, many of the manufacturers, desirous of a bigger piece of the "health" pie, are stretching the envelope on those claims. Both sides are nibbling at the law, slight tweaks of which can make huge differences depending upon how

those laws are interpreted. How this will shake out is anybody's guess. There will continue to be plenty of changes.

6. One thing is for certain: The supplement industry is now mainstream. We have already seen the "if ya can't beat 'em, join 'em" stance in the "health" industry. An industry once largely composed of small businesses founded by individuals who truly held to natural principles is now immersed in all the trappings of large industry.

Resources
Back to Eden, by Jethro Kloss, 1939
In our opinion, Kloss' premise is foundational. We do not see the value in taking a bunch of "health" products without first and foremost returning to as natural a way of living as possible.

Prescription for Nutritional Healing, by Phyllis A. Balch, James F. Balch, MD, 4th edition, 2000
This encyclopedia-like volume has a lot of information on how dietary supplements are used.

The Way of Herbs, by Michael Tierra, 1998

Herbally Yours, by Penny C. Royal, 1993

Health at Gunpoint: The FDA's Silent War Against Health Reform, by James J. Gormley, 2013
This book, written by the former editor of *Better Nutrition for Today's Living*, gets into the nitty-gritty of the war against the supplement industry. Frankly, it is upsetting reading and even the more so because many of the claims are verifiable. While I would much rather only talk about the positive, for the benefit of those who think "this can't happen here" I have included this resource.

Chapter 21
Some Principles for a Healthy Diet

"All things are lawful for me, but not all things are profitable. All things are lawful for me, but I will not be brought under the power of any." Paul

If we keep this maxim, we will eat to live, not live to eat. Our food will serve us; we will not be slaves of our appetite.

Since the diabetes epidemic has already spread to a third of the US population,[375] and since most diabetics or so-called "pre-diabetics" are older, it could be said that there are only two classifications of people in the US: those who have an abnormal and potentially dangerous blood sugar condition, and those who have a good chance of developing one. For this reason, diet will be discussed in this chapter from the standpoint of prevention and reversal, not only of diabetes, but also of ill health in general.

> **What I share with you in this chapter, as in the rest of the book, is what we have found to be good practice and is based upon common sense. What the reader does with this information is entirely his or her responsibility.**

By discussing diet, I am not talking about any popular diet. I am not talking about vegan. I am not talking about vegetarian. I am not talking about low carbohydrate. I am not talking about low fat, etc. There may be some virtue in some of these approaches, but I do not believe any of these should be the guiding principle of our diet.

Our root dietary problem is that for generations now, we in the industrialized world have become accustomed to eating dead food, and most of us do not have a clue that **it is only life that gives life**. We are being destroyed due to this lack of knowledge.

As with every industry, there is a lot of window dressing in the food industry. In other words, deception. Many of the big fast-food chains, long known for their unhealthful wares, now claim to serve healthy food. But what is the point in setting our sights too low?

The reasonable choice, I believe, is to get away from all the hype and **just buy real, unprocessed food—as close to the way God made it as you can.**

Actually, some garbage foods *are* healthier than other garbage foods. However, when you go grocery shopping, if you take a look at the *ingredients* of prepared foods, and not at the front of the colorful box, you will see clearly what you are taking into yourself. If you think it matters, you will probably leave 95% of it right there on the store shelf and not take it home with you.

Lifeless food, food void of vitality, is a thief. It steals stored nutrients from the body. One of the reasons we eat too much is that we do not get adequate nourishment from what we eat. Furthermore, our digestive system works far too hard because of the assault we make upon it when we eat too much or we eat heavily processed foods. This is a vicious cycle, and we can stop it.

Getting your diet right may not be easy. But getting on the right track is.

Besides returning to a diet of foods as close to the way God made them as possible, we would do well to **simplify**. Historically (and naturally), man's diet was not anywhere close to as complex as we have made it. A meal of a single fruit can be most nourishing. So can a meal of vegetable stew, perhaps with a small amount of animal flesh thrown in. Stews, simmered for a long time, have been part of mankind's traditional diet for millennia.

In past generations, a meal of gruel, made from grains high in protein, could be most nourishing. People lived on gruels and pottages for centuries. However, because of seed manipulation, balanced, high-protein wheat, barley, rye and other common grains are now hard to come by. You may want to try amaranth, kamut, and quinoa. Human hands have not had as much experience in making them into unbalanced foods. For extra vitality and flavor, save your vegetable and animal broths and use them instead of water to cook your grains in, or use them to start your stews. If you want some rice with your meat dish, cook the rice in the broth of the meat. (You may want to skip the broths from the cabbage family of foods and from kale, as those will make you gassy.)

A meal of raw **seeds or nuts** can be very nutritious.[376] However, we need to be careful with seeds and nuts because they can be constipating. To avert this, they can be sprouted, soaked overnight, or ground in a coffee grinder and the resulting meal soaked for a few minutes so the meal does not dry out the intestinal tract. Eating the same with celery or an apple is also good. Chew well—a great part of digestion takes place (or does not take place) in the mouth.

It is crucial to understand that we not only need calories for fuel, but just as importantly, we need food fiber for cleansing. Before putting something into your mouth, consider how you are going to get its waste products out. Fiber is not only needed to slow down the metabolic rate and complete the burning of certain fuels, it is also needed to clean the digestive tract. If there is not enough **moisture, lubrication, and fiber** taken with whatever meal we eat, be assured that the waste products are not all coming out. Some of that waste is staying inside of us, being putrefied, and making us ill. The colonic tube doesn't lie.[377]

Burn slow! You may not have a blood sugar problem—yet. But with such a very high percentage of the population prone to this condition, and the fact that it usually takes decades to develop before it is recognized, I don't think it will not hurt anyone to eat slow-burning fuels. In other words, proteins with vegetables instead of sugars with simple carbohydrates.

Always be in balance! If we go heavy on the non-starch vegetables, we are more likely to have a proper balance.

There is a tremendous amount of flexibility for a healthy diet, because different people do better with different foods. For example, Deborah gets a lot of energy from eating kale; I get none. Some people do very well with grains; others don't. Etc.

In turning to a healthy diet, you will find out a lot about yourself. If you have a sugar addiction, you will certainly find that out. One of the things I discovered when I determined to eat in a healthy way was how much I used my body as a trash can. That remaining food on the plate after I was satisfied—why did I put it into my mouth? It took me a while to break that habit. I was taught not to be wasteful, and I respect that, but now I am more concerned about not wasting my health.

As we straighten out our diet, we will also find out about **urges**. If we have an urge to eat that we think may be unreasonable, it probably is. Sometimes, urges to eat are really our body telling us that we need to exercise. Our body's "juices" are stagnant and need to get on the move. This is easy to prove to yourself.

Cravings
Cravings are urges gone berserk. We can crave *anything*. Cravings are almost always destructive in nature. If you have a yeast/fungal/candida problem, those guys will yell for the foods that sustain them. They love sugars and meat but can't live on non-starch vegetables. Because of that, there will be an uncomfortable withdrawal period if you change your diet to reduce their populations, but those and other cravings do not have to be our masters. In Chapter 14, I explained how to break the sugar habit. Other cravings are mastered in much the same way.

Are you tempted to eat bad food? For some people, it's pretty simple. They go right to the source of the problem and turn off the TV. Then keep it off. The junk food industry spends billions on television advertising because it is very effective. But it doesn't have to be effective on us.

You can never learn to play the acoustic guitar well unless you build up calluses on your fingertips. Likewise, you can never get your diet straightened out unless you build up calluses in your mind against junk food. It does not take long to do either, but it is a little uncomfortable at first. In both cases, **the key to success is a little understanding and a lot of desire.**

Eat Locally Grown Fresh Food as Much as Possible
Eating fresh produce in season helps us not eat too much of the same food, which can cause allergy. Also, a fresh picked, fully ripened peach or plum is infinitely more nutritious and better tasting than one that was picked before it was ripe, took three days to get to the distribution center, another four days to get to the grocery store, spent another day on the loading dock, sat in the cold storage room for a week, then was on the store shelf for a day, and

then was in your refrigerator for three days before it was eaten. So it is with all produce, not just fresh fruit. Also, the longer food is stored, the more reason there is for man to mess with it and the more opportunity there is for contamination. The farther food is shipped, the farther we are away from our natural environment, and again there is more opportunity for man to mess with it. All those fresh fruits we see in the winter that are flown in from South America may seem heaven-sent. But how are they kept from contamination on the way to market? Among other things, by the use of fungicides.[378]

Don't Like Fruits and Vegetables?
I think there can only be two reasons. First, if we are addicted to junk food, we cannot taste the flavor of good food. Thankfully, our taste buds can be re-educated—usually within a month. Second, if someone does not like fruits and vegetables, they have probably never had *fresh* fruits and vegetables. What I mean is this: The apples that you buy from a vending machine have been handled by people who deal in dead food. They are handled with all the care given to a can of soda pop. This is an extreme case, but many grocers do not understand real food much better than that. There are many grocery stores where I would rarely purchase a food item. These stores are great for supplying us with toilet paper, laundry soap, and dishwashing sponges, but not much in the way of food.

Vegan and Vegetarian
The vegetarian and vegan proponents have an excellent point: **We eat too much meat!** But to cut it all out does not work for everyone and may not be a good idea for a lot of people. We have several friends and acquaintances who have taken the vegan/vegetarian route. Two friends of ours were vegetarian or vegan for seven years. Both found out the same thing: They needed animal protein. Both developed potentially serious health problems, both added a little animal flesh to their diet, and both solved the problem.

We know many other people who likewise were vegan or vegetarian for shorter periods of time. Eventually they could not function well. I am not saying that is always the case—certainly it is not—I am only stating that it is the case with many people we know.

For those who cannot have a diet high in fruit, starches, grains and beans, a vegan diet is probably not workable. Without a large quantity of these foods, which someone with a blood sugar problem will not be able to handle, being vegetarian or vegan may not be a good idea at all.[379]

The bottom line is this: If you can't function well on a vegan diet, what's the point? If you function well and have plenty of strength when only eating a moderate portion of meat once or twice a week, why eat more of something that is so hard to digest?

Raw Foods
I should also address cooked versus raw food. Today there are many raw food proponents, and they, like the vegan folks, have a good point. The benefit of plenty of raw foods is very great. But I caution against the extremes that some have taken this to by saying that we should only eat raw foods. Cooking of food has been done for millennia in almost every culture, and I don't believe our ancestors were lacking in intelligence. Yes, we can cook a lot[380] of the vitamins out of our foods—especially by using high heat—but that cannot be the whole story.

Some Principles of Food Combining
Different people seeking to eat in a healthy way have come to slightly different conclusions on food combining. However, in the various discussions on food combining by people who have paid attention to this, there is a lot of common ground. The goal is simply better digestion.

Scientists explain the reasons for these principles of food combining; I'll just say you will likely feel better if you abide by them. You can prove all these things yourself and be just as smart as the scientists.

Fruit
Fruit should be eaten by itself. Exceptions: Papayas and apples. Papaya enzymes are good for breaking down proteins. Apples have a neutral pH and are okay to eat with many other foods.

Eat fruit in moderation. The fruits that we have available to us today are very high in sugars and relatively low in many other nutrients that are present in wild or less developed fruits. Too much sugar, if not burned off quickly, will ferment in the digestive tract.

Eat melons by themselves. Their enzyme action is incompatible with that of other fruits.

Eat citrus fruits by themselves. Their acids are incompatible with those of other fruits.

Allow at least an hour after eating fruit before eating another meal. You want to have your meal of fruit burned up before eating anything else.

Starches and non-starches
From what we understand, starches and proteins should be not eaten together. They burn at different rates—the starches fast, the proteins slow. If we eat them together, the proteins can be forced down the digestive tract too quickly, resulting in putrefaction of the proteins. In other words, "meat and potatoes" may not be a good thing. (That "lump" in the gut that you feel after such a meal is not normal; it is telling you something.) A small amount of animal protein with brown rice or potato skins is probably fine. Some cheese with whole grain crackers is probably okay too.

Eat starches by themselves or with vegetables.
Eat non-starch vegetables with meat. They digest well together.
Eat non-starch vegetables with anything (except fruit).

Fats
Olive oil, flax oil, and many other cold-pressed oils are excellent sources of healthy fats as long as they are not over-heated. Avocados are another excellent source of healthy fats. If we stay away from sugar-containing products, other junk foods, marbleized meats[381], and unhealthful oils[382], we have virtually eliminated the problem of unhealthy fats.

Fats, in limited quantity, are typically a good thing as long as sugar is not in the diet. If you take sugars with fat, your body will burn the sugars and store the fats. Therefore, fats should never be taken with sugar.

Animal flesh

We have found it good practice to always cook meat with herbs and eat it with plenty of non-starch vegetables. Animal flesh is hard to digest, and enzymes supplied by the vegetables help greatly.

Think in terms of the burn rate of fuels. Sugars burn fast, starches next, non-starch vegetables next, proteins next, and fats burn slowest of all. There is no problem eating non-starch, green vegetables with proteins and healthy fats. That is a good thing.

Other Basic Principles We Have Proven to be Helpful

We drink a full glass of water as soon as we get up in the morning. If taken alone on an empty stomach, water will immediately go to the bowel. Drinking on an empty stomach helps flush the digestive tract, especially the bowel, and consequently helps avoid having waste stay in the bowel too long and putrefying. If we do not have at least one full bowel movement every day, that is what is happening.[383]

Drinking too much water or other liquids with meals is not a good idea unless it is cooked in with the food, as it is with soups and stews. Water dilutes the stomach acids which are needed in the process of breaking down our meals.

Drinking plenty of water between meals is a good practice. Our bodies cannot metabolize nor cleanse themselves properly without an adequate supply. Most of us do not drink enough water, and many health problems—some of them serious—are simply due to this lack. (See Chapter 22, Water Treatments and Remedies.)

Sufficient protein at breakfast allows the brain to function better.

Be a nibbler. Many of us have found that frequent, smaller meals are easier on the digestive system than large meals.

We eat only as much as is needed to satisfy our hunger. We don't eat until "full." We want to be satisfied, not full. If we feel any discomfort after eating, our body is telling us something. We either ate too much, we cannot digest what we ate, or both.

We eat heavier meals early in the day so that the digestive tract can rest at night. It needs the rest, and we will feel the better for it.

It is not wise to eat a heavy meal before bedtime. It will sit in the gut and putrefy, destroying or overwhelming any healthy gut bacteria.

For a good night's sleep, stop eating fruit or any other sugars at least six hours before going to bed.

It is wise to refrain from eating when we are nervous, upset, or cloudy headed. We are toxic when this is the case, and our digestive system will not appreciate any more stress. Do drink water at those times. Some herbal teas may be better yet.

We eat raw food frequently—as fresh as we can get it.

Don't forget the value of stews and soups that have been slow-cooked. High heat kills enzymes and can negatively affect other nutrients.

Keep it simple. Every day should not be a feast day.

Help your bowel out. If our bowel cannot discharge waste, it will back up and poison us. We can help our bowel out by eating flax or olive oil sparingly, eating plenty of non-starch vegetables, eating other fibrous foods that are moistened, and of course, drinking an adequate amount of water between meals.

Fasting
The benefits of an occasional fast, or a partial fast, cannot be overstated. Abstaining from food for a period of time resets the body and the mind. Cravings are adjusted, toxic buildup is discharged, the digestive system is rested, intestinal flora can be made healthier, and perhaps most important, our attitude toward food can be realigned by this discipline. After you have fasted, you will understand what is meant by these statements.

Fasting occasionally is the natural way. For millennia, people had to fast from time to time due to an inconsistent food supply. However, for a fast to be healthy, **a few warnings are necessary**:

1. NEVER stop drinking water! Dehydration can be serious.
2. I think it is wise to start slowly, with one day fasts,
3. And always recover adequately before fasting again.

4. We think that if the fast is for more than one day, or if you have a blood sugar problem, harm can be done if the fast is done incorrectly. You may want to get professional help. By all means, stay away from the fads![384] Let others make the mistakes. After a method is well proven, over decades, then consider it—but never if it goes against common sense.

Because of poor eating habits or simply because of nutrient deficient food, our bodies have become unnatural and deficient in healthful nutrients. So there are certain things we must maintain when we fast that our ancestors did not have to maintain when they fasted. We can put fancy names on them—electrolytes, vitamins, enzymes, etc.—but basically we need supplementation while on a fast, especially if we are fasting for more than one day. This is why juice fasts, with <u>fresh</u> vegetable juices, can be helpful. In other words, what I think is beneficial is a partial fast.

You can easily find out the value of live foods by comparing freshly juiced fresh vegetables with those juices that are pre-prepared and pasteurized. There is no comparison!

Fruit juices should be kept to a minimum—yeast and candida love the sugars.

Juicers are a pain to clean, and none do both celery and spinach well, so I just throw veggies in the blender with a little water. The result is more like a smoothie and not quite juice, and the vitality is infinitely greater than that of pasteurized juice.

Warning: During a fast you may get cranky. This is common enough; laugh it off. This is why Deborah and I fast together—it is easier to laugh at it.

Warning #2: During a multi-day fast, you may not think as well as you need to. When we fast, we structure our work accordingly. For example, if you write contracts for a living, you may want to only write the rough drafts instead of proofreading and approving the final drafts. (!)

The V.E. Irons supplements can be most beneficial during a fast. Their Greenlife, Beet Extract, and Natural Source Vitamin C tablets, when combined with probiotics, enzymes, and oils, we have found to be excellent aids to a successful fast. Their products are expensive, but when averaged out, the supply of products purchased costs little more than what we would pay for the food that we are not eating on our fast days.

If a fast is longer than a day, we think it should be done **during warm weather**. We need the heat, and if we are not taking in the calories, our bodies will have to work hard just to keep us warm. That can be counterproductive to the rest that we are attempting to give our body through fasting.

Fasting is a time of rest. We will not have all our strength. If we usually run, it may be better to walk instead. We find that it helps a great deal to keep our minds active (and away from food), but rest when our body tells us to. When we fast, we are treating our body to a rest. We think it is best to keep it that way.

Suggestions for Eating Out
This is not a theoretical book. We do have to be practical. There are times when we need to eat and don't have the best food available. So, if I have to get a hamburger, I order it without any condiments and throw away the bun. Mustard may be okay; ketchup and other condiments are mostly sugar. I think it is wise to make this kind of eating a rare exception.

Stay away from sauces. They always have something bad in them— sugar, MSG, modified food starch, monoethylborboltate (I made that last one up, but you get the idea).

Time
A change to healthy eating will take an investment in time, especially when you are starting. **To find the time**, turn off the TV. Once you begin to make the switch to a healthy diet, you will find the strength to do so. For more time, get away from useless drivel on the computer. If you do these two things, you will likely find adequate time to plan your dietary project. There are plenty of resources in this book to help you get started.

Potpourri
People who eat less live longer. If we want to eat less, we cannot have **yeast, fungus, candida, or other parasites** eating up our

food. Therefore, it is prudent to avoid mushrooms[385], too much fruit, and undercooked or uncooked animal flesh or fish.

New diet plans: The question to ask is: "Are the basic rules of good nutrition being followed?" That will probably eliminate nine out of ten diet plans.

Soy: Poor George Washington Carver! He spent much of his life proving what a truly wonderful food the soybean is, and in less than a hundred years we have ruined it. At this time, virtually all commercial soybeans are genetically modified organisms (GMOs). Many people in the health community are avoiding soy for that reason. Some people, myself included, were able to eat soy until a few years ago. If this is because of a change in the soybean produced or in our body chemistry, I don't know.

Grains: Grains are not the balanced foods they once were and probably can't be the mainstay of a healthy diet for most people. (See Chapter 18.)

Fish: There is a big debate in the health community over fish. It could be that nearly all the world's fish are contaminated with mercury. Our oceans and waterways are. Fish are very good for you; mercury is not. I eat fish sparingly and stay away from the large predator fish. Deborah does not eat fish at all. With a history of mercury poisoning, she cannot afford to.

Liver: See the discussion of USDA Choice in Chapter 18.

Pork: Why eat *anything* that is so full of parasites?

Recent immigrants to the US: You may want to stay on your native diet if it is of natural foods. In other words, do what your momma says—she knows best.

Resources
V.E. Irons, www.veirons.com, PO Box 34710 N. Kansas City, MO 64116. Irons has excellent supplements to help with a fast.

A Short Course on Dietitians and Nutritionists

Teachers of nutrition and degree programs at the major universities and colleges adhere to the AMA/FDA, or government and medical/food industry, line of thought. They must, because that is where their funding comes from. Those who disagree are not welcome.

Registered dietitians (RDs), therefore, must practice according to that industry line of thought. A *practicing* "nutritionist" is *commonly* associated with "alternative medicine" and may be a member of the American Nutrition Association or similar group. They can include naturopaths, acupuncturists, chiropractors, and others. They typically are more in favor of natural foods. Both kinds of practitioners can be called "nutritionists."

A medical doctor may send you to an RD, but probably would never send you to a (natural-leaning) nutritionist. A registered dietitian is the one who oversees the menus at hospitals and care facilities—where they serve ham and sweet potatoes for dinner and chocolate cake for dessert. A practicing nutritionist would typically warn against that kind of a diet. The dietitian does not administer the insulin after such a meal; that's the nurse. The nutritionist is likely to advise a diet and lifestyle which, if followed, would make taking insulin unnecessary.

Natural-leaning nutritionists are not found working in hospitals. Dietitians probably would not be found in a health food store. Nutritionists are typically big on fresh vegetables, tend to recommend vitamins, and often discourage consumption of refined sugar. Dietitians often recommend Jell-O and similar foods, and discourage the drinking of "too many" sodas.

The Association of Registered Dietitians is in lockstep with those they serve; and those they serve are constantly lobbying for regulations that seek to secure a monopoly on "nutritional advice," thus eliminating competition. (See Appendix IV.) Nutritionists are backed by the pocketbooks of people who are not enamored with modern medicine and simply choose to eat in what they perceive to be a healthier way.

Part IV

More Lessons Learned,

Conclusion

Chapter 22
More Stories and Lessons Learned

This chapter is a collection of stories that have been selected to show the principles behind what we have learned. I think it is far better to grasp the principles than it is to lay hold of details. Detailed help may get us get through a crisis, but may not be of much lasting value. As the old Chinese proverb says:

"Give a man a fish, and you feed him for a day;
teach a man to fish, and he will feed himself
and his family for a lifetime."

There are some success stories in this chapter, and equally important, there are also accounts of some things that did not work. There is no theory here—I have only listed cases from our family's experience or the experience of people we know. All have been written only for the benefit of those who take full responsibility for their own actions.

> **Before reading this chapter, please re-read the warning at the beginning of this book that is located right after the preface. Thank you.**

I have put these stories and lessons learned into several categories and provide at least a few stories in each category. Several of the cases in this chapter were life-threatening; most were not—at least in the short term. I have classified them as follows:
  A. Chiropractic, Reflexology and Similar Stories
  B. Prescription Drugs
  C. Dietary Treatments and Remedies
  D. Water Treatments and Remedies
  E. Home Remedies
  F. Vitamin and Mineral Remedies
  G. Herbal Treatments and Remedies
  H. Work
  I. Surgery
  J. Hospitalization

Before going to the various categories, I want to tell you two stories from our family—one that is humorous, at least on the surface; the other was quite serious.

Concerning sweets and taste buds

As mentioned earlier in this book, in Chapter 5, we raised our children in a sugar-free home. That being the case, our children never developed a taste for that poison. Baked apples with cinnamon, or pears with nut butter, were the sweetest foods they ate while growing up.

In the sixth grade, while at school, our daughter was offered a Coke. Unlike at other times when she had been offered sweets, this time she accepted it. She took a sip and immediately spit it out. "That's gross!" she exclaimed. Yes, as a matter of fact, such is the *normal* reaction of anyone not addicted to "white death."

A dangerous spider bite

I mentioned in Chapter 1 that when our son was young, he got ill easily and his body reacted negatively to many things. When he was about six years old, he was bitten on his belly by a spider or insect while playing in the back yard. He came into the house to tell his mother, and she saw the red spot that had formed. Within about two minutes, a bright red line, in appearance as a blood vessel, had formed on his torso extending out from the site of the wound. Over the next few minutes it advanced significantly, traveling in the direction of his heart. My wife, thinking quickly, got out some yogurt and added her usual fortifiers to it—desiccated liver, cod liver oil, vitamins C and E, and a mashed-up vitamin B complex tablet. By the time she applied it, the red line was about four inches long and had come close to his heart. She applied it, and I'm sure we prayed. Within twenty minutes the red line had disappeared. Nothing remained except our thanks to God for sparing our son from any harm.

Note 1: From our son's reactions to bug bites and bee stings, we assume this was probably an allergic reaction, not a black widow or scorpion bite.

Note 2: The reaction was so fast that Deborah and I both felt it was necessary to treat immediately and not risk the time it would take waiting to be seen at the hospital emergency room.

Note 3: Again, I am merely a reporter of what we have experienced. Neither of us are medical professionals and I am not qualified to advise anyone what they should do in a similar situation. I have also given credit where credit is due.

A. *Chiropractic, Reflexology and Similar Cases:*

Career-ending back pain cured

I have a client, I'll call him Bob, who is a professional golfer. Over time, Bob developed a sore lower back. It kept getting worse, and eventually he could no longer swing a golf club. The doctors told him that the only solution was to have surgery and fuse two vertebrae. But that would be the end of his golf swing. He told me about it, and I told him, "You need to see my chiropractor." Well, Bob had heard the typical AMA line about the evils of chiropractic—how "those people hurt you" and how the whole thing was quackery, etc. By that time, I had heard that kind of talk dozens of times before, so when he brought it up I said nothing. But from day to day, Bob would ask me questions and I answered them the best I could. I told him of my own back injury, at age twenty-seven, and of my experience going to different chiropractors. He kept asking, and I told him of some other cases that I knew of firsthand. Eventually, backed against the wall of losing his career forever, Bob went to see my chiropractor. After two or three visits, Bob was out playing golf again. The chiropractor showed him how to do some exercises that, if done daily, would maintain good body structure and a healthy back. I saw him ten years later and he told me—with the biggest smile you can imagine—that he was still playing golf and doing his exercises every day.

I have often wondered how many needless back surgeries are being performed. People are shown X-rays that "prove" that they have a "slipped" or herniated disk, a degenerated disk, or some such problem, and are told that surgery and pain pills are the only options.

Not so, says another friend of ours who was shown such X-rays decades ago. She began doing stretching exercises after being given that diagnosis and has never gone back to the doctor about her back.

Maybe somebody reading this knows of someone who has had back surgery and does not have to take pain pills. I don't.

Different chiropractors, different methods
I mentioned my own back injury when I told you about Bob. I lifted something incorrectly once and my lower back has not been the same since. Like millions of others who had only gone to medical doctors all their lives, I also had heard of the evils of chiropractic. But I was desperate. I too was losing my career because I couldn't work at times. And I had two small children and a wife to feed.

I visited about five or six chiropractors before finding one who had the skill to solve my back problem. I think it is worthwhile to tell you briefly of the different approaches these chiropractors had.

The first chiropractic adjustment I had was from an old Mexican laborer at work. He had helped many people at the company I worked for, and I was in a lot of pain, so I finally gave in to at least give the chiropractic idea a try. He had me lie on my stomach, then lifted my leg and pushed on my back some. It didn't help much, if any, but at least it warmed me up to the idea of chiropractic. Next, I went to a Palmer School practitioner and he performed the standard adjustments for my case. I got some temporary relief and saw him a few times with the same results. Next, I got a referral to a fellow who specialized in manipulating only the top two vertebrae just under the base of the skull. He as much as told me that all problems could be solved by his technique. I thought the guy was a quack, and he didn't help me at all. (By the way, we avoid anyone who acts like they know it all or who talks too much. A helpful health practitioner spends his energy understanding the patient, not boasting about his talents.) Next, I went to a fellow who told me that my back "got out of alignment by force, and it will take force to get it back into alignment." It didn't work. (We think that is a bad approach too. It does take some force to perform certain adjustments, but for a skilled doctor who will work *with* your body, it does not take that much.) Next, I got a referral to Dr. David Bundy. This man was as methodical as an engineer, but was also very intuitive. He looked at his patient's spinal alignment carefully, then put them on the table and began checking pressure points in various places. He was picking up data. Then he knew exactly what he wanted to do. Sometimes he would press on a point for a while or briefly massage a particular area. He was Palmer School trained and used those basic methods, but he had greater skill than the others we had seen. He was gentle, did not over-adjust, and worked only on what he felt was most important. He understood the body as a whole better than anyone we have ever met and was our family doctor for more than a decade until he retired. What a Godsend!

Oh, and he solved my back problem. I still had to see him now and then, but as time went on, those visits became only about once a year.

[My wife and I lovingly refer to the Palmer Method as the "snap, crackle and pop method." In some chiropractic offices, the treatment is almost as standardized as a hamburger at McDonald's. At least you know what you are getting. However, when different chiropractors perform the same adjustments, the benefit of those adjustments can vary greatly. There is a lot of good to say about the Palmer Method, but we have found that in itself it is very limited. The best chiropractors we have seen also understand the body's muscular system and energy fields, have a good touch, and above all are intuitive. The body is far too complex to be successfully treated by method alone, and the intuitiveness of the practitioner may be more important than all the methods put together.]

Cranial adjustments
Yes, the subtitle is correct. Dr. Bundy was a craniopathy specialist; that is, he was skilled at moving the bones of the skull. That's pretty scary stuff and not the kind of thing I would usually go for on an average day. However, when our son fell off the swing set, hit his face on the ground, and got up with the shape of his face all distorted and couldn't see straight, we thought we needed to do something. Deborah took him to Dr. Bundy who fixed him right up, and both of them came home all smiles.

Actually the bones of the skull do move quite a bit, especially in children. But cranial adjustments should be approached with great caution. (I would think!) Very few chiropractors do this procedure and probably far fewer adequately understand it. As I said before, what a Godsend Dr. Bundy was!

Note: Before this incident, we had taken our son to Dr. Bundy for his eyesight, and Dr. Bundy had adjusted his back and cranial bones, so the idea was not new to us. Deborah says that was the beginning of stabilizing both his eyesight and his overall health.

Gallbladder dump
Once, for a couple of days, I had sharp soreness on the bottom of my right foot. At first it was occasional, but as time progressed it became aggravating. I was also feeling increasingly toxic. Eventually the condition had my full attention, so I looked on the reflexology chart and determined that the site of the soreness corresponded to the gallbladder. I applied pressure to the point[386] on a couple of occasions perhaps two hours apart. It was *very* tender. A little while later I had the most horrific smelling bowel movement and instantly felt much better. The soreness did not come back. This may have been a blockage in a duct of the gallbladder.

Hand injury
A carpenter I know developed a chronically sore hand. The two middle fingers as well as the bones on the back of his hand were not happy. Numbness, soreness, and just plain pain. I sent him to Dr. Bundy, the best chiropractor we have ever known. Even with several visits, he could not help the condition.

My point in telling this story is threefold. First, no health practitioner really knows that much—we are far too wonderfully made. Second, we have found chiropractors very helpful for back, neck, shoulder and hip problems, but less helpful for other problems. Third, looking at this from what I now know, I think the problem was largely muscular and located in the shoulder or neck.

Fibromyalgia
We know a woman with fibromyalgia who was in a progressed stage of the disease and was on her deathbed. The doctor's twenty-plus prescriptions had not helped and she had only become worse. Somehow, her husband found out about a chiropractor in the Lake

Tahoe area who was treating the disease successfully. They traveled to Tahoe and stayed for several treatments. She has been up and functioning well since that time.

There needs to be a "disclaimer" on this story. She also went off all of her medications, which undoubtedly helped.

> **A common problem in trying to determine what works and what does not, is that we often need to try multiple treatments at the same time. When we improve, we then do not know for certain which factors were effective and which were not. We are only given one body and do not have the luxury of pulling out additional lab rats to make this determination.**

Severe middle back pain, especially when coughing
We have an elderly friend named Jim who fell and shortly afterwards developed a constant nagging pain in his middle back. When he coughed, the pain was severe. As is typical for probably all of the back pain cases I have heard of (and that is plenty—I was in construction for more than thirty years), the medical doctors were of no help whatsoever. All they could do was what they do—they gave Jim some Vicodin for the pain. Jim called me and told me about his situation, and I took him to my chiropractor. Jim was in pain, and I was glad we did not have to wait long to see the doctor. I went into the exam room with the two of them, and Jim told the chiropractor of his constant pain since shortly after his fall. The doctor grabbed his leg in the middle of the calf, applied pressure to a point and asked him, "Where is the pain now?" In shock, Jim replied, "It's gone!" "You've got a cracked rib," the chiropractor told him, "and unfortunately it is going to be painful for a couple of months or so." He took his hand off the pressure point and the pain returned, then put pressure on the point again to show Jim what he needed to do if he needed temporary relief.

By the way, Vicodin may well have its place, but it is prescribed with great frequency and is severely constipating, and that is never good.

By the way #2: I have known two other men who had cracked ribs from falls in the workplace. In both of those cases the back pain did not come until the third day, then was constant just like Jim's. Same song, third verse.

Stiff neck: See Acupressure in Chapter 8

Sciatic nerve (down the back of the leg)
The sciatic nerve extends from the pelvis area of the back, down the back of the leg, to the bottom of the heel. It can become unhappy. Find the pressure point in the middle of the heel, about an inch in from the back of the heel. It is not too hard to find if the nerve is acting up. Use your knuckle, or better yet, a pencil (eraser end) or similar blunt object, and start probing with firm pressure. You may have to dig in. When you find the pressure point, you will know it. It will be *very* tender. That's how you know you are on a "pressure point." Keep the pressure on for a few minutes. I have done this successfully a few times. Something in this procedure resets the memory of the nerve, and the pain simply goes away. Of course, it is easier if someone can do this treatment for you.

Lower back injury
Our daughter played basketball in college. In her sophomore year, during a game, she went up for a rebound and came down on another player who had moved under her. Something happened in her lower back, and that was the end of her college basketball career. The pain was almost constant for years, sometimes debilitating. Chiropractors were no help in this case, and being raised in our home, she knew better than to use pain pills. X-rays showed nothing, and the medical doctors were of no help either.[387] Hot and cold packs sometimes eased the pain a little, but not much. She eventually had **prolotherapy** (injections of collagen), but that too had little effect. She lived in this condition for seven years. Later, while traveling in Mexico, she told an old Mexican folk healer about her back injury. He looked at her, felt her back, had her lie down on her stomach, and began massaging, then digging his fingers into the injured area. As if moving a taut rubber band, he **repositioned the ligament** to the correct position on the vertebra. Her back has caused her very little trouble since.

B. *Prescription Drugs*

New to drugs? Look out!

I have a neighbor whose elderly father I had the privilege of knowing. "Pops," as I called him, was a very pleasant old man. Although he could not speak a word of English, and I could not speak his language, we enjoyed each other's presence very much. Pops was in his eighties when I met him, and he was in great shape. He was from the old country and lived in a healthy manner.

When he was in his early nineties, he had some problem for which my neighbor took him to the hospital. The doctor there prescribed four medications and wanted him to take them immediately. Pops didn't like the idea. He had never taken medications of any kind and was concerned. But my neighbor was also concerned because Pops was not in good shape, and it seemed like the doctor knew what he was doing. So my neighbor told his father, "Dad, I trust him, you should take these." Eventually, the old man reluctantly agreed and took the pills. Pops died twenty minutes later.[388]

[Prescription drugs are one of the leading causes of death in the US. Very seldom is this cause written on a death certificate, however. See Resources for *Our Daily Meds.*]

Bipolar disorder

See Chapter 3.

Diabetes meds

Deborah had a **diabetic** friend who otherwise seemed to be in very good health, but she suddenly began failing. First, she lost her equilibrium and had to start using a walker, then she began having great difficulty remembering anything. She went to her doctor, but he refused to change her medications. She eventually ended up in the emergency room. The doctors there realized she was B-12 deficient and gave it to her intravenously. She recovered quickly. The ER docs told her that a diabetes drug she was on, M____, depleted vitamin B-12 and that there was nothing wrong with her other than that deficiency. She is taking B-12 now and has been fine since.[389]

Blood pressure meds

I have a friend, about fifty years old, who was put on blood pressure medication. As many people who go on those medications, he felt terrible while on them. He could not sleep, and using his term, he was "useless" during the day at work. He cut the dose down but was no better for it. His doctor could not help, and eventually he had "had it" and stopped the medication altogether. He then talked to a mutual friend who understands health from a natural perspective. This friend asked him if he drank coffee. "No, I gave that up; that helped for a while." "Good; how about soft drinks?" "Gave those up too." "Do you eat spicy food?" "Yes, all the time." "Spicy foods and stimulating herbs can raise blood pressure." My friend cut all spicy food out of his diet and in less than a week he was greatly improved. His blood pressure is now normal, and he tells me that he has not felt so well for a long time. He also purchased a copy of *Prescription for Nutritional Healing* so he can better understand how to take care of himself.[390]

Warning: High blood pressure can be <u>very</u> dangerous and needs to be kept in control in one way or another. I am **NOT** advising you to drop your meds. I am merely a reporter telling you what my friend did. Please read the warning at the beginning of this book, right after the preface; and thank you for understanding why I have to repeat this.

High blood pressure and high blood sugar often go together. It is very common for a medical doctor to "help" a patient get one of these under control by prescribing a medication, but in the process of doing so send the other condition out of whack. This is part of the diabetes medications roller coaster that millions of Americans are riding.

Fungus

When in my mid-thirties, I suffered from "jock itch" every summer. One summer, I also had athlete's foot and oil pockets, like little pimples, on one hand. I went to a dermatologist, and he told me it was all the same thing—a fungus—and should be treated with Lamisil (terbinafine hydrochloride). So I purchased the prescription and started to use it. It didn't do much for my fungal problems, but I did start to grow breasts. Now, if I was a woman, maybe I would have liked that, but I'm not, and I didn't. I stopped the use of the medication, but by that time a hard lump had developed in one breast. So I was told to get a mammogram. It showed nothing, and after a while the feminine features disappeared. But I have had hormonal problems since. A direct correlation? I don't know. I am just reporting what happened.

Lesson learned, #1: I applaud the doctor for recognizing that all three problems were in fact one. That was helpful.

Lesson learned, #2: All those scary possible side effects written in small print on the piece of paper inside the prescription box— they're for real.

Lesson #3, that was eventually learned: Certain foods support fungus. The worst is mushrooms, then sugars, then other acidic foods, including fermented foods such as vinegar and wine. Removing those foods from the diet and eating plenty of green vegetables can often get fungal populations in check. Garlic helps too.

Fungi are always present in the system and can become a problem at any time. If the population of fungi, molds, yeast, or candida in the intestinal tract becomes too great, it may take drastic measures to restore a proper balance of healthy bacteria. That can mean cutting out all fungus supporting foods for an extended period of time. Many illnesses (typically with a large number of symptoms) that "don't make sense" actually do. They are simply the result of unhealthy intestinal flora. In some cases, fungus becomes so saturated it can be found in the blood and in the tissues.

Shingles

When Deborah had shingles on her face, at her jaw, she felt that she should take the antiviral medication recommended.[391] The infection can spread fast, and we believed the risk of losing an eye was too great to take the time to try natural methods. We are not purists in our largely anti-medication stance. We simply believe that they are grotesquely overprescribed and overused. (See also Vitamin Treatments later in this chapter.)

Thyroid; thyroid medications and helps

The thyroid is part of the endocrine system, which plays a large part in controlling the entire body. Many disorders including diabetes, hypoglycemia, and autoimmune conditions and diseases, to name a few, may have a significant thyroid component.

Thyroid problems are very common now. Excessive radiation is often the root cause. X-rays, especially CT scans and MRI scans, can in fact be very harmful. This is well known in the industry.[392] Heavy metals in the body, including amalgam dental fillings and other metallic dental materials, also commonly disrupt thyroid function. **Iodine imbalance** is another cause of thyroid dysfunction.

We intimately know several cases of hypothyroidism and have followed them closely for decades. Our observations tell us that **thyroid dysfunction should be taken seriously.** Quality of life is hanging in the balance. Thyroid function is a very complex matter, and as with nearly any other condition, physicians are quick to prescribe medications for the condition.

Someone with **hypothyroidism**, that is, someone whose thyroid gland does not produce enough thyroid hormone, may eventually need to take a thyroid medication. The medications come in different forms: the glandular form, which is actual thyroid gland derived from swine, or a synthetic form that takes the place of the glandular or components of it. Once a person goes on one of these medications, they may not be able to get off of it. If there is a problem with the supply of the drug—and there is from time to time[393]—those dependent on the drugs can be in a bad way if they have to switch medications. We know.

Our decision (not someone else's) of how to treat a thyroid condition, or not treat it, could greatly affect us for the rest of our lives. In Deborah's case, she feels that going on thyroid medication was the right thing to do. In another case we know, it probably would have been better to try other means of treatment first.

Before going on any thyroid medication, you might want to get your **iodine level** checked, and with your health practitioner's help, see if the condition can be adequately addressed by maintaining proper iodine levels.

There are also naturopathic remedies available to help strengthen and balance thyroid function. For example, Metabolic Advantage makes a product for boosting thyroid function. The product may be effective enough for some people so that they can avoid prescription medication. It is a multimineral compound with L-tyrosine (an amino acid) and glandulars. Unfortunately, many people use these kinds of products for weight control instead of changing their diet. They are playing with fire, and some may be doing themselves harm.

Herbal remedies, some known for centuries, or other naturopathic means such as mentioned in the last paragraph *may* be a safer way to go *if* prescribed by someone knowledgeable who can monitor you carefully. In our opinion, if we have this condition, we *also* need to learn how to monitor our thyroid function. A physician who sees us for fifteen minutes cannot know what we know about how our body is functioning, but he or she probably knows some things that we don't know. I think it is prudent to get a good understanding of the condition *and* have professional help on this one. The consequences of not doing so may not be good.

Some doctors prescribe a thyroid medication as a preventive measure for people with a family history of heart problems. Again, once on the medication, it may be for life. Consider well.

Hyperthyroidism—when the thyroid produces too much thyroid hormone—we have no experience of, so I will not comment on it.

The Bottom Line on Prescription Drugs:
Medical doctors know how to medicate. If you want to take meds, go to those professionals—they are good at telling you which ones to take. If you do not want to take meds, you probably will need to go to someone else.

C. Dietary Treatments and Remedies

Two sad, but telling, sugar stories
Perhaps the saddest case I know of the dangers of a sugared-up diet is that of my own father. He died of diabetic complications at age

sixty-six. Often, when someone is talking to me about blood sugar problems, they tell me that something or another that they eat is not sweet. They are almost always referring to one sugared-up product or another, whether it is coffee cake or a "trail mix" containing mostly dried fruit. I always reply that my dad's famous last words were, "It's not sweet." Actually, those were not his last words, but he said them often enough, I am making a point, and I am trying to save someone else from what took my dad. My, how we all miss him!

From time to time for over a decade, both Deborah and I saw the medical doctor who put her on thyroid medication. He had a problem with his weight, which he had fought for nearly his entire adult life. He *hated* being fat but did not know, or at least did not address, what made him that way—sugar. When I began to have blood sugar problems, I went to see him a few times. One time, he told me about some new "health bars" he had started taking. He passionately told me, "If you put a cookie on the counter next to one of these, you will not want that cookie!" The fact is, I had given up on sugar before that time and had no desire for any cookie whatsoever. However, I did try his "health bar" and found it sickeningly sweet. The poor man never broke the sugar habit and went to his grave having hated himself for being fat for most of his life.

Alzheimer's

We have observed firsthand the effect of diet on people with this disease. Eating chocolate is the worst. The negative results (anger, irritability, incoherence, etc.) can often be seen in less than a day. Eating a healthful diet helps significantly. The results can be seen within weeks. We also know people with this disease who improved considerably after starting a regimen of vitamin B-12 and/or coconut oil on a regular basis.

Crohn's disease; diseases of the bowel

Diseases of the bowel are becoming more and more common. Thirty or forty years ago, few people had heard of Crohn's disease. Now it seems everyone knows some people who have it, and it is common in young people. (The effects of diet are accumulative not only over years but also over generations.)

My wife has a friend whose daughter has Crohn's disease. This young woman has suffered greatly. She discovered that if she does not eat chocolate, she is fine. In the long run, if she is to have any quality of life, her entire diet will need to be straightened out.

The increase in bowel diseases is not a mystery. They are typically the result of eating heavily processed foods, and our medical system is too compromised to address this squarely. Therefore, a dietitian will probably suggest more processed foods. A qualified nutritionist will take a considerably different approach. (See the end of Chapter 21.)

Migraines

One of my brothers had trouble with migraine headaches for years. When he told us, my wife asked him, "Do you eat broccoli?" "Yes, just about every night." "Cut it out of your diet, and also any other cabbage family foods." The migraines disappeared.

> **When we have reached a saturation point with any food, or group of foods, our body will tell us about it. It does not mean that we can never again eat that food. That may be the case, but more likely it is not. It simply means we have gotten out of balance, and a proper balance needs to be restored.**

Hormonal headaches

This may not be a technical term, but it is a factual one. My wife used to get headaches that she described that way. Cauliflower, broccoli, and the cabbage family foods stimulate the production of estrogen and can be the cause.

Sleep deprivation

This is a common problem, and it is very often linked to diet. Here are some cases I have seen.

A friend of ours told me that he suffered greatly from not getting enough sleep. He also told me that he had suffered from this condition for decades and that he was surviving on about three to four hours of sleep. I had been at some evening social functions with him and knew that he commonly ate desserts at that time. I told him to stop that, and to avoid anything sweet after midafternoon. He took my advice and almost immediately began sleeping about an hour and a half longer.

> **Eating sweets after dinner is a part of our culture. It is also the reason why so many people have trouble sleeping. We cannot have a stimulant in the evening and expect to have a good night's sleep. Besides sugar, spicy foods, coffee, tea, and chocolate are also stimulants.**

Not eating enough protein later in the day can cause some people to wake up too early. Also, eating a large meal before going to bed can cause a restless night. Give a meat meal at least three hours to be digested before going to bed; otherwise, it sits in the gut undigested, and your gut, unhappy with you for doing that, may wake you up to tell you about it.

While on the subject of sleep deprivation, I will mention a few other common causes, having experienced all of them myself.

Watching television and surfing on the web are also stimulants. If you do either of these before you go to bed, it may prevent you from having a full night's sleep. If you watch the "news" in the evening, unknown to you, the anxiety and stress from that stimulus can keep you awake *or* awaken you during the night. Instead, read a relaxing book or pray. Nothing calms the heart and mind like giving thanks to God and casting all our anxieties on the Lord.[394] I have been the beneficiary of many good nights of sleep due to this habit.

Going to bed too early, without being sufficiently tired, or staying in bed when you can't sleep can both lead to a lousy night's sleep. If you can't sleep, it may be best to get up and do something until you are sufficiently tired out.

The need for a full night's sleep, instead of fragmented sleep, cannot be overemphasized. The deep sleep that we have when we first fall asleep repairs and restores the body, but without the later dream stage of sleep, the mind will not be "defragged." [395] That is, it will not be reset properly. I have proven this, and many others have as well. After a good night's sleep, I am sometimes amazed at how sharp my mind is. New ideas are prolific, difficult problems have been solved in the night, and prospects are bright. That is not the case when full sleep is not experienced.

These are some of the simple mechanics behind an infinitely complex process.

Sleepwalking

Here is a case that freaked out these young parents. When our daughter was in first grade, she began sleepwalking after she had been in bed for a couple of hours. We would find her walking down the hall or sitting in the corner of her room talking to the door jamb. There was no waking her up. Deborah read in one of Lendon Smith's books that this was caused by not having enough protein at dinnertime. From then on, if she did not want to eat enough meat, Deborah would give her cottage cheese. The episodes stopped. Whew! Sometimes school is stressful for kids, and at that time, it was for our daughter. This probably played a role in the condition.

Typical diabetes cases

A business associate once told a friend, "If I'm spacey, it's okay, I'm diabetic." Lack of mental clarity is a common blood sugar problem, the effects of which can be debilitating. That is serious stuff when you are in an important business meeting!

Beth, a friend of ours, is diabetic. As with countless other diabetics, the disease is advancing, and she has had a miserable time of it. She called Deborah and told her of the trouble she was having. She said she was off sugar and was taking medications, but she was continuing to feel worse and worse no matter how her medications were adjusted. Deborah asked her: "Are you eating grains?" "Yes." "Stop." "I thought grains were good for you." "Grains are good, but not for you." Beth cut the grains out of her diet and immediately knew she had done the right thing. She felt much better.

The problem with diabetes is that by the time it is diagnosed, a lot of damage has already been done. There are clues all along the way, but they are commonly ignored, not taken seriously, or the sufferer genuinely does not know what to do.

In telling Beth's story, it is important to state clearly and emphatically that diabetes is a very serious disease and is almost always the result of decades of improper diet. (Whether of the diabetic, the diabetic's parents or grandparents, or all of these.)

The inability of Beth's doctors to "get her medications right" to compensate for the disease is a common complaint. Yes, we know of some diabetics who, for a time, seem to "have their meds right." But from what we have observed, that condition usually does not last, and there are periods—long periods for many—when diabetics are absolutely miserable, if not incapacitated. If they go the way of medications and do not get their diet straightened out, according to what we have seen, there is only one sentence for them—more and more medications and the medication roller coaster.[396][397]

The simple solution is to get the diet straightened out before the disease gets worse. Someone's case may or may not be too far advanced for them to get off medication, but it is unlikely they will hurt themselves by eating a proper diet—free of sugars, free of simple carbohydrates, and full of green vegetables, adequate protein, and a proper balance of other healthy low-glycemic, unprocessed foods.

In our opinion, it is diet and exercise—don't bother looking elsewhere.

Once again, I am only a reporter. I am only telling you what I have observed for four decades. I believe people with the condition need professional help. I also think it is prudent to get a health practitioner who will help you avoid the pathway of medications if at all possible.

The biggest disaster is that today people are becoming diabetic at a younger and younger age. Many children—like our own—are born with a glucose tolerance problem.

Another diabetic case, now common: young people
A person with blood sugar problems will need to be strong mentally if they want to be strong physically. They cannot behave in the way that other people do. They cannot eat what other people eat, they can't "party," and they will be the "odd person out" at times

because of it. The alternative is to suffer the consequences. We know a young diabetic woman, who, while in college, was shooting insulin so she could drink with her friends. That was many years ago. College is over for her now. I don't know if her life is, or if she is alive, what further weakened condition she has to deal with.

[For more diabetes cases, see the discussion of diabetes medications in the section titled Prescription Drugs earlier in this chapter. Also see Vitamin and Mineral Remedies later in this chapter.]

Glucose intolerance
When I was thirty-seven, I lost my health. Things had been going downhill for years, and I thought it was just because I was getting a little older. But at age thirty-seven, it was obvious to me that something was really wrong. I went to the doctor, who examined me and ordered the normal battery of tests. After the results came in, I went back to see him and was told, "It's all in your head. You're a healthy guy—look at these blood tests!" Yep, there it was in black and white—all great numbers. I should have been proud, I suppose. But I had no strength and just felt lousy all the time.

At my wife's prompting (I was ready to listen to her by that time), I switched to a hypoglycemic diet. It took a while, but within two or three months I could tell I was going in the right direction. At that time, my blood sugar did not test low, and we did not know the term "glucose intolerant." Now we know that if you have the symptoms of hypoglycemia, it is prudent to treat yourself as if you have it. What could be going on is that the body may be pumping too much insulin, which balances the blood sugar but greatly stresses the adrenals, the pancreas, and other glands and organs.

D. *Water Treatments and Remedies*
Other than improper diet and lack of exercise, perhaps the biggest cause of ill health is that we simply do not drink enough water. I mean water. Not sodas, not tea, not coffee, not milk. Water. Good water. This lack of water can cause a lot of problems and even lead to a diseased state of just about any form. What is enough water? Two quarts a day for a 128 pound person or three quarts for a 192 pound person may be a good rule of thumb, but saying that does not take into account heat and relative humidity, so

we need to adjust accordingly. If we have good water available, we will drink more of it. By the way, coffee, tea, and diet sodas have a net dehydrating effect.

Constipation

Constipation, **OR slow transit of waste from the bowel**, should never be taken lightly. **Either of these conditions can, in themselves, be the root cause of disease**.

Many people we know have been helped with constipation simply by drinking water. Can't go? Have a large glass of lukewarm water on an empty stomach. (Hopefully if you are constipated you have not eaten in a while—that is adding insult to injury.) If you don't go within ten minutes, have another glass. If you still don't go, and it's not too much, after another ten minutes have another glass. In almost all cases that will do it. If not, it's enema time.

Then, after being relieved, we need to understand how we got that way in the first place. It was one of two things, or a combination of both: Either we did not eat correctly, or we simply did not drink enough water at the proper times. If we eat heavily processed foods, we probably cannot eliminate adequately. White flour is the worst. We must eat enough lubricating and fibrous foods to carry out the fecal matter. If we don't, we won't.[398]

Just don't feel well?

So many people have told us this, and we testify of the same thing: Don't feel well? Feel a cold coming on? Just don't feel "right?" You might want to give yourself an enema. There may be nothing more effective. Grandma was right.

We just use water. Some people who are, or who have been, very toxic use coffee and swear by it. If you are going to use something other than water, it would be wise to know exactly what you are doing, because you can harm yourself.[399]

Colonics and cleansing

Colonics were discussed in Chapter 8, and if you have not read that section, please do so before reading this. In this section, I want to take the thought of cleansing and colonics further. We know several people who have been helped by colonics, and we are convinced that many others could also be helped enormously by the treatments. I will tell you of two cases here.

I know a man who became extremely toxic from eating too much meat. He was hypoglycemic and could not tolerate grains or legumes. His doctor advised him to eat a lot of meat to get the protein he needed. Eventually he realized that what he was eating was poisoning him. First he stopped eating meat altogether and just ate vegetables and seeds. Then he had a few colonic treatments. They were so helpful that he decided to go on an eight-day fast and cleanse. He went off all solid foods for those eight days, drank a lot of water, and took vegetable juices and vitamins. This regimen was complemented with a colonic every day for eight days. What came out of him was astounding—over fifty lineal feet of a thick, black, tar-like substance called mucosal plaque. On the sixth day of the fast he passed six feet of brown feces. The man was hardly overweight to begin with. This story is kind of graphic, but don't tell me—like many medical doctors do—that our bowels empty themselves perfectly well and there is no need to ever have colon irrigation. I know differently. I am that man.

[Note: In our opinion, no fast or radical cleanse like this should be done without competent professional guidance. You can hurt yourself if you do not know what you are doing.]

Many years ago, in the early stages of Deborah's health problems, we had a friend whose health was also unraveling. He was exhausted all the time, was falling asleep on the job, and had become extremely reactive to just about everything. It got so bad for him that if he was in a room with someone who was wearing deodorant or cologne, he would have to run out of the room. He also had a history of severe constipation. The effects of this condition really wore him down physically and mentally. We lost track of him long ago, so if he is still living or not, we don't know.

At the time, we did not understand what we do now. He was a classic case of auto-intoxication and was unquestionably toxic to the core. The bowel was backed up and loaded with extremely toxic matter that had even gotten into his bloodstream. Dr. Bernard Jenson (see Chapter 1) and Dr. Kellogg (see Chapter 8) were very successful in treating cases like this. The treatment begins with a radical change in diet and a radical cleansing of the bowel. In other words, stop putting the poisons in, and get the accumulated poisons out. The solution to many such problems may be no more complex than that.

The process of colon cleansing, as it is described in Dr. Jensen's book, *Tissue Cleansing Through Bowel Management*, cannot be spoken of highly enough. See Resources.

The plague of the elderly—dehydration
I have a friend whose mother, when in her seventies, was progressively declining in health. Her symptoms were so numerous that it is not worth taking up the page writing about them. She eventually fell down and was taken to the hospital. They ran nearly every test known to man on her. They gave her an MRI, kept her in the hospital for a few weeks, and found nothing. The most obvious thing was ignored.[400] She was eventually advised that she had been dehydrated.

It is no mystery that she was dehydrated. That is a *very common* problem among the elderly. Elderly people don't like to drink water because it is difficult for them to get up to go to the bathroom, or they don't have the bladder control they once had, and that's not pleasant either. So they don't drink water, and after a time their organs dry up, and they have a serious problem.

Dry eyes
Someone we know recently told me that she had been on different medications for years for dry eyes. She told me, "Eventually, I found out that when I drank enough water, the dry eyes disappeared."

By the way, she works for the government and has "good insurance," so all the medications and doctor visits were paid for without any co-pay. Another obvious case of "health care" that is in fact contrary to healthfulness.

The importance of water quality
Enough good cannot be said about unpoisoned water that is rich in healthful minerals. Distilled water or water deficient in minerals

will pull minerals from the body, which can eventually cause health problems.

Some municipal water supplies are much healthier than others. Chlorinated or fluoride treated waters can have a poisoning effect. Even bathing in highly chlorinated water is unhealthful.

Shortly after we installed a whole-house, carbon filter water system, our son stayed overnight for a couple of days. He was astonished by how much better he felt after he took a shower. At home, after he took a shower, he always felt drained. He now purchases those filtering devices you put on the showerhead. They have to be replaced every three or four months to be effective, but he swears by them.

Another chlorine story:
When I was growing up, I could not learn to swim. When I got in a pool, I was always short of breath and simply could not get enough air to perform normal swimming strokes. Also, in the summertime, I would often be short of breath and was unable to get a full breath of air. I thought it was the smog—which almost certainly played a part. It was not until much later, when we moved to an area where we had to buy bottled water, that my shortness of breath in the summers went away. Sometimes now, when I have to drink chlorinated water, I feel the same shortness of breath and tightness in the chest. Like many other people now, I try to always have bottled water with me.

E. *Home Remedies*

"Keep it simple."

Athlete's foot
This is what I have done: Apple cider vinegar applied topically gives immediate relief. I use a raw, unpasteurized product, which is more effective. When I had a bad case, I soaked my feet in a diluted solution.

Now, how I prevent it:

This is a fungal condition that can be very persistent, so think systematically. Fungi and yeasts love sugar. They hate garlic. They love damp and hot; they hate dry and cool. They love stale air; they hate fresh air. They thrive on unhealthy organisms; they don't have much of a chance on healthy ones. Like all fungi, this one lies dormant and waits for an opportunity to proliferate. So the key is to not give it an opportunity if you can help it.

Hot moisture is the enemy, so I put cornstarch in my shoes to absorb the moisture and take my shoes off at home.[401] Our feet were not designed to be in an enclosed environment surrounded by synthetic materials that cause sweat.[402]

This is the same condition as "jock itch," and an infection in one area can easily spread to the other. Dilute the vinegar if applied to the groin. (!) I wash socks and underwear in vinegar to kill the fungus if I have a persistent case. White vinegar is fine for laundry, not for food.

Concerning the over-the-counter preparations of Desenex, Tinactin and Micatin: These have different active ingredients, one of which may work for you (according to your body chemistry), while the others may not. In past decades, I used Desenex in the summertime and Bacitracin if it got out of control. These are "band-aid" fixes and do not address the root problem.

Note: A fungal infection can become systemic if allowed to persist.

Backache
We have found nothing nearly as effective as going for a long walk. (Walk upright with good posture and let the arms swing naturally.) Sitting for long periods of time is not only bad for the back, it is also bad for the gut. When desk-bound, I get up to walk around as often as I can. This practice helps a great deal.

Bronchitis
Some folks we know steam it out. They tell me a towel over the head with hot water running in the sink works well.

Burns (minor, skin not broken)
What we do is **immediately** run cold water on the burn for at least several minutes. (We don't use ice—it will stick!) After that, we pour on, or soak in, apple cider vinegar, and repeat if necessary. We have had astounding results with this method of treatment.

Coughs
I used to use lemon and honey in a hot herbal tea. The combination is very effective. Alfalfa tea is great if you need to go to sleep. It is very calming, so it is not a good idea in the middle of the day. After developing a glucose problem, the honey caused me problems, so I switched to a saltwater gargle, which is not as effective but does help.

Constipation
See Water Remedies, Vitamin and Mineral Remedies.

Depressed? Angry, on edge?
You may want to go for a run. Otherwise, it's enema time.

Eczema
Diet and skin contact are the most common causes. If skin contact, we will probably know what it was that caused the outbreak. The outbreak should be taken seriously, as we will likely react with less exposure in the future. The offender could be your laundry soap or other chemicals or, sorry, your dog or cat.

If food is the cause, find the offending food or foods (they will be different with different people) and eliminate them. This is trial and error. Listening to your intuition will cut down the error factor greatly. If you *truly* don't have a clue and you have already eliminated heavily processed foods, try eliminating wheat, dairy, eggs, and tomatoes.

Infection
Apple cider vinegar. We use raw, unpasteurized, if we can get it. I have used a teaspoon in a glass of water three times a day and found it helpful. Later, after developing blood sugar problems, I switched to vitamin C, which may be even more effective. See the next section, Vitamin and Mineral Remedies.

Jock itch
See athlete's foot.

Leg (calf) cramps, when lying in bed
With legs straight, point your toes up to your head, heels down, away from you. If you do the opposite it will make the cramp worse. It took us a while to figure this one out, but for us it works every time. The condition may be caused by a lack of minerals. You may want to take a multimineral.

Muscle aches and pains
Apple cider vinegar and a little red pepper applied topically worked wonders for Deborah.

Prostate (enlarged)
Pumpkin seed kernels (raw, not salted). I eat these as a preventative measure. They are also a good source of protein.

Rashes, hives
Apple cider vinegar bath. This is what Deborah has done when having an allergic reaction. They were very effective.

Sinus infections
Deborah uses a neti pot with plain water and swears by it. It is very important to have good, clean water and a clean pot. Deborah pours boiling water in and over the pot, then adds the water she is going to use.

Sore throat
Salt water gargle. Before we switched to a healthier lifestyle, I used to use commercial products. After using salt water, I don't believe any product can beat its effectiveness. Spit the stuff out and rinse the mouth, don't swallow all that salt!

Sunburn
For us, nothing works like aloe vera gel. And no commercial product is as effective as getting it straight from the plant itself. We get it on as quickly as we can and apply it frequently. We have had phenomenal success with this treatment.

Toxicity, general
See Chapter 8.

Toxic liver
Radishes open the bile ducts. This was effective for Deborah, but not nearly as effective as the Liver Chi tea. See Herbal Remedies.

F. *Vitamin and Mineral Remedies*
Of course, it is best to get our vitamins from eating healthy. But sorry to say, that alone is not adequate for many of us. The reasons are covered in Chapters 17-19. (By the way, I don't think you can supplement your way out of a bad diet or lack of exercise.)

Before I give specific examples of how vitamins supplements have been helpful for us, I should tell you what depletes our vitamins; that is, what steals our body's reserves.

The worst vitamin depleter of all
Sugar

The second worst
White flour

Another depleter
Many medications [403]

Another common depleter
Chlorine in the water. Of course, we understand the necessity of a safe water supply, but we shouldn't be drinking chlorinated water unless we have to. Even bathing in the stuff can deplete us. (See Water Treatments earlier in this chapter.)

Another depleter
For some people, mineral oil is a vitamin depleter, specifically of the oil or fat-soluble vitamins, which are A, D, E and K. (The others are water-soluble.) For this reason, we don't use products with mineral oil in them. Deborah makes her own products with a beeswax and olive oil base, or we purchase similar products from a good health food store. We avoid pharmacy store products. In our opinion, pharmacies are fully given over to the chemical approach, so even when they "come around" and add non-mineral oil

products, we will not buy them. Look at the ingredients and you will see why.

Vitamin and Mineral Remedies for Various Conditions:

Bipolar: See Chapter 3.

Constipation or insufficient bowel discharge, chronic

If water intake is adequate, as per the previous section titled Water Treatments, the condition is almost certainly diet related. If we eat heavily processed foods, we probably cannot eliminate adequately. If our foods do not contain enough **fiber, oils and moisture**, slow transit of waste, or constipation, or both will result. "**Constipated**" **means having less than one thorough evacuation a day. The transit time of waste through the bowel is crucial. The longer the waste stays in, the more we are poisoned by it.** If we can move the bowel fully every 12 hours or so, we can be kept from a lot of toxicity and consequently a lot of ill health.

In cases where constipation cannot be corrected by proper water intake and proper diet *as per Chapter 21*, it may be good to try magnesium and/or vitamin C. I have taken both because the magnesium buffers the acid in the vitamin C. I emptied a capsule of each in a glass of water once or twice a day. Magnesium by itself takes 12-18 hours to work. Vitamin C works in half the time. I do not think it is wise to stay on magnesium for too long because there is a calcium/magnesium balance that must be maintained.

Diabetes

See the discussion of diabetes medications and vitamin B-12 in the Prescription Drugs section earlier in this chapter.

Foggy Head? Don't feel right?

Probably a toxic condition. Vitamin C in a glass of water will often help within 45 minutes. I have used bentonite clay (with plenty of water) and achieved similar results. I repeat if necessary. If that does not do it, it's enema time.

Infection and the vitamin C miracle

We have found taking extra vitamin C (sometimes with echinacea) to be effective to combat just about any infection. We attack with doses of 1,000 to 2,000 mg of C about 4-5 times a day, and continue at least one day after we think we are clear. We buffer the C with magnesium (or it will burn like the dickens on the way out.) We also stop taking the C in the early afternoon so it does not keep us up at night. Loose stool is a common result of taking so much vitamin C, but it will almost always clear the infection, and usually within a day or two. We have been doing this for more than three decades now, and I don't think we have ever had a case where it did not work. This is what we do; what you do is your responsibility.

Memory fading?
My mother-in-law was becoming very forgetful. My wife told her, "Mom, here's some vitamin B-12, you need to take it." A couple of months later she was worse. "Mom, are you taking your B-12?" "No, Dr. _____ said I didn't need it." "Mom, take the B-12 or I'm not going to call you." Mom called back a week later and my wife could tell from talking to her that she was taking the B-12. She was coherent and the conversation was normal. "Are you taking your B-12?" "Oh, yes! I'm doing much better!"

And she was fine for about a year. Then the same thing happened— she couldn't remember anything. "Mom, are you taking your B-12?" "Oh no, I went to Dr. _____ and she told me I really didn't need it, so I stopped." "Mom, take it or I'm not going to call you." She did, and she was fine again.

By the way, Dr. _____ had her on eight prescription medications.[404]

See the discussion of Alzheimer's in Dietary Treatments.

Shingles
Shingles are caused by stress, so the best treatment is to back way off of whatever brought the condition on and rest as much as possible. The body needs to be allowed to heal itself. The consequences of not doing so can be serious. This is no condition to mess around with.

Shingles can come on with a fury, or the case can be mild. They can strike anywhere. Deborah had it on her face at the jaw (her weakest place after the dental work). Due to the closeness to the eye, and the fact that blindness could result if it spread, she took an antiviral medication. We are not purists who say there is never a time to use medications. Deborah also took drip infusions of vitamins B and C in addition to what she took orally. Further, she had two or three acupuncture treatments. Some would argue that some of these treatments could cancel the effectiveness of others. I don't know. Her physician was okay with the treatment combination. Deborah cleared up relatively quickly but has not regained all her strength.

Smell, lost sense of
Most likely a zinc deficiency. We have observed this at least a few times in different people. Warning: Too much zinc can cause nausea and vomiting.

Urination, painful
This can be a serious condition but usually is not. You will have to decide if it is or if it is not. Infections at the end of the urinary tract are common enough for women, and men can get them too. The cause is frequently the spread of bacteria from the anus to the end of the urinary canal. The usual symptom is a burning, cutting pain that varies in intensity. We have found that by far the biggest need is to flush out the infection with water. In other words, drink a lot of water. This may be uncomfortable, but that is how we have solved the problem. We have also found taking extra vitamin C to be effective. See Infections earlier in this section.

Others we know use apple cider vinegar—a teaspoon in a glass of water three times a day.

We get on any infection early, and it will usually go away in a couple of days.

What you decide to do for your case is entirely your responsibility. I am just telling you what we have done. Read the warning right after the preface. And thank you again for understanding why I have to repeat this statement.

Warts
Vitamin E attacks the virus that causes warts. We poke a gel capsule and squeeze out the oil onto the wart, then keep the wart moist with oil and use a Band-Aid if necessary to keep from wiping it off. We refresh the oil daily and keep it up for 3-4 days. In about two weeks the wart will fall off. If this does not work, we extend

the treatment longer. As I recall, this has worked every time for our family and for others we know. Typical burning off of warts with liquid nitrogen may or may not keep them from coming back.

A vitamin medicine

When our kids were small, Camy, our duck, became very ill. One of the children found him one day lying down on his side all twisted up with this head under his body. He was panting hard, had a high fever, and was all but dead. On a hunch, Deborah fixed up what she calls her "power pack, illness fighting recipe." It is a vitamin/medicine brew of vitamin B complex, vitamins C and E, cod liver oil, and desiccated liver in a base of yogurt. She thinned it with water, held the duck's bill up, poured it in, and rubbed his throat to get it down. She may have repeated it, I don't remember, but within hours Camy was up and about. He recovered to a very healthy state, lived many more years, and sired healthy ducklings, although after this bout he was slightly lame in one leg.

A mineral supplement case that went wrong

When our son was a baby, he had trouble sleeping. My wife read in an old Adelle Davis book that potassium would be helpful. She gave it to him. Then he was sleeping all the time. She took him to the doctor and they almost called the authorities.

The point in telling this story is fourfold:
1. We make mistakes.

2. A little knowledge can be dangerous. This was early on our path to a natural way of living, and it was a big lesson. We have since learned to consult more than one resource. We have also learned not to apply the common thinking with supplements—that you can just take something and then you will be all better. That may be the way we grew up to think, but it is contrary to all the principles of a healthy way of life.

3. Vitamins and minerals always have to be in balance. The potassium/sodium balance is crucial. So is the magnesium/calcium balance. The B vitamins also need to be in balance, which is why they are commonly sold as a complex. If we take one of the B vitamins without considering the others, that probably is not wise.

4. Adelle Davis took her comments on potassium out of the next edition of her book. Just like the medical mainstream people make mistakes, so do the alternative folks. We all do.

G. *Herbal Treatments and Remedies*

Adrenal problems

Adrenal problems have become *very* common. They go hand in hand with blood sugar problems, and both can become serious if not addressed properly. The conditions are hormonal, and one hormone affects another.

I have known several people who could not control their emotions. At times they seemed to get excited for no reason. Some of them ran out of energy at seemingly odd times and withdrew from social contact. Some of these people probably knew they had a physiological problem; others probably didn't have a clue. These symptoms are indicative of an adrenal problem.[405]

Adrenal problems are a huge subject, and in this book I deal with them in detail in Chapter 4 from a blood sugar and dietary standpoint. If that is not the source of the problem, it is so closely related that to take care of the one is for the most part going to take care of the other.

Besides taking care of the diet, there are also many herbal combinations that people take for adrenal support, some of which also contain a bovine adrenal glandular. I tried two or three preparations and did not find them helpful. All produced a worse adrenal reaction. Many of the herbs in the herbal preparations will affect the blood sugar. It is wise to be very careful using ginseng or licorice root, for example. These herbs, as well as many others, can cause a large release of insulin, which may in turn dump the blood sugar. If you have, or suspect, a blood sugar problem and you try any of these, you may want to cut the dosage way down to begin with. The last thing you want to do is get on the blood sugar roller coaster. If you can get an adrenal glandular by itself, without the herbs, you may want to try that; but again, the recommended dosage may be considerably too high for many people.

It is wise to take any adrenal problem seriously. We may not be able to undo the damage that has already been done, but we may be able to prevent further damage.

With adrenal problems, equally important as proper diet is to not allow yourself to get too excited. Leave a reserve. You may need it.

Arthritis

Deborah suffered from arthritis. For more than three decades now, she has been using **burdock root** and has been having no problems whatsoever. When she was in crisis with the problem, decades ago, she took 3-4 capsules a day.[406] She now only takes one capsule a day, and it keeps the problem under control.[407] Burdock is an excellent blood purifier, and that is what is needed to get toxins out of the joints.[408] Again I am a reporter, nothing more. I am not prescribing anything.

[Interesting note: While I was working on this chapter early one morning, Deborah woke up and came out to the kitchen. We said "good morning" to each other, and she mentioned that she had missed her burdock yesterday and that her joints were really telling her about it.]

Arthritis, 2

I put this story here because it fits well, even if it is not about an herbal remedy.

I once walked into a seminar class early and took a seat up front. The speaker was there, and I noticed that he had a copper bracelet on. Since he was relaxed and was just waiting for the time to begin, I asked him if he wore the bracelet for arthritis and if so, if it was effective. He said, "Yes, I was suffering from arthritis for some time, but I started wearing this two years ago and haven't had a problem since." He paused for a few seconds, then he added with a shrug, "But then, I'm a sucker for infomercials."

He had a technical presentation to deliver and others had come into the room by that time, so I suppose he had to cover his lack of "scientific" prowess. Anyway, I thought he gave a great answer!

Arthritis, 3

If you have a problem with arthritis, you just may want to check out what *Our Daily Meds* says about arthritis medications and the dangers of using them. (See Resources.)

Blood sugar getting a little too high? You may want to use a *little* **cinnamon**. Be careful! Using too much can cause your blood sugar to drop too low. If you have low blood sugar tendencies, it might be best not to use cinnamon at all. It is probably best not to start using cinnamon if you are already on diabetes medications unless you let your physician know about it. Cinnamon can throw the meds off, and the meds may need to be adjusted accordingly.

Colic

Our son had a bad case of colic after he was born. A mild chamomile and peppermint tea worked wonders.

Garlic

Who can say enough good about garlic? Garlic is good for *almost* anything. I mention it here because it is a good example to make a point: There are always potential downsides to any food or medicinal herb, so we need to have alternatives. Although garlic is excellent for a healthy gut and health in general, it also gives some people debilitating hot flashes, and because it is a stimulant, it keeps others awake at night.

Immune system boost

Echinacea. The *root* is for occasional use only. Some herbal books warn against using it on an ongoing basis.

Liver problems

Deborah used Liver Chi extract, and it helped greatly to get her liver enzymes back to healthy levels. It is a combination of three herbs: Schisandra chinensis, Bupleurum chinense, and Smixax glabra. Chi's Enterprise, Inc., Anaheim, CA 92807

Sleep

Having trouble going to sleep? First see Dietary Treatments and Remedies earlier in this chapter. If what is mentioned there does not work adequately, you may want to try some alfalfa tea. As a hot tea, alfalfa is very calming. It is not calming if the tea is not hot or if the alfalfa is taken in other forms. If I have had too much excitement during the day and I need a super knockout, I take alfalfa and/or chamomile teas.

[See Herbs in Chapters 8 and 20 for herbal principles.]

H. *Work*

This book is about taking a holistic[409] approach to health. Therefore it is needful to state clearly and emphatically that our work and our relationship with our work plays a very large part in our overall well-being. There is tremendous value in doing productive work and in taking responsibility for that work. From this we obtain a sense of usefulness, and from that we get a sense of well-being. Productive work gets the right juices flowing in us. This may be impossible to quantify, but it would be difficult to overstate its value.

Productive work is one thing. Having a job is another. Henry Ford was once asked, "How many people do you have working for you?" He answered, "About half of them." Having spent a good part of my life hiring people, I know exactly what he meant.

It does not matter if we are prune pickers or accountants, engineers or doctors, school teachers or school janitors—two people can be performing identical tasks, yet one can be working, the other just doing a job. The one is likely to have a healthy mind, the other cannot.

Whatever we do—take care of children, sell apples, or run a large corporation—it is good to do it with our strength. A healthy mind is necessary for a healthy body, and work has a lot to do with that.

I wrote a book on the value of work, and I'll put a plug in for it here. As a teenager, I worked on a farm. The experience was so positive and so educational I thought there was a worthy book that could be written about that time. Four decades later, I finally got around to it. The book title is *The Last of the Prune Pickers: A Pre-Silicon Valley Story*. It is a fascinating local history and a good farm story, and I receive many letters from readers who greatly appreciate the book. I think you will enjoy it. (See the back of this book for a preview.)

I. *Surgeries*

A dear old lady we know had surgery on her rectum to remove some hemorrhoids. She has had limited control ever since. Was there another way of treating her condition? Probably. But you may not hear it if you are talking to a surgeon.

One of our neighbors was not feeling well. He didn't think anything of it, but over the course of about a day and a half he became very ill. Eventually his wife said, "We're going to the hospital!" He had a ruptured appendix, and if you know anything about that condition, you know it was a good thing that they acted on it soon enough.

Another neighbor of ours has had 27 surgeries—at least that was the count the last time I talked to him. He had others scheduled; mostly joints. He thinks his doctors are doing a good job of taking care of him. I don't. From what he tells me, I don't think his doctors have the concept of finding the *cause* of the problem. My neighbor surely doesn't. When I have mentioned this to him, his comments were, "Oh, my doctors know how to take care of that."

His insurance covers everything, he gets paid whether he works or not, and he's willing to submit, so perhaps the judgment is skewed. The man is about fifty years old.

Actually, joint problems are very often caused by a buildup of toxins in the joint. That is pretty simple stuff from the standpoint of diet and detoxification as described in this book, but the odds of your medical doctor telling you that are probably nil.

Diet and detoxification may be worth an honest try. But how do you say that to someone who is so confident in his "health care"?

We know a young woman who had surgery on her two large toes. She was told that her condition was the same as what the basketball player Shaquille O'Neal had, and surgery was necessary for the same reason—worn out joints and bone spurs. She now thinks that the surgeries were a mistake and that she should not have gone for such a radical approach. But she was lured by the fact that they were paid for by insurance, and she was going to lose her coverage, so she went ahead with the surgeries.

I tell this story because I want to state emphatically that I think **having "good insurance" is the worst of all reasons to have a surgery.** She may never know for certain if her surgery was the best course of action to take, but she can't run anymore, and that is tough for someone who was an athlete.

Cataract surgery cases

One of my wife's colleagues had cataract surgery on both of his eyes. Both surgeries were "successful," but three months later both retinas became detached. He was without sight for about eight months, then had additional treatment, and it took about a year after that for him to regain his sight.

Another friend had cataract surgery. Her eyes were really okay, but she was told that there were cataracts and that eventually she would probably need to have surgery. For a year after the procedure she really struggled!

In stating these last two cases, I should also state that I know of some successful cataract surgeries. My point is twofold:
1. Cataract surgery, though much better than it was thirty or forty years ago, isn't always successful.
2. The least reliable person to tell you about the success rate of any surgery is the person who performs it. The second least reliable source may be the medical industry stats, unless you read the fine print. (See chapter 15.)

The bottom line is worth repeating. It is this:
Medical doctors know to medicate; surgeons know to cut.
If you want to do those things, go to those professionals.
If you don't want to do those things, go to someone else!

J. *Hospitalization*
I am thankful for hospitals when we need them, but...

Discomfort in the chest, 2 cases
"Get to the ER, I don't even want to talk to you about it," my doctor told me after I told him I had been having some slight pains in my chest from time to time.

I hadn't been feeling well for a while, so I asked my wife to drive me over to the ER. When we arrived, everybody in the place rushed over to me. I was a celebrity—everyone wanted to see me! I told them, "I don't think this is my heart, but I need to know what it is." They acted as if they didn't hear me. I got a little miffed and said sternly: "You can do this if you promise that you will tell me what you think this is when you're done." They ignored me. Who was I to ask them anything! Besides, they were too busy hooking me up to every machine they had. "You'll have to stay overnight for observation and have a stress test in the morning!"

I reluctantly agreed.

The next day and seven thousand dollars later, I was told that my heart was just fine and was shown the door. I was no longer a celebrity and couldn't get anyone to talk to me.

I'm glad I didn't have "good insurance." Maybe I would have gotten a "free" bypass if I did.

That was about eleven years ago, but a friend of mine recently had the same experience. Apparently, if you go to an ER and say that you have any pain in the chest, that is the protocol. From what we could tell, they were interested in two things: making money and covering their backsides. In our experiences, we were a commodity and were treated with the same regard as your car would be when you take it to the muffler shop.[410]

By the way, the hospitals that my friend and I went to both send out very nice, glossy brochures on a regular basis that show pictures of the happy people they are taking such good care of. They even have testimonials in those brochures. Why we got thrown out on our ears, I don't know. Maybe we were anomalies. But I doubt it.

[My mistake, as I understand it now, is that I did not differentiate between "pain" and "discomfort" as those terms are used in the medical profession. I have since been told that if it feels like an elephant has stepped on your chest, that is pain. If it's less than that, it's discomfort. Maybe your doctor can be more helpful in explaining the difference to you. Just ask him or her when you are not experiencing the problem, then maybe he or she will be a little more helpful than my doctor was.]

Staph infections

I think just about everyone knows at least one person who has picked up a staph infection in a hospital. Staph infections are very common and can be deadly. We know of two younger people—one in his thirties, the other in his fifties—who died of staph infections picked up in hospitals. Though downplayed in the industry, this has reached pandemic proportions. **Hospitals are not healthy places!**

One last hospitalization story

I recently went to visit a workmate who was in the hospital. As he ate his chocolate cake that came with his dinner, he told me that he was getting insulin in the IV he was hooked up to. "I didn't know you were diabetic." "I'm not, they give it to everyone." [411]

Oh.

Resources, listed in the order of the chapter contents

Back to Eden, by Jethro Kloss, 1939
Common sense was good in 1939. It is equally good today. Kloss had plenty of it. I put this resource first because it belongs first.

Reflexology Chart:
Pacific Institute of Reflexology, chart by Christopher Shirley

Prescription Drugs; Dangers of Medications:
Our Daily Meds, by Melody Petersen, 2008
A well-researched and documented book with many details and examples. In my opinion, a "must read."

Thyroid:
Hypothyroidism: The Unsuspected Illness, by Broda O. Barnes, MD, 1976

I'm sure there are newer books (which may or may not be better), but this one helped Deborah understand the condition.

Dietary Treatments, Water Treatments:
Tissue Cleansing Through Bowel Management, by Bernard Jensen, DC, PhD, 1981
In my opinion a "must read."

Detoxification Products:
V.E. Irons, www.veirons.com, PO Box 34710, N. Kansas City, MO 64116
Irons has excellent supplement products to help with a fast or detoxification cleanse.

Home Remedies:
Kitchen Medicine, by Ben Charles Harris, 1968. May be out of print. Get it used at abe.com.

Herbals:
The Way of Herbs, Michael Tierra, 1998
The best herbal we know of. But if considering a treatment, always check it with at least one other source. No one herbal is complete.

Herbally Yours, by Penny C. Royal, 1993
Another good herbal.

Herbal formula for liver support and detoxification:
"Liver Chi," Chi's Enterprise, Inc., Anaheim, CA 92807

Vitamins and Minerals Info.:
Prescription for Nutritional Healing, by Phyllis A. Balch and James F. Balch, MD, 4th edition, 2000. An excellent encyclopedia-like reference volume that is very strong on the subject of dietary supplements.

Vitamins for Bipolar condition:
True Hope www.truehope.com There are many other sources now; this is what our friend uses.

Chapter 23
It's Not Starbucks' Fault

The line extends down the street a good ways as it does here every morning just inside "The Beltway" that surrounds our nation's capital. Half-awake, bleary-eyed, professional-looking men and women—mostly younger—wait their turn. All heads are down, and no one is talking. These people are NOT happy. They need their morning stimulant, and they know it. The scene is repeated in hundreds of places all over the country every morning. Business is good.

After they have partaken, these people are no more alert at work than those who refrain from the habit, but for them to function at all they need what they need. It is not the fault of the businesses that provide these highly addictive substances; the coffee dens merely provide the stimulants of choice for many people.

The exponentially stronger caffeine doses of today were unthought-of just a generation ago. And the demand is for even stronger doses yet. Some of the people in the early morning power-caffeine line will have a "sports drink" (those marketing boys are slick, aren't they?) in the afternoon to help them get through the work day. Just as computer memory chips have become increasingly more powerful, so have the doses of caffeine and sugar.

A hundred and twenty years ago, the scene was similar, as it was common for people to say, "Let's go have a dope together," and head down to the soda fountain for a Coke. They knew what they were doing, and so do the people in the coffeehouse line.

But it's all good for business—look at the size of Coca-a-Cola and Starbucks today. They are world movers and shakers.

The diabetes epidemic came out of the refined sugar generation. What will come out of the mega-caffeine generation? We may not know yet, but it will be good for the economy. The diabetes industry is now $116 billion annually in the US. And that's not counting all the bypass surgeries—80% of which are performed on diabetics.[412] What diseases and other problems can we produce from high doses of caffeine?

As with the mega-dose caffeine items, there is only one reason that the majority of the grocery store shelves are full of products that should not be fed to a dog—people buy the stuff. It is not the grocers' responsibility to provide healthy food. They only stock what we demand that they stock. It is our responsibility to find good food and buy it, or grow it ourselves.

I'll tell you a story to underscore my point. When our town was young, thirty-five years ago, there was a small, local produce store that stocked the finest produce available. Their produce was fresh, they had a good variety, and word got around. As the town grew, that produce market grew exponentially, as everybody raved about all the wonderful fresh fruits and vegetables they carried. The grocery stores in town, which up until that time treated their produce departments as if they were unimportant, were really hurt, because people would not buy their produce anymore. They had been selling horrible quality produce, and now everybody knew it because they had something to compare it to. Hordes of us quit going to the regular grocery stores except for things that we could not get elsewhere. The grocers got the point. Without exception, all three grocery stores in town made a complete turnaround, and they also began stocking high quality produce.[413]

I think most of us know someone who broke all the rules of good health, and yet seemed to get away with it and lived a long and active life. I'll tell you what that is like with another story.

When I was in the service, I was in a unit of 60 men. One time, we were sent on a training mission to play war games in the desert near Las Vegas. After four days of eating dust and being awakened every night by simulated mortar attacks, our training was over and we were allowed to go into town if we wanted to. As I recall, the base even supplied a couple of buses for transport. Most of the men were very excited about going into Las Vegas and gambling, and the stories of how smart they were and how they were going to win big buzzed around like flies on the back porch. About 56 of the 60 men went into town that night, and all but one came back broke and very unhappy. They were not pleasant to be with for the duration of our assignment.

These men thought they were smarter than the people who built those expensive casinos. They weren't. And they paid the price for their arrogance. Likewise, if we really think we can beat the odds by living in an unhealthy manner, we (thankfully) are at liberty to do so. But should those who are responsible pay for those who are not?

We live in a culture that is ruining the health of its citizens faster than we can invent expensive ways to "care" for them. There is only one way out of the mess we are in, and that is the way of taking individual responsibility.

Many of us act as if we do not know about food ingredients and about taking care of ourselves and yet expect drugs and medical procedures to bail us out for the mistreatment of our bodies. But suppose we had to pay the bill ourselves.[414] If we had to pay for our foolishness, that would knock out a lot of nonsense—wouldn't it?

We got into the current "health care" mess by being lured away from taking care of ourselves. Is there any way out of it but to go back and do so?

Of course, we can spend our time blaming others for our ills. Avoiding responsibility and blaming others goes hand in hand, and it seems we easily fall into that frame of mind.

And some of us even end up blaming God.

Chapter 24
Why Did God Do This to Me?

This is a common question when it comes to human suffering, and it is fitting to address it here in this book, both from the standpoint of Deborah's experience and also in a broader sense.

Early on, at the time of her collapse, Deborah had this question. As one who had put her trust in Christ, she knew that God loved her and that He causes all things to work together for good for those who love Him. This was the promise made to her, and she was confident that the One who promised was able to perform. Her quest, then, became one of finding out, as she said, "What do I need to learn from this?"

One thing became evident to her early on: That is, she needed self-control when it came to eating. The limitations of health provided a means for her to become more disciplined, and it has carried over to nearly every aspect of her living.

Through the decades there have been times of sadness and longing to be well. I'll have her tell you about that:

"Yes, there have been those times, but I have had too much experience of God leading me to think that He will not continue to do so. I also know that the Lord is the Great Physician, so it is unreasonable for me to think that He will not help me through the rest of my life. The times of sorrow become prayerful."

What Deborah has learned, and I have too, is a practical, daily dependence upon our Maker and Savior. That dependence is in fact the larger issue.

In God's wisdom, we were born into this world as gods to ourselves. This is not to our benefit. Our great-grandparents were deceived into thinking it was, and they unwittingly passed this trait on to us. The story is recorded in the third and fourth chapters of the Bible. The effect of that turning away from God is perhaps the greater part of human history. It seems it is so easy for us to keep the Almighty right where we want Him—either pushed aside as much as possible, or relegated to the status of being our servant.

And then we are displeased with Him when He does not perform according to our view of things. We are so good at making gods according to our liking, in other words, at worshiping ourselves!

But God's wisdom is infinitely great, and beginning at the end of the third chapter of Genesis, God began to bring good news to us that there is indeed a way out of this condition of error and of being restored to the One who made us in His own image and for His own purpose. Nowhere is that good news more clearly stated than in the fifty-third chapter of Isaiah, where Isaiah says this of the Christ:

"Who has believed our report?
And to whom has the arm (strength) of the Lord been revealed?
For He (Christ) shall grow up before Him (God) as a tender plant,
And as a root out of dry ground.
He has no form or comeliness;
And when we see Him,
There is no beauty that we should desire Him.

He is despised and rejected by men,
A Man of sorrows and acquainted with grief,
And we hid, as it were, our faces from Him.
He was despised, and we did not esteem Him.
Surely He has borne our griefs
And carried our sorrows;
Yet we esteemed Him stricken,
Smitten by God, and afflicted.

But He was wounded for our transgressions,
He was bruised for our iniquities;
The chastisement for our peace was upon Him,
And by His stripes (whip marks) we are healed.
All we like sheep have gone astray;
We have turned, every one, to his own way;
And the Lord has laid on Him the iniquity of us all.

He was oppressed and He was afflicted,
Yet He opened not His mouth.
He was led as a lamb to the slaughter,
And as a sheep before its shearers is silent,
So He opened not His mouth.

He was taken from prison and from judgment,
And who will declare His generation?
For He was cut off from the land of the living;
For the transgression of My people He was stricken.
And they made His grave with the wicked—
But with the rich at His death,
Because He had done no violence
Nor was any deceit in His mouth.

Yet it pleased the Lord to bruise Him;
He has put Him to grief.
When You (God) make His (Christ's) soul an offering for sin,
He shall see His seed (offspring), He shall prolong His days,
And the pleasure of the Lord will prosper in His hand.

He shall see the labor of His soul and be satisfied.
By His knowledge My righteous Servant shall justify many,
For He shall bear their iniquities.
Therefore I will divide Him a portion with the great,
And He shall divide the spoil with the Strong,
Because He poured out His soul unto death,
And He was numbered with the transgressors,
And He bore the sin of many,
And made intercession for the transgressors."

This is what Jesus, the Christ, did for us, and it is—or more precisely, *He is*—the inheritance of all who put their trust in Him.

For thousands of years before His coming, the prophets spoke of Him; and His story is clearly recorded in the books called The Gospels at the beginning of the New Testament in the Bible.

When taken with prayer and with a true heart, there is no medicine as powerful as the Bible. There is a wonderful, living person behind the words of that Book, and if we will but take Him at His word, we will find that He is faithful. He heals the inward parts, and He, Himself, is the answer to *all* of our questions and problems.

Epilogue

Although Deborah is pleased that I took the time to write this book, it was difficult for her to relive some of the things she has suffered so that her story could be accurately presented. If those sufferings were limited to the physical ones, that would have been a heavy enough load to bear, but they were not. The added burden of dealing with a system of "health care" that proved to be contrary to health was almost unbearable at times. The fact is, Deborah was often the only sane person in the equation. It is a lonely place to be. And that was especially the case in earlier days before many of the illnesses described in this book became more known. Forty years ago, hypoglycemia, sensitivities to electromagnetic fields, severe food and chemical allergies, and many other conditions of ill health mentioned in this book—and all of which Deborah suffered from—were almost unheard of. Today, many of these ailments are much more common.

We found out about Deborah's mercury poisoning in the spring of 2006. At the end of that year, I told Deborah that I thought it would be good to share what we had discovered in our annual letter that we send to friends and family at Christmas time.

She was very hesitant at first, as talking about health—especially her own health—is one of her least favorite subjects. That is more than understandable. But I told her, "Deb, there are plenty of people out there who are suffering from this, and they don't have a clue as to what the problem is."

She knew it was the right thing to do and consented.

We sent out about fifty letters, and within a short time, we received two phone calls. One was from a friend of a friend to whom we had sent the letter. She was suffering greatly from mercury poisoning. The other call was from someone who had a relative who had a mercury problem. That was the beginning. More calls and more questions followed—and not just about mercury poisoning. People with different health problems simply did not know what to do, and their doctors were of little or no help.

We were accustomed to calls and inquiries about health matters, as mentioned earlier in the book, but a new wave hit, and we were not prepared for it.

As I said in the preface, quick answers to health problems are rarely good ones, and eventually it became obvious to me that I should write down what we have learned. There are simply too many people who could receive help from reading about our experience, and to ignore them would not be right.

Mercury toxicity is at the center of this book, and there is the need not only to sound out a warning about it, but also to provide a *practical* understanding of the subject matter. However—and this is a huge "however"—metals toxicity, and any other health condition for that matter, should not be looked at as something separate from the way we take care of ourselves. I hope I have made that clear in this book.

Our hearts ache to see so many people who simply do not know how much damage they are doing to themselves by going against the principles of healthy living.

So, now you have this book in your hands. Sharing our story is meant to encourage and empower the reader, and I hope it has been a help, and will continue to be a help to you and to others you know.

Concerning Deborah's current health status:
It would be nice to say that Deborah is now eating any food she wants, is always robust, and is a perfect picture of health, but that is not the case. I know health books are supposed to resolve everything and have a completely happy-ever-after ending, so I am sorry to disappoint anyone who expected that.

As I said at the end of Chapter 13, Deborah is in the repair and maintenance phase of a lengthy healing process. The residual effects of long-term mercury poisoning, as with many serious conditions, requires the repair of damaged tissues and the resetting of the body's autoimmune system response, and that could take several years. Further, it is likely that some damage from the mercury poisoning will not be repairable.

After we went through the process of getting the mercury out of Deborah's body and she had pretty well recovered, Deborah contracted shingles. Twice. Shingles are brought on by stress and an impaired immune system. The first episode was when her mother became very ill. The second, which was much milder, was when her mother passed away. The shingles episodes were severe setbacks for Deborah's health, and her stamina has not been the same since. So, she is not a perfect lab rat from which we can draw flawless "scientific" conclusions regarding her mercury detoxification. But then, life itself does not take place in a lab and does not allow us to derive more than a general understanding of many health matters.

Deborah can eat about fifteen foods now—mostly vegetables in addition to chicken, sunflower seeds, and pumpkin seeds. She was up to about twenty-five foods shortly after chelation began, but after a while she began re-reacting to several of them. As is common in detoxification (see Chapter 8), when a toxic burden is removed from the body, the body often rejoices in such a way that one can think all is well. As time goes on, however, it becomes apparent that there is another layer of healing that needs to take place.

Deborah enjoyed eating cauliflower again, but apparently ate too much of it, reached a saturation point, and now gets a headache when she eats it. So she doesn't. Ditto with beet tops, bell peppers, an occasional rice cake, one egg a week, and a few other foods that she had added back into her diet.

For Deborah, a headache is the usual symptom that tells her to "back off" of a certain food; at other times she just doesn't feel well.

Maintenance detoxification, which we believe is a helpful lifelong practice, Deborah handles with various herbs and a monthly colonic. She exercises every day and avoids stress as much as possible. She is well aware that the virus that causes shingles does not leave the body and will manifest itself again if given the right conditions.

Like the rest of us, Deborah is simply weak at times and needs to rest. At other times she is stronger. But for the most part she lives a normal life. She adapts to what she can handle, and avoids what she cannot.

In Deborah's journey, and in mine, nothing is more helpful than a living hope in the One who put us here in the first place, who has shepherded us up to this point, and who will complete that work which He began in us. If any suffering we have gone through helps someone else come to a living knowledge of Him, we have been well compensated.

Appendix I
Principles of Healthy Living

1. No one else can know our body as well as we can, so taking full responsibility for our own health is number one.

2. We want to eliminate those things which poison us:
    a. Start with unhealthful foods
    b. And unhealthful water. Chlorinated or fluoride treated waters have a poisoning effect. Some municipal water supplies are much healthier than others. Even bathing in highly chlorinated water is unhealthful. In those places, a whole-house carbon filter may be helpful.[415]
    c. Curb unhealthful thoughts. Nurture a positive attitude.
    d. Avoid any and all unhealthful practices of the body, of the mind, and of the spirit.

3. We cannot avoid a toxic environment. Therefore, detoxification is imperative.

4. Maintain a healthy bowel.
    a. As stated earlier, the bowel is not a pipe; it is part of the digestive system, and nutrients and toxins are being absorbed from it into the bloodstream. A tremendous amount of health is lost because of a toxic bowel. Keep it moving. One *full* movement per day, minimum. For proper elimination, think of foods in terms of fiber, lubrication (oils), and moisture.
    b. Enemas can be very helpful. Learn how and when to use one.
    c. If we have ever eaten a typical American diet containing processed foods, or if we have ever had a period of time when we did not have full bowel movements on a daily basis, there is a high probability that we have an impacted bowel. Therefore, it may be beneficial cleanse the bowel to remove the old, impacted, putrefied, highly toxic material. (See Chapter 8.)

5. Exercise. Walking or running, stretching, moderate lifting. "Use it or lose it."

6. Practice deep breathing, especially when in good air. The lungs are huge filters—clean them out! This also cleans the blood.

7. Sweat. The skin is not a wrapper, it is an organ—the largest of our body. It absorbs what it comes into contact with, and if given the opportunity, it also eliminates toxins from the body.

8. Fortify. Eat for your health. (Only.)

9. Drink water.
   a. Drink enough of the best quality water you can get. Many recommend a minimum of 64 ounces a day for a 128 pound person; 96 ounces for a 192 pound person. More is needed on dry or warm summer days; maybe less on cool, rainy days. We will find that we drink more water if it is of good quality and the supply is unlimited.[416]

10. Rest.
   a. Sleep allows the body to repair itself. Get enough. We are more productive if we have adequate sleep.
   b. A day of rest allows the mind to do the same.

11. Our intuition is a safeguard. We are better off when we pay attention to it.

12. Listen to your body, but not to its cravings.

13. Learn. Feed your mind with good things.

14. Love your Creator. Turn away from every form of evil.

15. We pass our strengths and weaknesses on to our children. Live for them.

16. Be thankful and give thanks. Giving thanks cures covetousness, which is a great destroyer. This practice also builds a healthy attitude.

Appendix II
Dietary Comments for Blood Sugar Disorders

The optimal diet for high blood sugar (diabetes), for low blood sugar (hypoglycemia), and for those who are simply glucose intolerant is essentially the same. In any of these cases, to gain or maintain health we must take personal ownership of our diet and learn to listen to our body.

> **The diet is very simple:**
> **We need to change from eating fast-burning fuels to eating slow-burning fuels, and do so in proper balance.**

I am a reporter only. I am not a professionally trained nutritionist and am unqualified to give any nutritional advice. What is stated here is simply what we as a family have found to be good practice, having lived an accumulated 120 years with hypoglycemia. It is also based upon a long family history of diabetes, and upon our speaking with other people who have hypoglycemia or diabetes and have learned to control their condition. **For your diet, you may want to consult a qualified health practitioner. This is an imperative if you are on diabetic medications. Above all, take responsibility for yourself!**

By the time most people realize that they have a blood sugar problem and decide to act on it, a lot of damage has already been done to the organs and glands. That's the bad news. The good news is that in most cases, we can minimize the effects of that damage, and slow down or arrest the progress of disease.

I have assumed for the purpose of this chapter that the reader does not want to go on diabetes medications. If you do, you probably did not read this far in the book. Therefore, having that goal, this is what we and others we know who have controlled the disease do:

<u>**The first thing**</u> **we believe is necessary is to get sugar intake under control.** In order to do this, we need to get off almost all highly processed foods.

Almost all highly processed foods have sugar or some sweetener added to them. **If we have a blood sugar problem of any kind, we are wise to consider that nearly all prepared foods are a poison to us.** Besides being loaded with sugar, these foods are also loaded with modified food starch and other highly refined carbohydrates that burn almost as fast as sugar does.

Just a little sugar, modified food starch, or a sip of wine can cause great havoc for someone who does not metabolize them well. The need for a diabetic, hypoglycemic, or someone with glucose intolerance is to burn slow-burning fuels at an even rate so that he or she can maintain relatively normal blood sugar levels. This is done by eating an adequate amount of protein with *complex* carbohydrates. It cannot be done eating sugars and simple (fast-burning) carbohydrates. These will spike the blood sugar level; then it will crash. These spikes can be a serious threat to health. Unless we are temporarily in a *very* low blood sugar condition, **fast-burning fuels are our enemy.**

Second, we look at metabolism as a whole. With metabolism we are not just looking at blood sugar, but at the entire matter of how we process our food.

The diet we have found most helpful for someone with a blood sugar condition is as follows:
Sugar and other refined sweeteners are excluded [417]
Finely ground or bleached (white) flours are excluded [418]
Seeds and nuts are plentiful.[419]
Grains are whole and limited in quantity [420]
Beans and other legumes are limited in quantity
Protein *must* be adequate. Animal flesh is probably needed.[421]
Non-starch vegetables are plentiful
Starchy vegetables are very limited or eliminated
Fruits are very limited and eaten whole (not taken as juice)

Third, it is good to understand that after the above, **everyone's dietary program will be a little different.** No two people are alike. No two hypoglycemics will have the same optimal diet, and no two people with diabetes or glucose intolerance will have the same optimal diet either.

Some hypoglycemics and diabetics can eat fruit sparingly. Some cannot even eat beans or grains, because even these foods metabolize too quickly for their bodies to handle. Some can drink a limited quantity of milk or eat (plain) yogurt. Others can only have cheese. Some can eat a limited quantity of carrots or onions (which are high in sugars). Others can have nothing sweeter than celery.

Getting the diet straightened out is a project, and it is all trial and error. If you have a blood sugar challenge there will be plenty of error. Keeping a diary helps. **Desire to be well helps more than anything else.**

Fourth, after we have proven to ourselves that we are on the right track by getting sugar consumption somewhat under control, it is better not to tease ourselves but rather get it over with and get sugar out of the diet. After a while the desire for it will go away. Many of us have proven this.

We have seen many hypoglycemics and diabetics flirt with sugar and refined foods and do not know any who are healthier for doing so. We do know many, however, who have worsened their health by compromising with sugar. That is why we strongly disagree with the medical establishment's compromising stance on this point.

Fifth, we who have a blood sugar problem will eventually discover that eating too many **natural sweets** is not a good thing. For example, many of us have found out that it is not wise to replace a refined sugar habit with a dried fruit or fruit juice habit. Both natural and refined sugars will likely damage the pancreas if we take too much. Both fruit juices and dried fruit (and I loved them as much as anyone on earth) are super-saturated with sugars and are not a good choice for a diabetic or a hypoglycemic. Eating whole fruits, rather than fruit juices, slows the burn rate. Take fruit sparingly, if you can tolerate it at all. If we take too much, the time will likely come when we won't be able to eat fruit at all without feeling ill. Honey can be used sparingly, if we can tolerate it. Use a *little* cinnamon with it, and that will lower the effect of the sugars.

Sixth, cravings (even of wholesome foods) are a warning. We can crave *anything*. If we crave a food, it may be good to avoid it for a week. If we feel better, that food was not good for us. It may be fine, in limited quantity, after a period of abstinence.

Seventh, if we have any blood sugar challenge, it is wise to avoid **alcohol**. Nothing is sweeter and nothing will tear us down faster. If we want any quality of life and do not want to be forced onto the medication treadmill, we will give it up.

Eighth, eat plenty of non-starch vegetables. We may find it beneficial to avoid **starches** altogether or have a very small portion of whole rice (brown rice), potato skins, or zucchini[422] at most once or twice a week.

Ninth, eating **smaller meals** and **eating more frequently is beneficial**. Many people with a blood sugar condition eat five or six small meals a day. The goal is to keep the blood sugar from going up or down too much.

Tenth, when you need to eat, eat! Do not wait. Once the body gives the signal, we do not have long before bad things start to happen. If we do not eat on time, our adrenals will start pumping. This MUST be avoided! Although adrenaline will temporarily buy us some time before we need to eat, that habit will eventually damage the adrenal glands, and we do not want that to happen. It can lead to a potentially serious condition. If we are in a social situation, we say "excuse me," get up and leave if we must, and eat. It is our current and future health that is on the line.

Eleventh, **if our blood sugar goes low**, or if we have the symptoms of low blood sugar and…
1. We know we should eat *soon* but can't: We may snack on some raw sunflower seeds. Chew well.
2. We are in trouble: We eat a piece of string cheese or some almonds. I melt the cheese in my mouth and chew the almonds well. The mixing of saliva greatly speeds and enhances the digestive process.
3. We are really in trouble: In times past, Deborah did what the doctor said to do and licked some hard tack candy, taking just enough to get her out of trouble until she could eat properly. For decades she has done fine without resorting to candy simply by

catching the situation earlier and eating string cheese, nuts or seeds instead. Our son, who is also hypoglycemic and has no minor case, has never taken candy, nor have I since developing the condition. I have taken a bite of apple with cheese at those times and it has worked well. Although candy is routinely recommended for the purpose of raising blood sugar, this should be done in an emergency situation only. From what we have observed, it is not prudent to make a habit of this, because in time the practice will make the body weaker overall.

Note 1: If a medical doctor does not suggest fruit instead of candy in an emergency blood sugar situation, that is probably evidence that he or she is sold out to a ruinous diet. Granted, a piece of hard tack is easier to have with you when away from home, but the failure to mention fruit as preferable is inexcusable.

Note 2: The sunflower seeds, nuts, or string cheese will probably only buy us about thirty to forty minutes before we need to have a *balanced* meal. If we try to stretch it past that, we will likely pay for it—maybe dearly.

Note 3: Eating is not always the way out of what appears to be blood sugar trouble. The symptoms of auto-toxicity are essentially the same as those of low blood sugar. Sometimes the need is not to eat, but to detoxify—NOW. If you suspect this is the case, you may want to take a capsule of vitamin C and empty it into a glass of water, stir it in, and drink the full glass. I use 1000 mg of vitamin C.

Twelfth, whether we tend to high blood sugar (diabetes) or low blood sugar (hypoglycemia), it is relatively easy to identify immediate responses of the body to a low blood sugar condition. It is not so easy to identify **next day responses**. So, we have to look for those too. The effects of diet, exercise, stress, adrenaline rushes, and other behaviors or factors may not manifest themselves in the blood sugar level until the next day. If we are not feeling well and do not know why, we look back at the previous day.

One good example: Our son is hypoglycemic and loves to run. And he feels great afterwards. However, it took him quite some time to realize that he must stop before he feels he needs to or the next day is shot. In other words, if he does not stop soon enough, he will spend the next day in a low blood sugar state. **A hypoglycemic must always keep a measure of energy in reserve. He cannot afford to empty the tank however good that may feel. The same is probably true for a diabetic.**

Thirteenth, always have emergency food with you. Sunflower seeds, high protein nuts, such as almonds or walnuts, and string cheese are good choices. **Also, always have good water with you. Remaining properly hydrated is crucial** for everyone, but especially for someone with blood sugar problems. If we don't have good water, in an emergency, we drink the chlorinated stuff. Whatever we do, we do not allow ourselves to become dehydrated.

Fourteenth, understand that the effects of any blood sugar abnormality are accumulative. Our body's health is a bank account.

Fifteenth, in many cases it is best to pack our own lunch and take it to work with us. We may have no choice if we want to avoid a worsened condition.

If we must eat out—and we all must at times—it is wise to always have our emergency food with us. There may not be anything on the menu that we can safely eat. After making ourselves sick a few times, it is very easy to follow these suggestions. I know; I've done it, and I do.

- Order a green salad with the dressing on the side. Head lettuce (iceberg) is useless; romaine, green leaf, and spinach are infinitely better. Dressings with sugar will bite you. That eliminates almost all of them. Plain vinegar and oil may be okay. Some blue cheese dressings are okay in moderation. Hardboiled egg and cheese can add needed protein. Skip the bacon bits, chunks of ham, and croutons.
- Non-starch cooked vegetables are okay if they are not cooked in a sauce. If they are cooked in a sauce, you can be sure there is sugar in it. Steamed vegetables, such as broccoli, cauliflower, etc., with cheese can be hearty.
- Skip the potato and rice, and substitute a double portion of steamed vegetables. I've never been charged for making this substitution. If the vegetables are squashes, they are a little better than potatoes or rice, but not much. Best not to eat

much of them. You may want to eat the skins and leave the rest.

- Sauces nearly always have something in them that are unfavorable to someone with a blood sugar condition. Modified food starch, sugar, MSG, and a thousand other similar products will take the strength away from a hypoglycemic or diabetic. **It is NOT normal to feel depleted after eating a meal,** yet someone who is glucose intolerant frequently does because he or she has eaten improperly—and this is one of the most common culprits.

- Sorry, tomato sauce and pasta—even the healthiest of them—may not be a good idea for people with a blood sugar condition. We may "get away with" them for a while, but if we find ourselves craving them, we can be assured that they are not good for us. The (natural) sugar content in tomato paste and sauces is very high. The pastas—even if they are made of spinach or artichoke—are heavily refined and tend to convert to sugars very rapidly. (I loved these two foods also, but I like being able to function much more.)

- Fish, if not fried, may be a good choice.

- Chicken will almost always be prepared with sugar. (Go figure!) If you see it on the menu you can ask about that, but our experience has been that we cannot trust what we are told. In a restaurant, it will invariably have something on it that will make us sick, even if it's just lemon juice.

- Besides fish (see chapter 9), about the only safe main course we have found is steak—if it is not marinated. Anything marinated will certainly have sugar in it. Avoid all lunch meats—they are all loaded with sugar.

- If a hamburger is all we can get, fine. We can throw away the bun and leave off all the condiments except the mustard. Obviously, we don't want to have this meal often, but we may be able to get by in a pinch.

And last, but really first of all, give thanks for what you can eat. This cures the ill of self-pity, and your digestion will be the better for it.

Some substitutes you may find helpful
Instead of _____, have _____

Bread[423]
Sprouted whole grain breads (without honey or sweetener)

Jam or jelly
Honey with cinnamon (go sparingly and find the ratio right for you)

Apple pie
Baked apples with cinnamon (Romes are great!)

Pumpkin pie
Pumpkin pie filling, made using a little honey to sweeten

Ice cream
Plain yogurt with apple bits and cinnamon

Pasta
Rye crackers (made with course ground flour) with avocado

Tomato sauce
Fresh tomato (sparingly)

Gravy
Juices from cooking the meat (pour off the fat)

Rice (white)
Brown rice

Breakfast cereals (prepared)
Rolled oats (lightly roasted if you wish) OR,
Ground sunflower or pumpkin seeds. Let the meal soak for 5-10 minutes in water or vegetable juice. You may want to add a cooked vegetable such as bok choy or cabbage.

Butter
Avocado

Potatoes
Potato skins, OR minimal tiny potatoes with a steamed green vegetable

Starch vegetables (potatoes, squash, etc.)
Kale, bok choy, broccoli, cauliflower, etc. (add cheese for protein if needed)

Fruit juice
Green vegetable juice (without fruit juice added to it)

Eggs
Omega 3 eggs (from chickens fed flax seed)

Fruit (various other fruits)
Apple (a tart or moderately tart variety)
Or, papaya (they contain very helpful enzymes)
Or, celery

Note: Everyone with a blood sugar problem is different. Some will be more limited than others and cannot have some of these items.

Building the Diet

An abnormal blood sugar condition should be approached systematically, as a project. We handle our project well. It is our quality of life that is at stake.

The world is full of foods. We just need to eat the ones that allow us to function optimally, and avoid the ones that make us weak or sick. On a base of non-starch vegetables, we build the diet that is right for us.

The crucial thing is to know the rate at which we burn various fuels and adjust accordingly. The combinations of foods are important and we need to find out what combinations work well for us. For example, I usually eat avocado with chicken because that fuel mixture burns better (lasts much longer) than when they are eaten separately. In other words, I digest better.

Some diabetics and hypoglycemics will be able to tolerate very limited quantities of **beans and brown rice**. Normally, these foods in their natural state can be very healthy. However, for someone with abnormal blood sugar metabolism, they may turn to sugars too quickly. It is the same with other grains and legumes.

If we cannot eat grains or beans, **we must get our protein** from somewhere. Seeds and nuts (raw, not roasted or salted.[424]) may not meet the entire requirement, but that is a good place to start. If seeds, nuts, and a limited amount of cheese don't fulfill the protein requirement—that is, if we are too weak—we probably need animal flesh. We think it is wise to keep animal flesh to a minimum. (You will find out what that minimum is.) We always cook the meat with herbs and eat it with plenty of hearty non-starch vegetables. This helps digestion greatly. In our family, every one of us needs meat almost every day in order to function optimally.

Note: After an extended fast, we often find that we feel better eating less meat. I think that is telling us we were eating too much.

Each one of us with an abnormal blood sugar condition must figure out what works for us. **Adjust as your body changes. It will.**

A Few More Points:

1. The **Nutritional Facts Chart** in the next appendix gives a basic understanding of the protein, carbohydrate, sugar, and fat content of some foods. We have found that information very helpful. The chart has also proven to us that there is more to metabolism than merely understanding the ratio between these components of a food. We have not found the **glycemic index** very helpful.[425] A person with a blood sugar condition *must* learn to do what their body tells them to do, not what some chart or index says to do.

2. Taking a multiple vitamin may be a good idea. If we have a blood sugar abnormality, we *are* depleted.

3. We take only as much coffee or other stimulants as we do arsenic. (That's a joke—we avoid stimulants.)

4. If you are very limited and are allergic to a lot of foods, it may be wise to get tested for heavy metals—especially mercury, nickel, and copper. (See Chapter 9.)

5. If you are having trouble knowing what is causing an allergy problem, you may want to reset your digestion by going on a

vegetable juice fast for a few days. Then **keep it simple** by adding back in one food at a time.

6. Make your **herbal reference book** your friend.

7. Understand that no book has the right diet for you and all of us writing on the subject will say something different. That is because we have all found that we are different. We all need to find out what is right for our optimal health. Hopefully you won't deceive yourself about sugar in the process. That is very easy to do. I know, I've done it.

8. Eating natural foods in the proper balance for your condition is what is important.

9. We use **moderation** in everything except the avoidance of sugar.

10. Armed with some basic knowledge, *and with sugar out of the way*, our body will tell us what to do. We listen to it. All the doctors in the world cannot be as helpful.

Once again, I am not a health professional and cannot tell you what you should do in your particular case. You must figure that out yourself. And you can! Here's to your health!

Resources:
Breads:
Ezekiel 4:9 bread: Food for Life http://foodforlife.com/our-products/ezekiel-49
Julian Bakery: http://www.julianbakery.com/

See other resources in Chapters 4, 14, and 21.

Appendix III
Nutritional Facts Chart
(As per USDA required labeling of various foods)

This chart follows Appendix II because a person with an abnormal blood sugar condition must understand the protein, carbohydrate, sugar, and fat content of the foods they eat. Such a person must eat foods that are high in proteins, moderate in carbs, and low in sugars. Healthy fats are highly beneficial if sugars are minimized and carbohydrates are balanced with protein. What is important is to understand the ratios between the proteins, carbs, sugars, and fats in any given meal. Therefore, the only relevance of the numbers is their relationships with one another. This abbreviated chart shows the principle of the matter. For example, compare the last two items on the chart: vegetable juice and apple juice. I listed mostly high protein foods, as these are so vital for someone with a blood sugar condition. All numbers were taken from food labels.

US law requires putting this information on the labels of foods. The ratios tell a lot, but they do not tell the whole story.

Food item	Protein	Carbs	Sugars	Fat	Fiber
Chicken, canned in water, breast	12	0	0	2	0
Chicken broth, low fat	5	0	0	1.5	0
Eggs	6	1	0	4.5	0
String cheese (Mozzarella)	6	1	0	6	0
Monterey Jack cheese	7	0	0	8	0
Cheddar Cheese, med	8	1	0	6	0
Yogurt, nonfat, plain	11	18	14	0	0
Cottage cheese, 2% fat	13	4	3	2.5	0
Milk, whole, pasteurized	8	11	11	8	0
Buttermilk, low fat	9	13	13	2.5	0
Almonds, raw	6	6	1	14	3
Pecans, raw	3	4	1	21	2
Peanuts, Spanish, raw	8	6	1	14	3
Filberts (Hazelnuts), raw	4	5	1	18	3
Cashews, raw	5	8	2	14	3
Walnuts, English, raw	4	5	2	19	1
Brazil nuts, raw	4	4	1	19	2

Food item	Protein	Carbs	Sugars	Fat	Fiber
Almond butter, raw	7	6	2	16	4
Almond butter, roasted (1)	7	6	2	16	4
Peanut butter, raw	8	6	3	16	2
Sunflower seeds, raw	8	8	0	16	1
Pepitas (Pumpkin seeds), raw	9	4	0	15	2
Sesame seeds, raw, with hulls	6	8	0	17	4
Rice, brown, long grain	3	37	0	2	3
Rice cakes, brown rice	1	14	0	0.5	1
Rolled oats, Quaker	6	27	1	2.5	4
Quinoa	6	30	0	2.5	3
Amaranth	7	32	1	1	8
Barley	5	32	1	1	8
Wheat, whole grain	7	31	0	0	5
Wasa whole grain rye cracker	1	10	0	0	2
Soy beans	13	11	3	7	3
Kidney beans, canned	8	19	1	0	4
Pinto beans, not canned	7	22	1	1	14
Garbanzo beans, not canned	6	18	3	2	5
Lentils	8	19	0	0	9
Green vegetable juice (2)	3	5	3	0	0
Apple juice	0	30	24	0	0

1: This is a good example of how this chart does not tell the whole story. The raw almond butter gives far more energy to someone with blood sugar problems than the roasted. Yet the ratios on the chart are the same.

2: This juice was a pasteurized product and contained celery, spinach, parsley, cucumber, kale, romaine, wheat grass sprouts, sunflower greens, and clover.

Most meats are not listed. They are all high in protein. Fat content varies. All have essentially no carbs, sugars, or fiber.

Vegetables are not listed. They fall into three categories: non-starch vegetables, such as leafy greens, celery, etc.; vegetables with high glycemic index, such as beets and carrots; and starch vegetables, such as potatoes, squash, etc.

Appendix IV
A Very Brief History of the AMA

This brief history is intended only to give a basic timeline and highlight some important issues and behavioral patterns in the organization's long history. Some of the issues listed here would never be mentioned by the AMA in its historical recaps. They are given here to provide a balance to the typical AMA histories.

1847: AMA founded by Nathan Smith Davis, who had served in the Medical Society of New York. His intent was to "elevate the standard of medical education in the US."

1849: The AMA studies quack remedies and begins to advise the public about the same.

1850's: The AMA becomes the prominent US medical association.

1858: The AMA forms a Committee on Ethics.

1892: The American School of Osteopathy is founded in the US as a protest against the medical system of the day, which by default meant the AMA. The founders believed that the AMA was corrupt and that it emphasized treatment of effects, instead of causes, of disease. The AMA took them on, labeled them as an "unscientific cult," and declared it unethical for a medical doctor (MD) to associate with an Osteopathic Doctor (DO). This was the beginning of a hundred-year war between the two groups that was of David and Goliath proportions.

1930's: The AMA prohibits its members from working for the newly formed health maintenance organizations (HMOs) that sprang up during the Great Depression. (Kaiser and others.)

1943: AMA conviction in AMA v, US, 317 U.S. 519 (1943) for violating the Sherman Antitrust Act in not allowing member doctors to work for the early HMOs.

1950s, early 1960s: The AMA vehemently opposes Medicare.

Mid-1960's: Seeing that the battle was lost, that public opinion and the political tide was against them, and having lobbied successfully to shape the system so that it was favorable to its cause, the AMA becomes a staunch supporter of Medicare.

1961: The AMA finally begins to publicly discourage smoking. The organization had turned a blind eye for decades even when cigarettes were added to the rations of GIs during World War II, thus creating millions of new addicts among young servicemen. Henry Ford, with the collaboration of Thomas Edison, wrote his classic book, *The Case Against the Little White Slaver,* in 1914, nearly fifty years before the AMA acted.

1962: In California, The California Medical Association (a branch of the AMA) spends about $8 million to try to end the practice of osteopathic medicine in the state. The CMA sponsors a statewide ballot initiative, Proposition 22, for this purpose. The measure passes, and the CMA offers to issue MD degrees to all the DOs in California for a nominal fee. 86% of the DOs agree and become MDs. The newly founded University of California at Irvine College of Osteopathic Medicine becomes the UCI School of Medicine.

1966: The AMA backs proposed new FDA regulations on vitamins and dietary supplements. Under the regulations, vitamins in dosages above the US Recommended Daily Allowance would have required a prescription from a medical doctor. A ten-year legal battle ensued culminating in a 1976 law, Public Law 94-278[426] signed by President Gerald Ford, in which the FDA lost on every major point of contention. The FDA, backed by the AMA, then redoubled its efforts (essentially to destroy AMA competition), which culminated in the Dietary Supplement Health and Education Act of 1994. The Act was sweeping in its scope and again instructed the FDA to "back off" on nearly every point of contention. The war is not over. (See the end of Chapter 20.)

1974: In Osteopathic Physicians and Surgeons of California v. California Medical Association, the California Supreme Court rules that licensing of DOs in the state be resumed. There were similar cases in other states which resulted in different rulings.

The AMA was successful in keeping osteopathic competition out of many states. Where they could not outright ban osteopathy from a state, the AMA attempted to absorb osteopaths into its fold. Where they have been successful, the results of the absorptions have been similar to what happened in California—most DOs, tired out or bankrupted from fighting, gave in, and osteopathic practice in general has been compromised.

1990: In <u>Wilk v. the American Medical Association, 895 F.2d 352</u> (7th Cir. 1990) the court rules against the AMA for its practice that held it unethical for medical doctors to associate with an "unscientific practitioner." Wilk was a chiropractor, and the AMA code of ethics, to which its members must comply, had labeled chiropractic as an "unscientific cult."

1990s to today: The AMA, forced by the Wilk Decision to be at least somewhat cooperative toward those outside its fold, and in more recent years, aware that the tide of public opinion has turned against its attitude of exclusion, has become quite friendly toward osteopaths. Some DOs are now in medical groups with MDs.

2010: The AMA supports President Obama's Affordable Care Act.[427] Is this any wonder? With the new mandates, more people will have access to the wares that represent more than 17% of the US Gross Domestic Product. We can be certain that the bill's 2,000 pages are full of the lobbying efforts of the association and of the pharmaceutical companies that it supports.

2013: The AMA has yet to denounce the typical sugared-up American diet that is made up largely of heavily processed, unhealthful foods. That it will eventually have to do so is obvious on two counts: 1) The AMA is losing its customer base. Too many people have come to the conclusion that the chemical approach to health is unhealthy. As with the smoking "controversy" of fifty years ago, too many people have seen past the deceptive claims of the pharmaceutical and processed food industries, and know in their gut (if not in their head) that this diet is ruinous. 2) An elementary understanding of mathematics tells us that the days are numbered for our government to continue to pay for what is currently called "health care." When this money source finally dries up, there will be no choice but to admit the obvious.

Appendix V

International Organization of Oral Medicine and Toxicology

IAOMT Recommended Procedures and Guidelines for Safe Removal of Amalgam Fillings
(re-printed from website by permission)

Dentists all over the world remove millions of amalgam fillings every day, with no regard for the possible mercury exposure that can result from grinding them out. Much of the time, a new amalgam filling goes back in place of the old one. The dental establishment claims that amalgam is a stable material, that emits little or no mercury, but then turns around and blames the mercury–free dentists for "unnecessarily exposing patients to excess mercury" when removing amalgams electively. Well, which is it? Stable, or mercury emitting?

We know beyond any doubt that amalgam emits mercury, as elaborated in the related articles, "The Scientific Case Against Mercury Amalgam" and "Understanding Risk Assessment for Mercury From Dental Amalgam." Finished amalgam on the bench at 37°C will emit as much as 43.5 µg of mercury vapor per square centimeter of surface area per day, for extended periods of time.[1] Samples of the leading brands of amalgam kept in water at 23° C released 4.5 to 21 µg per square centimeter per day.[2] Cutting the amalgam with a dental bur produces very small particles with vastly increased surface area, and vastly increased potential for subjecting the people present to a mercury exposure. In fact, in a recently published experiment, volunteers with no amalgam fillings swallowed capsules of milled amalgam particles, and, sure enough, their blood mercury levels increased.[3] These authors concluded that "the GI uptake of mercury from amalgam particles is of quantitative importance." Molin, et. al. demonstrated a three to four fold increase in plasma mercury the next day, and a 50% rise in urine mercury for a month following amalgam removal in ten subjects, after which their mercury levels began to decline.[4] Snapp, et. al.[5] showed that efforts to reduce mercury exposure during amalgam removal resulted in less uptake of mercury than that cited in the Molin study.

Less well studied than mercury vapor is the problem of amalgam particulates. Taking out fillings with a high speed dental bur generates a cloud of particles, at least 65% of which are one micron or less in size. These are fully respirable, get deep into the lungs, where the microscopic particles are broken down and the mercury is systemically absorbed within a few days. This mercury exposure can be as much as a hundred times greater than that from the vapor. [6, 7]

Stories abound concerning patients having adverse reactions – getting sick – following removal of amalgam fillings, whatever they are replaced with, although there is no established scientific literature on the subject. The mercury free dentists of the world have been acutely aware of the excess exposure problem, and have devised a number of strategies for reducing the amount of mercury exposure to both patients and dental staff during amalgam removal. This article will cover the physical methods, the barrier and ventilation techniques, that can be used in any dental office. The techniques in this chapter have been checked with the aid of the Jerome mercury vapor detector by IAOMT members, and found to reduce mercury vapor in the air that the patients and dental staff breathe. Even though it has not been tested experimentally and published in peer reviewed journals, experience indicates that when the dentist fastidiously reduces mercury exposure while removing amalgams, the patients report fewer episodes of feeling sick afterwards.

However, please bear in mind that the material presented here is intended strictly as a set of suggestions. A licensed practitioner must make up his or her own mind concerning specific treatment options.

Cut and chunk, keep it cool

Most of these suggestions are simple and obvious, common sense physical means of reducing exposure. If you remove an old amalgam by slicing across it and dislodging big chunks, you will aerosolize less of the contents than if you grind it all away. If you keep it under a constant water spray while cutting, you will keep the temperature down, and reduce the vapor pressure within the mercury.

Suction!

Your best tool for removing mercury vapor and amalgam particulates from the operating field is your high volume evacuation (HVE). Keep it going next to the patient's tooth until you are finished with the removal and clean-up process. But check to see where in your office it discharges! If the vacuum pump discharges into an open trap or through its own base, you could be pumping mercury vapor into your utility room or lab.[8] (See also the Environmental articles on this website for information concerning mercury separators for your suction system, to remove the amalgam particulates and dissolved mercury before they are discharged into the wastewater.)

A highly effective HVE adjunct is the "Clean-Up" suction tip, which has an enclosure at the end that surrounds the tooth you're working on. It dramatically reduces the spatter of particles, directing them efficiently into the suction tube. "Clean-Up" is available from the IAOMT, through the online store, or at (863) 420-6373.

Rubber dam or no rubber dam?

Some dentists hate rubber dams, while others can't live without them. Amalgam removal with reduced exposure can be done either way. A rubber dam will help contain the majority of the debris of amalgam grinding, among its many other benefits. Berglund and Molin [9] demonstrated, as a follow-up to Molin's 1990 study, that the use of a rubber dam eliminated the spike in plasma mercury one day after amalgam removal, as well as the spike in urine mercury ten days afterward: evidence of its protective benefit. Of course both amalgam removal groups, dam or no dam, showed 50-75% reduction in blood mercury levels a year later.

But you must know that mercury vapor will diffuse right through the dam, and some of the particulates will often sneak past it, too. So:

- Always use a saliva ejector behind the dam to evacuate air that may contain mercury vapor. Nitrile dams are better vapor barriers than latex.
- Rinse well as you go, especially under the rubber dam clamp, because amalgam particles left on the used dam

will emit mercury from your garbage can. (If you wipe your dirty mirror on a gauze square or the patient's bib, that gray smear also emits quite a lot of mercury vapor!)

- As soon as the amalgams are out, remove the dam and thoroughly rinse the patient's mouth before placing the new restorations. It can take as much as sixty seconds of rinsing to fully remove the mercury vapor. Search for gray particles. If there are particles on the back of the tongue, have the patient sit up and gargle them out.

- Post-removal rinses can be used to scavenge mercury from the patient's saliva. Some of the substances that can be suspended in water and used for this purpose are activated charcoal, chlorella, or n-acetyl cysteine.

If you don't use a rubber dam, you must be vigilant with the HVE, and take frequent breaks to thoroughly rinse the field. Either way, the "Clean-Up" suction tip reduces the dispersion of particulates in the area.

Cover the skin

Covering the patient's face with a barrier will prevent spattered amalgam particles from landing on the skin, or the eyes. The barrier can be as simple as a moist paper towel, or as elaborate as a surgical drape. [see photo on IAOMT site]

Rubber gloves

Mercury vapor will diffuse through latex and vinyl gloves, just as it does through latex and vinyl rubber dams. Nitrile material is a more effective diffusion barrier, and while there are no nitrile rubber dams available, nitrile rubber gloves appear to better protect the dentist's hands from a concentration of mercury vapor.

Controlling the breathing space

However efficient your HVE technique is, the air surrounding the operative field will fill up with a mercury vapor and amalgam particulate aerosol. Keeping the breathing space of the patient and dental staff free of contamination is the next priority.

Supplemental air

Provide the patient with piped–in air, so they do not have to breathe the air directly over the mouth during amalgam removal. A positive pressure respiration device such as a nitrous oxide nose hood, or a similar ventilation device, is probably the best way to provide clean air. A nasal cannula that admits ambient air won't help.

Respirators for the staff
The typical paper hygienic masks that are in everyday use are of no benefit whatsoever for removing either amalgam particulates or mercury vapor from the air we breathe. The best protection for the dental staff, from an industrial hygiene point of view, would be a positive pressure breathing system. This kind of system is certainly available from safety equipment suppliers. Much simpler to set up would be a Bureau of Mines certified, "half–mask" respirator, with mercury rated filter cartridges.
The IAOMT Online Store sells the MSA "Comfo-Classic" respirator for this purpose. The 3M company makes a similar half-mask respirator with mercury rated cartridge (#6009) and accompanying P-100 pre-filter which will remove particles as small as 0.3 microns, available from many industrial sources.

Maintain clean air in the operatory
Mercury vapor and amalgam particulates generated by removing amalgams disperse in the air of the operatory, leading to a background exposure throughout the office.
Beyond opening the window, here are some strategies for mitigating the problem:

- **Filtration:** Several manufacturers supply high tech room air purifiers that can effectively remove mercury vapor and particulates from the operatory. They use various methods of ultrafiltration together with negative ion generators, plus basic vacuum force to remove the air from the operative field. Dent-Air Vac, E. L. Foust, Smart-Air Solutions, and Tact-Air can be contacted and their products compared via the IAOMT Sponsors page.

- **Supplemental evacuation:** Simply moving air away from the operative field can be effective in reducing mercury exposure, and some offices have installed creatively designed mechanisms. One IAOMT member had the central vacuum cleaner in his office vented to the exterior of the building. The patients hold the vacuum hose under their chins as he removes their amalgam fillings, resulting in zero mercury vapor detectable in the room.

taking mercury vapor seriously while removing amalgam fillings
[see photo on IAOMT site]

references
1 Chew, CL; Soh, G; Lee, AS; Yeoh, TS. Long-term dissolution of mercury from a non-mercury-releasing amalgam. Clin Prev Dent. 13(3): 5-7. (1991)
2 Haley, BE, IAOMT website article
3 Geijersstam, E; Sandborgh-Englund, G;Jonsson, F; Ekstrand, J. Mercury uptake and kinetics after ingestion of dental amalgam. J Dent Res. 80: 1793-1796 (2001)
4 Molin, M; Bergman, B; Marklund, SL; Schutz, A; Skervfing, S. Mercury, selenium, and glutathione peroxidease before and after amalgam removal in man. Acta Odontol Scand 48(3): 189-202 (1990)
5 Snapp, KR; et al. The Contribution of Dental Amalgam to Mercury in Blood. J Dent Res, 68(5):780-5, 1989.
6 Richardson, GM; Inhalation of mercury-contaminated particulate matter by dentists: an overlooked occupational risk. Hum Ecol Risk Assess 9:1519-1531 (2003)
7 An extensive discussion of this issue is presented in Richardson's lecture to the IAOMT in October, 2004. A DVD copy of the lecture can be obtained through the Online Store.
8 Stonehouse, CA; Newman, AP. Mercury vapour release from a dental aspirator. Brit Dental J. 190:558-560 (2001)
9 Berglund, A; Molin, M. Mercury levels in plasma and urine after removal of all amalgam restorations: the effect of using rubber dams. Dent Mater 13:297-304 (1997)

Appendix VI
Using "Dr. Google"

The Internet has changed medical practice forever because many people now consult the Internet before they consult their doctors. This is a significant extension of consulting health reference books. One big downside of the web, when it comes to health, is that we can be improperly influenced by quick, readily accessible information. Another downside is that we can waste a tremendous amount of time searching for information. So, with these two things in mind, I have a few comments that may be helpful:

First, on using search engines: Google has (or at least had) a very good motto: "Don't be evil." The company's mission was "to organize the world's information and make it universally accessible and useful." They have done an excellent job of it. Google leadership understood that people would be relying on information that they were disseminating—even for health decisions—and that the handling of information could open the door to all kinds of evil practice. Contrary to what some people say, there is evil. The buying of "reports" and "news" items, as well as the political agendas of network owners, has rendered most of the mass media unreliable. The same happens on the Internet, and the founders of Google were well aware of the problem, hence the motto. The company is new; it was not incorporated until 1998, and its initial public offering was not until 2004. At least for a brief period of time, we have enjoyed access to what appears to be an objective and unbiased dissemination of information. However, knowing the character of mankind and human history, we cannot think that corruption will not work its way in at some point. In every big business, a large number of decisions are made every day. Only constant vigilance and the willingness to lose a buck will safeguard the company's reputation. [I also applaud Google for standing up to China. This cost them financially, but was the right thing to do.]

Thankfully, there are other search engines also. Sometimes I use different search engines for the same search, but I usually stay away from those that have an obvious political agenda.

Be aware that web content is constantly changing—usually according to pop culture. Whatever is "groovy" at the time will be all over the web. Hence the importance of books—especially older ones.

Concerning websites that require you to sign in: If the site is not a trusted site and you sign in, you can expose yourself to a lot of harassment, if not mischief. Even with trusted sites this can happen. Therefore, I usually get the information I want elsewhere.

Concerning subscription websites: I am happy to pay for information; I am not happy to have a security risk with my credit card or personal information. Therefore, if I see an abstract of an article I want, I'll either purchase a Visa gift card for the purchase, or print out the abstract, take it to the local library or medical library, and obtain the article there.

Concerning websites that ask you to enter personal information of any kind: Only to sites that I think are trustworthy will I give my contact information, nothing more. Any site that asks for other personal information, like health information, I avoid.

Wikipedia is a great place to *start* some searches. The site is not 100% reliable, but it is quite objective.

For scholarly work, Google Scholar is excellent; so is the government site PubMed.

Concerning websites with lots of ads and pop-ups: I have not found their information helpful. These sites tend to focus on metering out as little objective, practical information as possible, not on offering useful, reliable information. It seems to me that these sites are designed for people who want to get their health information in five seconds or less, and then purchase a product that will solve all their health problems.

Concerning nonprofit websites (.orgs): I am not one of those who thinks that "for profit" is a bad thing and that "nonprofit" is a good thing. Depends who is running the organization. I needfully put quotes around "nonprofit." Remember the United Way and Red Cross scandals? We found out through them that the rules for what is used for salaries for top executives, and what is actually given to charity are very lax. Also, many legally nonprofit organizations receive their funding from certain industries that have a great interest in the direction that the "nonprofit" takes. For example, The American Heart Association and the alphabet soup of similar organizations are joined at the hip with the AMA. (See Chapter 15.) Having said that much, I greatly appreciate many nonprofit sites. There are many honest, dedicated people behind a lot of them. There are also many honest, dedicated people behind many "for profit" businesses. Both types of organizations are businesses, and just like you and I, all of these people need to eat.

Concerning websites that try to wow you with their superior "scientific" knowledge: I am not impressed in the least and do not waste my time with them. Ditto with sites that essentially say, "Follow me, I know all the answers," or "We have a product that will cure everything."

The tough part of all this is that those businesses that are honest and present good information are copied and stolen from, and that can make it hard for them to make a living. Please reward those who are upright. Thank you!

Resources for Parts I, III and IV

Books:
Note: Some of these books are old or out of print. No problem, go to ABE.com and you can get most of them used for very little cost.

These are listed approximately in the order that they are referred to in the text of this book. **Additional resources are at the end of some of the chapters.**

Back to Eden, by Jethro Kloss, 1939
Common sense was good in 1939. It is equally good today. Kloss had plenty of it.

New Low Blood Sugar and You, by Carlton Fredericks, 1985
A "must read" for a hypoglycemic.

www.fred.net/slowup/hai185.html
This website is that of the Adrenal Metabolic Research Society of the Hypoglycemia Foundation and is the work of Dr. John W. Tintera, MD. He and his wife both had the condition. They know what they are talking about.

Is Low Blood Sugar Making You a Cripple? by Ruth Adams and Frank Murray, 1970
Similar in scope to Carlton Fredericks' book.

Banting's Miracle, by Seale Harris, MD, 1946
This is the biography of the discoverer of insulin written by a leading diabetes specialist who, after the discovery of insulin, identified non-diabetic hypoglycemia.

Know Your Nutrition: The Complete Guide to Good Health Through Natural Living, by Linda Clark, 1973.
Deborah got a lot of help from this book early on.

Kitchen Medicine, by Ben Charles Harris, 1968
This is a book of "old school" remedies. It shows clearly how far we have strayed from the natural way of true health care.

The Way of Herbs, by Michael Tierra, 1998
The best herbal we know of.

Natural Detoxification: A Practical Encyclopedia, by Jacqueline Krohn and Frances Taylor, 2000
Deborah says: "I cannot recommend the book highly enough. Everything they say is spot on."

Tissue Cleansing Through Bowel Management, by Bernard Jensen, DC PhD, 1981
In our opinion a "must" read.

The Healthy Liver and Bowel Book, by Sandra Cabot, MD, 1999
Deborah learned a lot from this book and recommends it highly.

Hypothyroidism: The Unsuspected Illness, by Broda O. Barnes, MD, 1976
I'm sure there are newer books (which may or may not be better), but this one helped Deborah understand the condition.

Prescription for Nutritional Healing, by Phyllis A. Balch and James F. Balch, MD, 4th edition, 2000
An excellent encyclopedia-like reference volume, especially for dietary supplements.

Our Daily Meds, by Melody Petersen, 2008
A very well-researched and documented book. If you are thinking of taking medications or are already taking them, a "must read."

Uninformed Consent, by Hal Huggins, DDS and Thomas E. Levy, MD, 1999
A discussion of current dental practice and its harmful effects. These effects are far greater than one can imagine. A "must read."

The Trigger Point Therapy Workbook: Your Self-Treatment Guide for Pain Relief, 2nd edition, by Clair Davies with Amber Davies, 2004

Primal Panacea, by Thomas E. Levy, MD, 2011
A very good book on the use of high dosage vitamin C. Like countless other health books, I think the author's claims go too far. But if one tenth of what he says is valid, it is well worth looking at. And we can vouch for much more than one tenth.

The Milk Book: How Science is Destroying Nature's Nearly Perfect Food, by William Campbell Douglass, 1994

Old, helpful, reference books you can see on Google Books or similar websites:

Concerning old books: We live in an age where history is being revised at a very rapid rate. Therefore, it is a good thing to have some old books and to compare them with current thought and with what is currently stated as historical fact.

Foods and Their Adulteration, by Harvey W. Wiley, 1907

The Food and Drugs Act; A Study, by Arthur P. Greenly, 1907

Autointoxication or Intestinal Toxemia, by J. H. Kellogg, MD, 1919
An invaluable work that many have since built upon.

Colon Hygiene, by J. H. Kellogg, MD, 1915
Bernard Jensen built much of his life's work upon what is discussed in this book. Jensen took it further, and many have now taken Jensen's work further without abandoning their teachers' principles.

The New Method in Diabetes, by J. H. Kellogg, 1917
This book is full of the common sense that is lacking in most of the current-day discussion of the disease.

Chart:
Reflexology Hand, Foot Chart © Christopher Shirley, Pacific Institute of Reflexology, 2002

Lab tests, medical consultations:
Life Extension, lef.org. To get the same *standard* lab tests (not heavy metals tests), from the same labs, for about half the cost, join this organization. Membership cost us $75 and paid for itself when we ordered our first lab tests from them. (We use Genova Labs for heavy metals testing.) A big benefit of membership is that you can call and talk to a physician at no charge. We have found these consultations helpful. They are pretty much mainstream medical doctors, but we have found them to be a useful resource.

Other Services:

Intravenous vitamin C infusions:
Institute for Progressive Medicine, Irvine CA (949) 600-5100.
Many other clinics on the periphery of the medical establishment
also do the infusions. I don't know of any hospitals that do. (You
can search the web under "integrated" medical practitioners.)

"Alternative" allergy testing: Center for Advanced Medicine,
Encinitas, CA. See Dr. David Nelson, a nutritionist.

Colon hydrotherapy (colonics):
For practitioners in your area, contact the International Association
for Colon Hydrotherapy, www.i-act.org

In Orange County, CA: Embrace Health, Costa Mesa, CA
(949) 642-3424

NAET (Nambudripad's Allergy Elimination Technique)
Dr. Mala Moosad
6714 Beach Blvd., Buena Park, CA 90621
(714) 523-8900

Resources for Part II, Mercury!

A. General Information on Mercury, Mercury Toxicity:

"Toxic Effects of Mercury on the Cardiovascular and Central Nervous Systems," by a panel of authors in the *Journal of Biomedicine and Biotechnology*, 2012
http://www.ncbi.nlm.nih.gov/pmc/articles/PMC3395437/
This is the best summary of mercury toxicity I have seen.

"The Three Modern Faces of Mercury," by Thomas W. Clarkson, 2002
http://www.ncbi.nlm.nih.gov/pmc/articles/PMC1241144/pdf/ehp110s-000011.pdf
A scientific paper from the Department of Environmental Medicine, University of Rochester School of Medicine, Rochester, NY. Clarkson is a leading mercury toxicologist. The paper deals with fish, dental amalgams, and vaccines and does an excellent job. Nearly free of bias.

On the EPA website: You may want to read the following articles and perhaps some of the referenced articles:
"Organic Mercury TEACH Chemical Summary," 2007
"Inorganic Mercury TEACH Chemical Summary," 2007
"Elemental Mercury TEACH Chemical Summary," 2007
The EPA website is far more objective than the "public health" websites when it comes to health matters.

www.mercurypoisoned.com A very helpful site. This site is that of an individual who had mercury poisoning. If you want professional credentials on everything you read, you gain only an academic understanding of the subject and often a heavily biased one at that. Where the rubber meets the road and the b.s. stops is when you, yourself, have to deal with a practical problem. Many of the links on this site are excellent.

PubMed, http://www.ncbi.nlm.nih.gov/pubmed is a government source for biomedical literature. Allows access to 22 million "scientific" papers.**

For "scientific" papers** on mercury toxicity or chelation, go to PubMed or Google Scholar and do a specific search there.

** **"Scientific" needs quotes.** Some "scientific" papers are far more objective than others. Please understand that only articles that have been sanitized to conform to the positions of industry will appear in the major medical journals. Therefore, in researching a health issue, it is wise to look equally into less guarded sources, especially those not so tied to US medical practice.

B. Information on Dental Amalgam and Thimerosal:

To see one side of the amalgam and thimerosal stories, see:

CDC websites: http://www.cdc.gov/ ;
http://www.cdc.gov/vaccinesafety/Concerns/thimerosal/

FDA websites: http://www.fda.gov/
   For amalgam, see:
http://www.fda.gov/MedicalDevices/ProductsandMedicalProcedures/DentalProducts/DentalAmalgam/default.htm ;
http://www.fda.gov/MedicalDevices/ProductsandMedicalProcedures/DentalProducts/DentalAmalgam/ucm171094.htm ;
   For thimerosal, see:
http://www.fda.gov/BiologicsBloodVaccines/Vaccines/QuestionsaboutVaccines/ucm070430.htm

Also see American Dental Association websites:
http://www.ada.org and http://www.ada.org/1741.aspx

To see the other side of the dental amalgam story, see:

US Agency for Toxic Substances and Disease Registry (ATSDR) "Public Health Statement for Mercury"
http://www.atsdr.cdc.gov/phs/phs.asp?id=112&tid=24

It's All in your Head: The Link Between Mercury Amalgams and Illness, by Dr. Hal A. Huggins, 1993
Good to its title, the book is highly informative. Whether we wanted to or not, through Deborah's experience we certainly proved many of the claims made in this book.
A "must read" in our opinion.

Uninformed Consent, by Hal A. Huggins, DDS[428] and Thomas E. Levy, MD, 1999
The typical dental patient has no idea of the risks involved in various dental procedures. The health dangers of root canals, of bio-incompatible dental materials, and the frequency of dental-related illness are discussed. The title is most appropriate.
A "must read" in our opinion.

The Toxic Time Bomb: Can the Mercury in Your Dental Fillings Poison You? by Sam Ziff, 1984
Ziff and Huggins were very instrumental in bringing this matter to the forefront.

International Academy of Oral Medicine and Toxicology www.iaomt.org This nonprofit organization has significant information on its website. IAOMT recommendations for amalgam removal are in Appendix V.

Dental Amalgam Mercury Solutions (DAMS) www.amalgam.org
Another nonprofit whose website is full of information.

www.mercurypoisoned.com This site has a lot of helpful links, including a link for videotaped testimony at the December, 2010 FDA hearings on amalgam where top professionals—dentists, research scientists, etc. spoke. See also:
http://www.youtube.com/user/mercurymatters

Symptoms and Differential Diagnosis of Patients Fearing Mercury Toxicity from Amalgam Fillings, by S. Stenman and L. Grans, 1997
(Published on PubMed) www.ncbi.nlm.nih.gov/pubmed/9456068
This is a Scandinavian study and is preliminary in scope. I believe it is more objective than US "public health" sources. Foreign sources, in general, are more objective on the subject. (They may not have as much built-in conflict of interest.) The Swedes banned amalgam in the late 1990's. A few other countries have banned it as well.

To see the other side of the vaccine story, see:
"Limiting Infant Exposure to Thimerosal in Vaccines and Other Sources of Mercury," by Neal A. Halsey, MD, *Journal of the American Medical Association*, Nov. 10, 1999

"Balancing Risks and Benefits," Halsey and Goldman, *Pediatrics*, 2001, 108:2, pgs. 466-467

Evidence of Harm: Mercury in Vaccines and the Autism Epidemic: A Medical Controversy, by David Kirby, 2005
This is a big subject and the author gives an excellent and thorough (as possible in 460 pages) presentation both of the history and of the issues. The book is well documented.

C. Information on Heavy Metals Chelation and Detoxification:
"A Comprehensive Review of Heavy Metal Detoxification and Clinical Pearls from 30 Years of Medical Practice," by Dietrich Klinghardt, MD, PhD
www.klinghardtacademy.com (909) 899-1650
This paper was the best information Deborah found on chelation before her treatments. Until I set out to write this book, we did not know of most of the other resources listed here. Some of it did not exist at that time. (See next refs.) Klinghardt's 20-page paper with more than 100 references has been removed from the Klinghardt Academy website. I called to see why and was told that it, and a lot of other information, was removed from the website because health practitioners and patients tried some of these things on their own, hurt themselves or their patients, and then sued Dr. Klinghardt. I mention this to underscore two points: 1) We like to sue, and 2) Chelation of mercury is nothing to attempt without knowledgeable, experienced professional help. What is posted on the site as of this writing (11-6-12) is very short. I disagree with Klinghardt on the DMPS Challenge Test. I think it can be much more dangerous. Nevertheless, I think this 20-page paper has great value if you can find it.
On the Klinghardt site also see:
http://www.klinghardtacademy.com/Articles/Mercury-Detoxification-Perpetuating-Factors-Problems-and-Obstacles.html

Mercola.com
Dr. Joseph Mercola, DO, has some of the best information on this topic that is easily accessible on the web. See his "Revised Protocol for Detoxifying Your Body from Mercury Exposure" and "Mercury Detoxification Protocol." The information is very incomplete and we do not agree with him on all points, but he has a holistic,

reasonable approach. Since our public health departments are mute on practical help and mainstream medicine denies the condition, I don't doubt that Mercola's work, as well as the work of the others listed here, has been a Godsend to many.

Amalgam Illness: Diagnosis and Treatment, Andrew Cutler, PhD, 1999

An excellent book written by a chemist who had the condition. If you suspect the condition, it is a "must read" in my opinion. Cutler's methods differ from Klinghardt's, most notably concerning intravenous DMPS. Due to the seriousness of the condition and of chelation therapy, if you are considering chelation, I believe it is best to read both of their works as well as what Mercola, IAOMT, and DAMS have to say. The information is empowering. You may also want to read the reviews of Cutler's book on Amazon. (I read all 59. All the reviewers were thankful for the book. Several criticize the presentation and organization of the material; none were critical of the content. Many people were helped, and some significantly.)

Cutler is a chemist and sees things like a chemist, so he has a different view than we have and a different approach than what we took. I disagree with the statement that heavy metal problems are easy to correct. We have not found that to be accurate, either in our case or in some other cases we know of. Deborah also thinks that the recommended dosages of DHEA and ALC are far too high. Though it is fourteen years old, I highly recommend the book as a resource. And thank you, Andy, for writing it!

Order it from Cutler directly for $35; pay twice that ordering elsewhere. http://www.noamalgam.com/ In his other book, he has more, and newer, protocols. See http://www.noamalgam.com/hairtestbook.html

Harrison's Principles of Internal Medicine, 1998

This medical textbook describes the DMSA test for mercury exposure. Your doctor is probably unaware of this and will most likely say that it is not covered by insurance. In fact it may be.

See "A" above for how to find scientific papers on chelation. **Scientific papers are necessary, but only tell half the story**. The other half of the story is testimonials. It is better to get these firsthand, but lacking that, you may want to do a web search for your questions and see what you can find.

http://www.dmpsbackfire.com The website is that of an individual who was harmed by DMPS treatment and has testimonials of many others who also were harmed, or at least claim to have been harmed, by intravenous DMPS treatments. The testimonials bear out the points of caution made in Chapter 12. Seeing both sides of an issue can be very helpful. I cannot emphasize enough the need to do your own research, prepare yourself, and not merely trust what someone says—*whoever they may be*. Between a government position that mercury in our mouths and in vaccines is no problem and the statements of those who can profit by "helping" us, the entire subject is very murky. It is ours to decide what to do, because we will be the ones who will live with the results of any action or inaction that we take or don't take.

http://mercuryandmore.weebly.com/mercury-story---illness.html
This is the story of a woman who had (has) a case similar to Deborah's. "Unscientific" real-life stories such as this are very helpful in diagnosing and understanding the condition. They tell what blood, urine, and hair tests cannot tell.

Concerning online groups such as Yahoo Groups, *Frequent Dose Chelation* and Yahoo Groups, *Adult-Metal-Chelation*: I am not big on chat rooms and the like, as I can't take the drivel or bear with people who can't spell, but there may be some value there. I could not navigate the sites. Warning: Every group has an owner or moderator, so information may be selectively presented.

D. More Good Books:
New Low Blood Sugar and You, by Carlton Fredericks, 1985
Fredericks discusses the hypoglycemia and mercury toxicity commonalities in some detail.

The Healthy Liver and Bowel Book, by Sandra Cabot, MD, 1999
Deborah learned a lot from this book and recommends it highly. A healthy liver and bowel are essential for removal of mercury from the body.

E. Products and Services:

Detox products:
Herbal formula for liver support and detoxification: "Liver Chi," Chi's Enterprise, Inc., Anaheim, CA 92807, (714) 777-1542

Dr. Bob Marshall, Quantum Nutritional Labs, (800) 370-3447
http://healthline.cc/
Marshall's clay baths were the most effective of those Deborah has used. His Nano-detox she also found helpful.

Dentist:
If you have no clue who to see, you may want to contact:
(Listed in alphabetical order)
Dental Amalgam Mercury Solutions (DAMS), (651) 644-4572
Huggins Applied Healing, (866) 948-4638
International Academy of Biological Dentistry and Medicine, (281) 651-1745
International Organization of Oral Medicine and Toxicology (IAOMT), (863) 420-6373
The Holistic Dental Association, (305) 356-7338
I have no experience with any of these folks, so can say nothing more. I hate to add, but must, that some dentists have merely jumped on the bandwagon of "biocompatible" or "holistic" dentistry. As always, "Let the buyer beware."

If you are in the Washington DC area, you may want to consult with Mark McClure, DDS, at National Integrated Health Associates, (202) 237-7000
If you are in Southern California, you may want to consult with Dr. Andrew Pallos, DDS, in Laguna Niguel, (949) 495-1659

Chelation:
Allan Sosin, MD, Institute for Progressive Medicine, Irvine CA, (949) 600-5100

Testing:
If your doctor does not know how to order testing for heavy metals:
Genova Diagnostics, gdx.net, (800) 522-4762

Notes

Chapter 1, The Setting

[1] Or Sta-Fresh. This product was common in the 1980s. What it was chemically, I don't know. I could not find any reference to it on the web in 2012 but did find other products used for the same purpose.

[2] Later in life, this drug adversely affected the hormone function in many female children of the women who took the drug. See Center for Disease Control website: www.cdc.gov/DES , National Cancer Institute's Facts About DES at http://dccps.nci.nci.gov/ACSRB/pubs/DES_Pubs/Facts , and www.desaction.org

[3] Increased levels of bilirubin in the blood. This is very hard on the liver, pancreas, and other organs and can lead to a diseased state.

[4] Medical professionals are greatly divided over tonsillectomies. Some, even today, think of the tonsils simply as unnecessary parts that are prone to infection. The argument is that if they are removed there will be less infection. This may be true, but why not find out what is causing the infections in the first place? The tonsils are part of the lymphatic system and produce protective antibodies that circulate in the bloodstream. The lymphatic system is in fact very little understood, which is probably why doctors greatly disagree on the matter of tonsillectomy. Whether we understand it or not, the tonsils, like all other members of the body, serve a function. No doubt, there are cases where tonsils need to be removed. To remove them routinely is another matter.

[5] If there was ever a case of reaping what we sow, the source of the plague of our culture—drug addiction—is no mystery. As a society, we sowed the wind and reaped the whirlwind.

[6] Smoking in films and on TV is unquestionably the most effective advertisement vehicle for hooking new smokers. US legislation has danced between the tobacco companies and public health for decades.

[7] Phenylephrine

Chapter 2, Collapse

[8] The main effect of Fetal Alcohol Syndrome is permanent central nervous system damage, especially to the brain. Developing brain cells can be malformed or have development interrupted if the mother drinks alcohol. This can create an array of primary cognitive and functional disabilities (including poor memory, impulsive behavior, and poor cause-effect reasoning) as well as secondary disabilities. From Streissguth, A.P., Barr, H.M., Kogan, J., & Bookstein, F.L. (1996), "Understanding the occurrence of secondary disabilities in clients with fetal alcohol syndrome (FAS) and fetal alcohol effects (FAE): Final report to the Centers for Disease Control and Prevention on Grant No. RO4/CCR008515" (Tech. Report No. 96-06), Seattle, University of Washington, Fetal Alcohol and Drug Unit. (See article in U of W FA&D Unit website) (from Wikipedia article on FAS.) FAS can occur at any time during the pregnancy.

[9] These pills do a lot more than merely prohibit conception. It is most telling that a doctor asks a woman if she has *ever* taken birth control pills. This is the way the question is phrased, and it is quite revealing. That we are messing with life itself when we take these or similar meds should be obvious.

Chapter 3, Nuts

[10] At that time, this condition may have been uncommon. Regardless, it is common now. Even the medical community has caught on that it is diet related. We have heard of the same kind of reaction to milk.

[11] Formerly called manic depression.

[12] There are many bipolar supplement formulas now. Our friend uses True Hope, www.truehope.com

[13] If a person is found by a court to be a danger to themselves or to others, they may (most likely *will*) be subject to involuntary treatment with various drugs. As of 2010, the individual states govern this for the most part. In addition to the successful lobbying efforts that have made these involuntary treatments law, the pharmaceutical companies have also lobbied successfully to have laws passed that require a large number of schoolchildren to take psychiatric drugs if they can be labeled as having one problem or another.

Psychiatric medications include: antidepressants, which are used to treat depression, anxiety, eating disorders, and personality disorders; stimulants, antipsychotics, and mood stabilizers, which are used to treat bipolar and other disorders; anxiolytics, which treat anxiety; and depressants, which are used as sedatives and hypnotics. How big this industry is depends upon what is counted. Conservative estimates are that it was a $40 billion industry in the US in 2008. By all accounts the industry is growing extremely fast. The untold part of the story is that the gold mine in the industry is with children who may become dependent upon these kinds of medication for their entire lives.

ABC Nightline did a piece on what foster care children are frequently being prescribed. It aired on December 1st and 2nd, 2011. I looked briefly at it on the web. If only one tenth of their findings are true, we have a huge problem on our hands.

[14] I am not a doctor and know almost nothing. I am simply a reporter telling you of cases we have seen and known firsthand. If you or someone you know has a similar condition, I think professional help is in order. I simply suggest that it might be wise if the health professional you choose is not a medication pusher and understands the value of a balanced diet *consisting only of natural foods*. Such a diet eliminates refined sugar, and natural sugars are taken in the form of whole, fresh fruits and not juices or dried fruits.

In my opinion, which is according to our experience, those trained in traditional American medical practice are too compromised by their training to be qualified to help with diet.

I am not saying that there is never an occasion to prescribe some of the psychiatric drugs that are used today. I will say, however, that there is a large and growing number of medical doctors themselves who are saying that these drugs are far overused. How far overused is the question. There is no need to get involved in the silly debate over this—about what I say or what anyone else says. The truth of the matter is simple enough to see—just follow the money. The billions of dollars spent on psychiatric medications in the US annually didn't just happen. That adolescent wards of the state, such as foster children and delinquents, are routinely put on several of these medications also did not just happen. That these drugs have invaded public schools did not just happen. And that many of these drugs are now prescribed by law didn't just happen either.

There may be only one question here: If faced with a mental health issue yourself, are you going to go along with the system that led to these abuses, or will you take another way?

The sad truth is that it often takes time to clean out all the poisons that contribute to, or cause, the conditions written about in this chapter. Many people feel that when faced with a similar case with a loved one, they don't have time to take a healthier approach than that of taking mind-altering drugs. In some cases they may be right. But that's the kicker. Once someone is on the medications, it is usually difficult and uncomfortable to get off of them.

Perhaps it is best to be proactive *before* you or someone in your family has a crisis.

[15] Like most people reading this, we know several people who are on, or have been on, psychiatric medications for various reasons. We do not know the whole story of most of these people, **but we do not know of one case where someone has truly been helped by psychiatric medications**. With one possible exception, of the cases that we have adequate knowledge of, the personality changes have been far from anything you would want to see.

[16] We know a man who was placed on psychiatric medications and lived in a near zombie-like state for more than a decade. He got off of the medications and returned to a normal state. When we saw him, we couldn't believe it was the same person. He was vibrant, well kept, and had his head about him. A few months later, we saw him again and he was back in his zombie-like state. We were told that he "had an episode" and went back on medication. I asked his wife what the "episode" was. She said he had been stressed out and became violent. His problem was eventually found to be a case of his thyroid gland not producing enough thyroid hormone. The man drank alcohol and apparently it reacted with the medication he was taking.

Chapter 4, Hypoglycemia, Hyperinsulinism, Glucose Intolerance

[17] Later edition is called *New Low Blood Sugar and You*

[18] The quote is from Seale Harris, MD, (1870-1957) and is in Fredericks' book. See note later in this chapter for more on Harris' work with hypoglycemia.

[19] If we wait too long, we may not be able to recover in the same day even after we eat. We need to manage the crisis before it manages us.

[20] If this is your problem, don't get into the stupid argument over which came first, the chicken or the egg. Just straighten out the diet and see if the problem goes away.

[21] It may be your diet, the diet of your parents or grandparents, or all of these. It is likely a combination in most of us.

[22] Fredericks, page 23. Fredericks' book, updated in 1985, is too old to be of much help on current statistics, but it is not too old to state the principle. Adams and Murray also put the estimate at 10%, as does Dr. Tintera. Our own observations, from more than 35 years of observing the condition, lead us to

believe that the cases vary so much in degree that it is very difficult to state this accurately. Some suggest that the figure is much higher. They could be right.

[23] American Diabetes Association, http://www.diabetes.org/diabetes-basics/diabetes-statistics/ I strongly disagree with the term "pre-diabetes," and a lot of MDs do too. These people have high blood sugar. A diabetic is a diabetic.

[24] American Diabetes Association , http://www.diabetes.org/diabetes-basics/diabetes-statistics/ ADA's figures are as of 2011 and do not account for hypoglycemia, or low blood sugar.

[25] See Chapter 14 for historical statistics and chart.

[26] See note on **Seale Harris** below.

[27] In more recent years, hypoglycemia became talked about a lot, but blood tests did not confirm it, so the baby got thrown out with the bath water. The word "hypoglycemia" was, and sometimes continues to be, misused when the correct term may be "hyperinsulinism" or "glucose intolerance." So, if your doctor has told you that those people who talk about hypoglycemia don't know what they are talking about, he may have some ground to say so. But he misses the point.

[28] Some MDs have gone so far as to define hypoglycemia as a blood sugar count below 40 mg/dl. (Example, *Total Nutrition*, edited by Victor Herbert, MD, 1995). With levels that low, the sufferer would be close to going into a coma. Normal levels are between 80 and 110.

[29] With the discovery of insulin in 1922, hypoglycemia, induced by excessive dosage of insulin, became common. A renowned diabetes specialist named **Seale Harris** recognized that this same condition was also in some of his non-diabetic patients. The conditions were identical. The treatment to bring the blood sugar up was to administer sugar. Harris, therefore, understood that these patients, instead of not secreting enough insulin, were secreting too much and that the surplus was constantly burning up the blood glucose, leaving the blood sugar low and the patient excessively hungry and irritable. This disease—hyperinsulinism with secondary hypoglycemia—which had long mystified doctors, was now understood. Without the isolation of insulin, this discovery could not have been made. Harris and other diabetes specialists also understood that this hyperinsulinism frequently exhausted the pancreas and led to diabetes. They further understood that if the patient's diet was controlled, this was not likely to happen.

Today, there is a large medical clinic in Birmingham, Alabama that bears Harris' name, but his work on non-diabetic hypoglycemia has been covered over by an enormously profitable diabetes industry. See *Banting's Miracle*, by Seale Harris.

[30] What "really low" is varies with the individual. We know a hypoglycemic who seemed somewhat normal when her count was in the 30s. That is a very dangerous condition. Most other people would be passing out by that time. For a non-diabetic, "really low" may be in the mid-50s. If you are diabetic, your count is normally high, so "really low" could be higher depending upon the severity of your condition.

[31] A good example of my point is this hypoglycemia diet advice written by an MD that I recently read: "Make complex carbohydrates—starchy foods such as

potatoes, pasta, bread, cereals, grains, peas and beans, and related foods—the mainstay of any meal." I give the MD credit for acknowledging non-diabetic hypoglycemia, but he is obviously not hypoglycemic himself and has no practical knowledge of the condition whatsoever. (SANR, CW, pg. 202)

[32] I was in his home many times while dinner was being prepared, and I saw what was being prepared. The meals were just as are recommended in this book.

[33] Page 277

[34] The quality of life of a person with a low count can be pathetic. Deborah has only tested under 50 mg/dl one time.

[35] This is a classic example of what happens when something gets written in a medical textbook—medical people throw out their brains and quote the book.

[36] I am referring to Type II, but if we look back a generation or more, probably Type I as well.

[37] Actually, it is probably much closer to a $200 billion industry. The American Diabetes Association website, http://www.diabetes.org/diabetes-basics/diabetes-statistics/ , states that direct medical costs are now $116 billion annually. Exactly what they include in that figure is not defined. If all the diabetes-related heart cases are not included, this number could be much higher.

[38] http://www.diabetes.org/food-and-fitness/food/what-can-i-eat/?loc=DropDownFF-whatcanieat 10-30-12

Please note: The American Diabetes Association, the American Heart Association, and other similar organizations, though "nonprofit," are so closely joined at the hip (pocket) with the AMA in philosophy that they are, for all practical purposes, one and the same.

Chapter 5, Taking Care of the Children

[39] Kloss, pg. 64

[40] This comes from the book in the Bible called Deuteronomy, ch. 30, v. 19

[41] From Proverbs, ch. 3, v. 5 and 6

Chapter 6, Living and Dying

[42] Don't think you can just take burdock root and all arthritis will go away. The need is to purify the blood. If you are poisoning yourself in other ways, the burdock will likely not have much effect. In other words, we need to get away from the concept of popping pills, and pick up the habit of a healthy lifestyle. A healthy lifestyle with mild herbs, when needed, can work wonders.

[43] See Part II

[44] The first thing I should say about food allergies I did not put in the main text because it would be too distracting. That is, that mainstream medicine is insane when it comes to this matter. They give variations of this theme: "Two out of five Americans believe that they have had adverse reactions to certain foods, yet when properly tested, less than two percent of the American population has true food allergies. Among adults who are properly tested, only five percent who think they have food allergies turn out to be correct." Obviously, their narrow definition of an allergy is correct and the rest of us are just stupid!

[45] For another alternative, see NAET in Chapter 8.

[46] Deborah's reaction was a classic autoimmune response. Such autoimmune cases are becoming more and more common. If you have this kind of condition, read the whole book and mark it up for a reference tool. This one is not so simple.

[47]The first thing to say about accepting thyroid medication is that you may be making a commitment to stay on it for the rest of your life. So, this is very serious. The second thing to say about thyroid medication is that doctors like to prescribe synthetic thyroid instead of the natural glandular. What they are taught is that this is because they can more accurately measure the dosage. For more than three decades, we have known several people who take thyroid medication—both synthetic and natural. The problems that we know of are all with the synthetic. There are two reasons the synthetic is pushed. 1) There was one occasion where there was a problem with natural thyroid, and it made a lot of press. 2) The synthetic can be produced much cheaper and can be sold at a higher cost. In light of the problems we have seen with the synthetic, the accuracy of measurement argument we simply do not accept. The third thing to say about thyroid medication is that the supply can, and does, get cut off from time to time. More on thyroid in Chapter 22.

[48] Often small press materials, but also some "best sellers."

[49] A medical insurance or employment application may require you to state whether or not you have ever filed a workman's compensation or disability claim. Employers and insurance companies don't like claims. If you were the one paying, would you?
To not file a claim was a good decision. However legitimate a claim would have been, we are better working if we in any way can.

[50] Typically called "peripheral neuropathy."

[51] The US government agency in charge of this is the Center for Devices and Radiological Health, which is a branch of the FDA. The government of France has been proactive about the ill effects of Wi-Fi. You can search the web for the latest developments.

[52] The increased number of brain cancers came from somewhere. According to a lot of health practitioners, here is a likely candidate.

[53] Think about it! Is not putting an antenna right next to our brain (which is electrical in nature) one of the dumbest things we could do?

[54] In California, tall buildings are built in such a manner that when the force of an earthquake hits them, different shock waves will be set in motion. Smaller waves cancel out the larger waves so that the frequency of a wave cannot continue to build up. It is the same concept with these devices. The electromagnetic waves can be canceled by something giving off a different frequency wave.

[55] Intuition is natural. It is NOT something you conjure up. If you do the latter, you cannot hear the former.

[56] She makes up for the lack of necessary oils by eating ground sunflower and pumpkin seeds.

[57] They are trained to ignore it if the entire gut is sore. This is probably one of the many cases in which they are taught to believe that the patient is neurotic.

Chapter 7, Raised from the Dead

[58] I contacted the center, but they told me that the "general clinic" had closed. They would not offer any information about the machines they use or used.

[59] Unfortunately, I could not find out what the herbs were.

Chapter 8, Detoxification; Alternative Treatments

[60] See Resources.

[61] I am responsible for what I do with my body; you are responsible for what you do with yours. It is with this understanding that I share the following with you:

I do an enema when my stomach is empty or nearly so. I always drink a tall glass of water first. This helps the bowel move, and if I am dehydrated will keep the water used in the enema from merely being soaked up and staying in the bowel.

The speculum is lubricated with a non-petroleum lubricant to make insertion easier. To insert, I lay on my left side with the right knee bent up toward the chest. I breathe deeply and insert slowly when exhaling. The rectal muscle involuntarily relaxes a little when you exhale deeply. Water should be close to body temperature. I try to avoid water with chlorine in it. Chlorine is a poison, and we should not be drinking it either.

I try to get in as much of the bag of water as I can and hold it for up to twenty minutes if possible. Filling slowly may be beneficial in this regard.

Sometimes I want to maximize the procedure. After I became comfortable with the process, I found that I could get up to two bags of water in.

Occasional deep breathing, belly breathing, gentle patting of the abdomen, and rubbing very lightly in the direction of travel helps distribute the water into the many folds of the colon.

The speculum is washed and sterilized after every treatment. Due to the possibility of pathogen transfer, never use a speculum that has been used by another person.

[62] Cornmeal was much different a hundred years ago than it is today. See Chapter 18.

[63] The story varies depending upon who is telling it, but when considering Dr. Kellogg's writings on health, what is stated here is by far the most plausible.

[64] See notes in Chapter 15, Unhealthy Secrets.

[65] Linus Pauling was a chemist and the recipient of two Nobel Prizes. He was quite outspoken about the virtues of vitamin C.

[66] Please don't take the freedom of choice for granted. All health-related issues are at risk to political lobbying efforts. The more we take the lazy way of shrinking from personal responsibility for our health, the more successful the lobbying will be and the more we open ourselves up to be taken advantage of. There is no mystery here.

[67] I am aware that many chiropractors want to get their patients on a regular program where they come in for adjustments three times a week for several weeks. This may in fact be helpful in a very few cases, but overall I don't buy it. It is worth noting that this practice of asking the patient to get on a "program" did not come into vogue until the insurance companies started paying for chiropractic

care. That came shortly after the verdict in the antitrust case brought against the AMA.

[68] We didn't know about Tiger Balm at the time.

[69] I believe many of them were designed to treat a condition, when what is perhaps more needful is to understand the underlying cause of the condition. In this, the practice of prescribing these products can be essentially the same as in mainstream medical practice.

[70] Lymphatic massage is a **very** light massage. Few practitioners are adequately trained in it. The idea is to get the lymph moving in an unimpeded way.

[71] Deborah's problem was largely electrical, and the treatments are electrical in nature.

Part II, Mercury! Chapter 9

[72] In 1997, the US EPA lowered what it calls the "safe intake" of methyl mercury by a factor of five, to 0.1 µg (same as micrograms or mcg) per kilogram of body weight, per day. That means that a 7 ounce can of tuna a week could meet or exceed the "safe" limit, depending upon an individual's body weight. USFDA says five times that amount, or 0.5 µg, is "safe." The US Agency for Toxic Substances and Disease Registry says 0.3 µg is safe. (Clarkson, pg. 1.) However, all cans of tuna fish do not contain the same amount of mercury. Averages are just that—averages.

[73] Heavy metals are a "hot potato" in the medical industry. No one wants to touch them, and most labs don't do the tests. This is why Deborah was on her own to find a way to get tested. Much more on this later.

[74] Nickel and cadmium are in cigarette smoke. Though she did not smoke herself, Deborah grew up in a home with heavy smokers.

[75] Exposure of children to lead has become a political darling, and is the exception. It is most certainly dangerous, but not more so than mercury.

[76] "Cause" is a problematic word. Usually there are multiple conditions that bring about an illness or diseased state. When the last of those conditions is thrown on top of the pile of other conditions, it is hardly accurate to say that it "caused" the disease. See next note. In most cases, we need to unload the camel, not argue over which straw it was that broke its back. In other words, detoxify as per Chapter 8.

[77] Heavy metals, especially mercury and aluminum, are highly suspect. Balch, page 169; Clarkson, pg. 1. I interviewed a medical doctor who runs a clinic and who has treated metals poisoning for thirty years for this book. On the subject of Alzheimer's and the possibility of it being caused by heavy metals, he said this: "We can't say it is, and we can't say it is not. It could be the added toxin that when added to insufficient oxygen leads to the disease."

[78] Mercury and other metals should be suspect in any disorder of the nervous system. The nervous system is electrical. Metals are conductors. Connect the dots! See Resources, Clarkson, pgs. 1, 7.

[79] If you have chronic fatigue syndrome or anything like it, and also have a root canal, dental crown, or similar device, reading Huggins is a must. See Resources.

[80] If you have or suspect MS, please read Huggins and Levy, pages 150-159.

[81] Mercury and other dental metals such as copper and nickel, as well as other heavy metals, are suspects. While writing this book, I spoke with a physician/researcher who knows quite a bit about the mercury/auto-immune connection. Unfortunately, due to the risk to his career involved in speaking about mercury, he did not wish to be interviewed for this book. See Huggins & Levy, page 174; Balch, pgs. 516, 545.

[82] Huggins & Levy, page 174.

[83] See the testimony of Benjamin Zander at www.Mercurypoisoned.com . Zander is a renowned orchestra conductor who had Meniere's, lost his ability to work because of it, got the metal out of his mouth, and fully recovered.

[84] See Clarkson in Resources.

[85] Enzymes use beneficial metals in their function, but mercury inhibits enzyme action thereby disrupting digestion. This is very severe in classic autism.

[86] None of this can be "scientifically" proven because not everyone reacts to the various metals the in same way. If you insist on perfect results, you will never get them. The body's function is simply too complex. Think of it this way: In a criminal trial, you need a 12 out of 12 vote from the jury to get a conviction. In a civil trial you only need 9 of 12 to agree. You will never get the 12 of 12 to "prove" that metal poisoning is a significant component of many cases of these diseases, but you may get 6 of 12, and with that there is good reason to be suspicious. Some who claim to be "scientific" consider this kind of thinking as anecdotal evidence. Regardless, if you or someone you know is suffering from one of these diseases, it might be a good idea to check for heavy metal poisoning.

[87] See "Epidemiological and Clinical Study and Historical Background of Mercury Pollution on Indian Reservations in Northwestern Ontario, Canada," by Harada, M. Fujino, et al. Published in *Bulletin of the Institute of Constitutional Medicine*, Kumamoto University, Kumamoto, Japan. By necessity, the Japanese toxicologists became experts on industrial mercury poisoning. When the Canadian tragedy came to light, they were brought in to help.

[88] Mercury from the mother's amalgam dental fillings, fish consumption, or shots can go right into a developing fetus. The CDC is big on warning pregnant mothers about the fish.

[89] See Clarkson in Resources. This is one reason that vaccines containing aluminum (and that may be most of them), especially in the volume they are now given, are potentially dangerous. Aluminum is a very common element and is much less toxic than mercury unless combined with it. However, if buildup occurs, with or without mercury, the effect can be quite serious.

How Do You Get Mercury Poisoning?

[90] Mercuro Chrome Merbromin Solution

[91] It can be argued, of course, that many crops that may have otherwise been lost have been protected from fungus by the use of ethyl mercury. Many of these mercury-containing products have been banned.

[92] Huggins and Levy, pg. 169. Different compounds have been used over the years, but mercury has always been the leading ingredient. Liquid mercury is

always mixed at approximately a 1:1 ratio (by weight) with a powder of the other metals.

[93] Common in the Roman era. Spanish mining operations in the Americas also used vast amounts of mercury.

[94] In California, during the gold mining era, a huge mercury mining industry was also booming. Although common enough in many of the Central California coastal mountains, the world's largest deposits of cinnabar ore, from which mercury is extracted, were found just south of San Jose, CA. The place was called New Almaden after Almaden, Spain, which was previously the world's largest mercury producer. The ore is crushed, then cooked to release mercury vapor. The vapor is condensed, and the resulting liquid is drained off. According to the US Geological Survey, about 200 million pounds of liquid mercury was produced in California between 1850 and 1981. It is estimated that about 26 million pounds of this total was used as an amalgam for gold recovery in California. A large amount was exported to Nevada, Colorado, and other Western states. The balance was exported all over the world, mostly for mining operations. The yield of liquid mercury from a ton of ore at the best mines at New Almaden was about 24 pounds. See "Mercury Contamination from Historic Gold Mining in California," by Charles N. Alpers and Michael P. Hunerlach, USGS Fact Sheet FS-061-00 http://pubs.usgs.gov/fs/2005/3014/ .

[95] Volcanoes do the same.

[96] According to Hightower, pg. 73, as of the year 2000, 53 of 62 US chlorine plants had eliminated the use of mercury in production. Many other plants have closed but have left mercury behind.

[97] The pigments are red or orange. Use of mercury in paints was banned in the US in 1991. Whether some mercury-containing dyes and paints have slipped through the regulations, I don't know.

[98] Other mercury-containing products used to preserve vaccines or other health-related products are Merthiolate and Bacteran. See product list in note below.

[99] This one will unquestionably come back to bite us. When these bulbs are broken, mercury vapor is released and is easily inhaled. Seemingly imperceptible amounts can cause great havoc in the body, especially in the central nervous system. Have you ever seen a warning with these bulbs to air out the house well if one of them is broken? In other words, don't think "green" is green.

[100] See the EPA site: http://www.epa.gov/hg/mgmt_options.html. A very short list of potential mercury containing products: many electrical switches, sensors and controls (tilt switches, mercury switches, flow meters, pressure controls, etc.); barometers, thermometers, thermostats, pilot light sensors; ultrasound equipment; glazes for some ceramic ware (never eat off of, or drink out of, ceramic ware made in Mexico); manganese, alkaline, zinc, and silver oxide button cell batteries (commonly used in watches, calculators, toys, etc.); electrical capacitors, LCDs, backlight display screens, children's light-up shoes; jewelry (especially from Mexico); any fluorescent light bulbs; fungicides (now banned in the US but not in many other places where our food is grown); dental amalgam, thimerosal; as a preservative for some contact lens solutions, diuretics,

ear and eye drops, ointments, nasal sprays, skin creams and salves, and antibiotics.

Note 1: The use of mercury in some, but not all, of these products has been banned. See EPA list called "Mercury in Drug and Biologic Products."

Note 2: Mercury will <u>not</u> be listed in the ingredients of these health and body products. The compound containing it will be. A good example of a hidden source of mercury poisoning is the epidemic of Pink Disease, or Acrodynia, in American children in the early part of the 20th century. At first the cause of the epidemic was unknown. Eventually it was traced to calomel, which is mercury (l) chloride. When this substance was eliminated from teething powders, in 1954, the disease all but disappeared.).

[101] Consequently our water supplies do too.

[102] Mostly from *Journal of Biomedicine and Biotechnology*, July, 2012, http://www.ncbi.nlm.nih.gov/pmc/articles/PMC3395437/.

[103] There is a separation of circulating blood and cerebrospinal fluid. Specialized cells allow certain molecules into the brain and keep others out. For example, bacteria are kept out; organic mercury is not.

[104] See "Toxic Effects of Mercury on the Cardiovascular and Central Nervous Systems," by a panel of authors in the *Journal of Biomedicine and Biotechnology* http://www.ncbi.nlm.nih.gov/pmc/articles/PMC3395437/ .

[105] The US Agency for Toxic Substances and Disease Registry, "Public Health Statement, Mercury, Cas #: 7439-97-6," 1999, pg.3.

[106] Now I understand why my chemistry professor freaked out when someone knocked over an apparatus in the lab causing liquid mercury to be spilled. Safety guidelines for handling mercury spills are on the EPA website.

[107] EPA's "Inorganic Mercury TEACH Chemical Summary," revision of 9-21-2007

[108] *Journal of Biomedicine and Biotechnology*, July, 2012

[109] Clarkson, pg. 12

[110] If you turned to this note, you must be asking, "How could that happen three times in fifteen years?!" Well, after the 1956 outbreak, most of the officials who had anything to do with the matter were killed in a revolutionary purge in 1958. Consequently, not many people knew much about it when more treated grain was ordered in 1960. Then more officials got the ax—many in the slaughter that took place between the Ba'athists and the Qassim (an Iraqi version of the Hatfields and McCoys). By 1971, Saddam Hussein's party was in power and had a proven way of getting rid of people they didn't like—such as the Kurds. So, guess where most of the treated grain was sent? (E. Hughes, "Pink Death in Iraq," *London Sunday Times,* Sept. 9, 1973. (The treated grain was dyed pink.)

[111] "The Three Modern Faces of Mercury." (See Resources.)

[112] Any kind of neurological disorder could have mercury as its root. See "Toxic Effects of Mercury on the Cardiovascular and Central Nervous Systems" in Resources for a short list of changes in the nervous system caused by mercury poisoning.

[113] Ditto. Like CFCs that destroy ozone in the atmosphere, a minute amount of mercury in the blood sets off a chain reaction that causes plaque to form.

[114] See "Toxic Effects of Mercury on the Cardiovascular System"; Cutler, Mercola. Many enzymes are manufactured by the pancreas and liver, and mercury in either organ may alter those enzymes.

[115] The immune system will react to metals in the body. How it will react is anyone's guess. See Clarkson, Klinghardt, Huggins & Levy, (pg. 174); Balch (pgs. 516, 545), and others listed in Resources.

Amalgam, Fish, Vapor, Vaccines

[116] Since the mid-1800s, mercury amalgam has been the dental restorative material of choice. But it was not always so. The use of amalgam was considered malpractice by The American Society of Dental Surgeons from the 1840s. Some dentists disagreed, however, and what became known as the first Amalgam War ensued. It ended in 1856 with the demise of the ASDS and the formation of the American Dental Association. From *American Journal of Dental Science*, pg. 170, by The American Society of Dental Surgeons, 1845. (See Google Books.)

[117] Since the early 1970s, we have been in what is called the third Amalgam War. All through the history of amalgam use in the US, many top doctors, dentists, and toxicologists have been adamantly against the use of mercury amalgam. See *California Dental Association Journal*, 2006, 34(3), pages 215-229, article by J.M. Hyson, Jr. for more detail. Even this industry-sponsored article cannot deny—and must address—the longstanding controversy among experts. Also see Resources for "The Three Modern Faces of Mercury," pg. 1, and the preface of *It's All in Your Head.*

[118] The fact is the stuff is very malleable, is inexpensive, and plugs the holes in your teeth really well. If it was not a neurotoxin, it might in fact be the perfect material for the job.

[119] This is no longer denied because several studies in the last 25 years have proven it, but government agencies now tell us that it is not enough to cause harm. However, concentrations of mercury vapor in the mouth have been shown to exceed occupational health standards. (See "The Three Modern Faces of Mercury" in Resources.)

[120] When you have an amalgam-colored stain on a tooth that does not have an amalgam filling but is directly above or below a tooth that does, guess where that stain comes from! Also, dissimilar metals in the mouth are subject to electrolysis, just like metals are anywhere else. By means of the saliva, electrons flow out of one metal into the other. When in electrical contact with another metal, it is the amalgam that dissolves. This action is increased by chewing gum and by drinking hot liquids.

[121] See US Agency for Toxic Substances and Disease Registry "Public Health Statement for Mercury."

[122] http://www.fda.gov/food/foodsafety/product-specificinformation/seafood/foodbornepathogenscontaminants/methylmercury/ucm115644.htm .

[123] Clarkson, pg. 2

Classifications of Mercury
[124] As measured in blood plasma. (Wikipedia)

[125] *Journal of American Medical Association*, Nov. 10, 1999, article by Neal Halsey, MD

[126] The "green" industry is as politically charged and corrupted as any other industry. The environmental industry is an industry, and a highly lucrative one at that. That industry is a blend of the public and private sectors. We typically don't think of industry as being in the public sector, but in fact it is and nowhere more than in the environmental industry.

There is nearly always an *environmental* downside to any decision made "for the environment." Those downsides are virtually never disclosed by leaders in the industry—certainly not if there is financial interest at stake. And there always is. An ignorant and unsuspecting public has become the prey of unscrupulous individuals in this industry just as it has been the prey of individuals in any other industry.

[127] http://www.epa.gov/cfl/cflcleanup.html

[128] By the way, our vaccines also commonly contain formaldehyde, aluminum hydroxide, aluminum phosphate, and phenoxyethanol, which is antifreeze. (See *Physicians' Desk Reference*.)

[129] CDC publication: "Understanding Thimerosal, Mercury, and Vaccine Safety," last updated March, 2012. Thimerosal is also still commonly used in the manufacturing process for sterilization. We should only be receiving "trace" amounts of it this way. I could not find any CDC statement about other mercury-containing products being used in vaccines besides thimerosal.

[130] Institute for Vaccine Safety, Johns Hopkins Bloomberg School of Public Health publication "Thimerosal Content in Some US Licensed Vaccines," updated May, 2012.

[131] "Recommended" is a nice word. "Mandated" may be more accurate. In many places, many or most of those vaccines are (or were) required before a child can (or could) be admitted into public school.

[132] National Research Council. "Toxicological Effects of Methyl Mercury," Washington, DC, National Academy Press, 2000

[133] What some of these officials thought was that the .01% represented a "trace" amount which would be 1 to 2 parts per billion. Thimerosal is used in sterilizing the manufacturing equipment, and some thought that was what was indicated.

[134] It is no wonder that many of these people were often described as mentally dull by early visitors to certain parts of California.

[135] Hightower, pg. 62-63. She cites a 1999 letter from the USFDA to vaccine makers. See Clarkson for the exponentially higher toxicity of mercury when combined with aluminum in the body.

Symptoms; Understanding at Last

[136] Some additional symptoms of mercury poisoning, not otherwise covered in this book, include: shakes or jitters, a metallic taste in the mouth, tics or twitches in facial muscles, elevated liver enzymes (AST, ALT), low thyroid numbers, profuse sweating or not sweating at all, feeling as if a tight band was around the head, and metabolism problems. Mees' lines, or white spots or lines in fingernails, are also a sign of either heavy metals toxicity or of kidney problems

or both. Cutler has a much longer and very helpful list as well as a self-diagnosis test.

[137] Use of dietary supplements and/or of medications can normalize conditions that would otherwise show up in medical tests. In other words, symptoms of mercury toxicity can be masked by use of these products.

[138] Klinghardt, Fredericks, pg. 214; Huggins & Levy, page 174; Balch, pgs. 516, 545

[139] I have used the terms "poisoning" and "toxicity" interchangeably because in different writings one or the other term may be used. There is in fact no difference. Some medical professionals try to differentiate the two, probably for liability reasons. Poisoning does not differ from toxicity any more than a donkey differs from a jackass. Mr. Webster agrees with me.

[140] Cutler, pg. 35 (See Resources.)

[141] Clarkson, pg. 2

[142] See *Evidence of Harm.*

[143] See Cutler's book *Hair Test Interpretation.*

[144] It is worth pointing out here that many dental professionals are heavily mercury toxic and that strange, seemingly unprovoked outbursts of anger are common with the condition.

[145] See the beginning of Chapter 4.

[146] Mary had injections of a drug for weight control purposes. The drug had mercury or a mercury compound in it, and Mary has not had a weight control problem since. Just a mercury problem. She told Deborah that the drugs were common in Europe fifty to sixty years ago.

[147] What data is given is skewed. The person who phrases a research question can get precisely the "scientific findings" they want to get. Never regard any "scientific" study without carefully reading the parameters given for that study. Often the parameters themselves can give a good indication if there is any true science involved or not.

Chapter 10, Amalgam Removal

[148] According to the American Dental Association, only 41 people have been reported to have had "true" allergic reactions to dental mercury since 1905. Hyson. (See next note.) The millions of other negative reactions, like Deborah's, I suppose are "false." The statement is a smokescreen trying to take attention away from chronic illness caused by amalgam. The FDA, in its webpage titled "About Dental Amalgam Fillings," concedes that there in fact can be problems but pushes them all off on your dentist. The ATSDR, in its "Public Health Statement for Mercury" also tells of increased risk when amalgam is removed.

[149] "Amalgam: Its History and Perils," J. M. Hyson, Jr., *California Dental Association Journal*, March, 2006, pgs. 226-7

[150] By the way, Deborah was fortunate to find a dentist who would work on her teeth without anesthesia. It was as hard on the dentist as it was on her.

[151] "Dental Fillings Facts," from the American Dental Association. They are quoting an FDA statement, perhaps to insulate them from liability. See Resources for what is being called invalid scientific evidence. The mention of allergy is a smokescreen to divert attention away from chronic illness.

[152] *American Dental Association Principles of Ethics and Code of Professional Conduct*, revised April, 2012

[153] This wording was adopted in 1986. I think the ADA was reacting on three fronts: 1) Some dentists were advertising that they had a "mercury-free" practice, and this made the other dentists and the association look bad. 2) They probably don't want people going to the dentist solely for the purpose of getting mercury out of their mouths. This would be tantamount to admitting that there is in fact a problem with amalgam. 3) Surely some of their advisors (at least the legal ones) knew or suspected that there could (or "would") be more poisoning cases as more people had amalgam removed. A sudden increase in toxicity cases would in effect confirm what they do not want to admit—that mercury in the mouth is toxic.

[154] At the same time, *The California Dental Practices Act with Related Statutes and Regulations*, 2012 edition, states: "It is unlawful for any person licensed under this division...to mislead or deceive because of failure to disclose material facts." (section 651.a,2)

[155] Some dentists have sued their state dental boards on the basis of the First Amendment over this matter. McClure v. Maryland State Board of Dental Examiners was slightly successful in that it (at least temporarily) stopped the boards from bringing up charges against mercury-free dentists, but the laws remain on the books. (From testimony of Mark McClure to the US House of Representatives, May 29, 2003.) From what I can tell, an uneasy peace has ensued in which many of the state boards are not filing charges as long as the dentists keep a low profile on being "mercury-free" and otherwise do not create a stink.

[156] Though the industry denies that mercury is a health hazard for the patient, in 1984 the ADA instituted new guidelines for handling dental mercury materials. They recommend a well-ventilated operating room (though I haven't seen an operable window in a dentist office for more than forty years), using single-use, precapsulated alloy, using a water spray, a high-volume vacuum, and wearing a facemask when removing old amalgam to help avoid breathing amalgam dust. They also advised against handling amalgam directly. The material left over and not placed in your mouth was to be placed in a tightly sealable container then covered with a sulfide solution. (*California Dental Association Journal*, March, 2006, article by J. M. Hyson, Jr.) Other than that and the EPA guidelines that are in effect before and after your time in the dentist chair, dentists who want to protect their patients are left to themselves when it comes to how to do that in the best way. Different dentists and other professionals have come up with different protocols. (See Appendix V.)

[157] Huggins discusses the importance of correct time periods between treatments, as does Cutler. See Resources.

[158] Deborah's liver enzymes were always in the normal range until about the year 2000, then they gradually increased to be nearly double what they should have been. It appears that this was due to increased mercury exposure. We were concerned that the liver would be overloaded by the dental work, and therefore had the enzymes checked about every six weeks during the dental work period to

be sure that the levels had not increased. If they had increased, we would have backed off on the additional exposure.

[159] Before the first amalgam removal session, Deborah was given a dose of DHEA (dehydroepiandrosterone). DHEA is a controversial compound and comes with serious warnings, so it is nothing to be played with. The dentist wanted to give her 25 mg. Deborah told him, based on thirty years of sensitivities, that probably the right amount would be about $1/10^{th}$ of that. The dentist muscle tested her again and again and eventually found that in fact about $1/10^{th}$ of the usual dose was right. (Muscle testing is a method used in applied kinesiology, which like many alternative medicine methods is considered quackery by the AMA. Nevertheless, many practitioners—including some MDs and DDSs—use it as an aid in their work.)

For the drilling work, a special vacuum apparatus to catch the drilled matter was used which was tooth specific. Nothing was to go down her throat, and the standard dental vacuum was also used as an additional precaution. A special air purifier was also a few feet away. The dentist wore a special gown with tight sleeves, wore gloves and a face mask and cap. Deborah had safety glasses on and a mask to cover her nose.

[160] The various materials have been approved by the dental industry, and many dentists don't give a second thought to the matter. Some dentists have seen the ill health effects of this attitude, and practice in a more holistic way, so now we have the terms "holistic dentist," "mercury-free dentist," and "biological dentist." No doubt, some have jumped on the "bandwagon" of these titles merely because they see a more lucrative approach to making a living. (Instead of getting $__ for replacing a filling, they may get a lot more.) Others are more genuinely concerned for their patients' health and actively approach their trade from a whole-body point of view.

[161] The whole tooth is alive, not just the pulp and nerve. Potential toxicity of dental materials is a thought rejected by mainstream dentistry. See previous note.

[162] Immediately after getting out of the dentist's office, Deborah made a chlorella paste and put it around the subject tooth. She was quite a sight with what looked like deep green lipstick on, and she hung her mouth slightly down to allow the saliva to drool into a cup all the way home. I told her, "I hope I don't get pulled over by a policeman, because I will never be able to explain what you are doing!" When we got home, Deborah removed the chlorella pack, washed her mouth out, and took a fresh dose of chlorella. She then got into a clay bath, and followed a specific protocol from a company called Health Line. After the clay bath, she was to be in the sun for a certain period of time. After that, she came in and put a camphor oil pack, on flannel, over her liver. My job was to keep the hot towels coming to put on top of the pack. Deborah followed up the next day with a colonic.

This protocol is a combination of Dr. Klinghardt's and Dr. Marshall's. See Resources.

[163] We strongly disagree with the common attitude that someone else bears the responsibility for our health. The victim mentality is not helpful or healthful, either for the individual or the society as a whole.

[164] In December of 2010, the FDA conducted hearings on the amalgam issue. Several dentists testified that not only did mercury go into the bloodstream but also into the jawbone and surrounding tissues. See www.mercurypoisoned.com for taped testimony.

[165] The great majority of people with whom I have shared this had no idea either.

[166] Teeth are living members of the body and are traumatized when worked on.

[167] www.Precious-metal-services.com/information-on-valuation-of-dental-gold/

[168] See Resources for Huggins' books.

[169] What may be compatible with our body now may not be compatible in the future. In other words, after we have done our best to get a compatible material, that does not mean it is in fact biocompatible. It is far better to avoid decay in the first place, which can usually be done simply by avoiding sugar.

[170] See Resources.

Chapter 11, Three Other Mercury Poisoning Cases

[171] Mercury will be part of a compound. It is the compound that will be named on the list of ingredients. The US EPA banned many mercury containing fungicides in the late 1990's. How much is currently used in the US, and how much is currently brought into the US with imported food and other agricultural products, I don't know. Less than one tenth of one percent of imported food is tested. And we can be sure that a producer will do just about anything to save his crop.

[172] See the warning on glutathione in Chapter 12.

[173] Autism Spectrum Disorders. There are now at least a few classifications. What is described here is "classic autism."

[174] For the supposed purpose of trying to prevent rare diseases, the toxic burden on these little bodies is greatly increased.

[175] Also known as Merthiolate. Ethyl mercury is used in the product. (See Clarkson, pg. 3.) Some sources state that the product used is an inorganic compound that converts to ethyl mercury as soon as it is in the body. For practical purposes it makes no difference. The substance also changes again— to elemental mercury—if it enters the brain. To extract it from the brain it must be chemically changed back into an organic form. I say this much here to show that mercury in the body is not a simple matter.

[176] Babies do not produce bile until after they are weaned, or at about six months of age. Bile is crucial for the removal of mercury (and other toxins for that matter) from the body.

[177] See the first note in Chapter 9. As with lead, lower concentrations of mercury were found to be more dangerous than previously thought. For this reason, in 1997, health authorities lowered the "acceptable" levels considerably. The EPA did by a factor of five.

[178] Autism is just the most glaring part of the story. Attention Deficit Disorder (ADD) and Attention Deficit Hyperactivity Disorder (ADHD) became household words at the same time. All three are neurological disorders and all became epidemic during the same time period. Are the disorders new? No. But talk to any older grade school teacher and they can tell you when the explosion of cases took place. More on ADD and ADHD in Chapter 14.

[179] The federal "Vaccine Court" (Office of Special Masters of the US Court of Federal Claims) is presided over by (politically) appointed judges who make all the rulings. The court was established by an act of Congress, The National Childhood Vaccine Injury Act, in 1986, after a large jury award against a vaccine maker.

[180] One group of three cases was decided in 2009, another group of three cases was decided in 2010. For the first group, see "U.S. Court Finds No Link Between Vaccines, Autism," in The Washington Post, February, 13, 2009. For the second group, see "Vaccines Court Rejects Mercury-Autism Link in 3 Test Cases," in The Los Angeles Times, March 13, 2010. The federal "Vaccine Court" ruled in all the cases that thimerosal does not cause autism. More than 5,300 parents had filed claims stating that their children had developed autism as a result of vaccinations. Six judges ruled on the cases.

[181] The FDA has stated that the product is safe, although they now do not allow it to be used in vaccines for children or pregnant women. In 1999, Public Health Services and The American Academy of Pediatrics agreed that thimerosal should be eliminated from vaccines given to children as a precautionary measure. The product has been used in various vaccines since the early 1930s. CDC says that thimerosal has been used in flu vaccines since 2001 (From CDC website).

[182] "U.S. Court Finds No Link Between Vaccines, Autism," The Washington Post, February 13, 2009.

[183] Statistics are difficult to establish partly because definitions and classifications have changed considerably. In the late 1960s, autism was established as its own classification instead of being lumped in with "mental retardation" or "schizophrenia." Today, the term Autism Spectrum Disorder, or ASD, is used. As of this writing (2013), the CDC says that one in 88 American children develop some kind of ASD. With the explosion of autism cases in the 1990s, classification became much easier. Classic autism, as described in Jean's story, obviously skyrocketed at that time and few professionals today would argue much with the one in 166 number for that era. The dark side of the statistics story is that now many new drugs are on the market for these individuals, making it a popular and profitable market for the manufacturers. The higher the numbers, the more their wares will be prescribed.

[184] One of the later "studies" frequently quoted is mentioned in Chapter 15 under the heading "Pseudoscience."

[185] Things may have turned out very differently had the events of Sept.11, 2001 not happened. Part of "Homeland Security" was the vaccine industry, and under the threat of the terrorist war, the government gave virtually complete immunity to vaccine makers for past and future sins. This was done in a deceitful way, by adding two paragraphs to the Homeland Security Act of 2002 at the last moment. Few signers of the bill were aware that these provisions had been slipped in, and many were quite upset when they found out about it later. This created quite a public stir. For details, see Evidence of Harm. The story is easily verifiable.

[186] See Evidence of Harm by David Kirby. The book is well documented, and plenty of the damning evidence he cites concerning the cover-up is public record.

[187] We know this phenomenon very well having dealt with it for decades.

[188] As stated in *Pediatrics*, February, 2001, pgs. 411-412

[189] Before autism became a household word, autistic children were typically categorized as "mentally retarded" or as "schizophrenic." However, classic autism is easily recognizable, and if these adult persons existed in anything close to comparable numbers they would have been easily identifiable.

[190] Today (2013), the CDC still claims, "We do not know all the causes of ASDs." That is a carefully worded statement that may serve commerce well, but it does not promote healthfulness. In fact, we do know some of the culprits that led to the epidemic, but instead of addressing two of the most obvious ones, the CDC now says that some people are more genetically disposed to autism. Seems to me that if public health is truly the concern, it might be better to focus on minimizing probable contributors to the disease rather than blaming our genes.

[191] This was based upon a study of 33 children who had received vaccines containing thimerosal and was reported in the *Lancet*, a British medical journal, on November 30, 2002. See "Mercury Concentrations and Metabolism in Infants Receiving Vaccines Containing Thimerosal," by Michael E. Pichicero, et al.

[192] The CDC has based much of its current stance on a few newer "studies." To see a good sampling of these "studies," go to the EPA site called Organic Mercury TEACH Chemical Summary. Read the article and see the appropriate references given there. Even a layman can quickly tell that a study of 40 children is not adequate to be called a study on the subject of autism; nor is a "study" that only followed the kids until their third or fourth birthdays. How about the "studies" written by people who receive much (or all) of their living from the pharmaceutical industry? For more on these "studies," see Chapter 11 in *Evidence of Harm*. See also Hightower, pg. 61, for comments on a later "study."

[193] See *Evidence of Harm*, pgs. 209-210.

[194] For example: Someone will work for a drug maker one day, then have a top post at the FDA, then essentially retire with a pension from their firm. See *Evidence of Harm, Our Daily Meds,* and *The Future of Food* for specific examples. To see more of how this system works, read Chapter 15, A in this book and the notes there.

[195] The parents of these children were injured in many ways. First, their children were greatly injured, causing them to live what most of us would consider a miserable life. Second, with a few exceptions early in the investigative process, the public health authorities would not help them. It became obvious to parents that the authorities were not only stalling, but were hiding something as well. Third, because of this lack of cooperation, the parents had to figure out what the problem was themselves. They did. (During the trials it became evident why the public health officials would not help the parents. They were too busy covering their backsides. Many internal documents were presented to the court showing that both the drug maker and the various public health departments knew of problems with thimerosal. Some of these documents are accessible to the public.) Fourth, the financial cost to take care of these children is tremendous. Nearly all the families were brought to financial ruin. Fifth, after the litigation began, they were blasted by comments from government agency spokespeople in the press

mercilessly. Many marriages broke apart under the strain. And it was all done in the name of "public health" and paid for by their (and our) tax dollars.

[196] I am not suggesting enormous payouts in lawsuits. I am advocating honesty. And the two do not have to be mutually exclusive.

[197] "US Government Asks Court to Seal Vaccine Records," *Reuters Health*, November 19, 2002. Senator Patrick Leahy challenged this but did not get far because at that time the country was in the immediate aftermath of Sept. 11, 2001. Facing the threat of biological or chemical warfare, the vaccine makers were, and perhaps are, a crucial part of our national defense.

[198] CDC publication "Vaccine Safety, Thimerosal," updated February 11, 2010; as posted on the web April 28, 2013.

[199] The thimerosal issue had touched the sacred cow of "public health"— vaccines—and logic was, and is, inappropriate in such a case. A $1.5 trillion part of the "health care" industry rests on the foundation of pharmaceutical drugs, and at the heart of the pharmaceutical industry is the vaccine policy. There would be no objectivity in the matter.

[200] Thankfully, other agencies, not in the direct line of fire, such as the EPA and the Agency for Toxic Substances and Disease Registry, are more forthright on the subject.

[201] See the first note in Chapter 9. Prior to 1997, the EPA's allowable maximum was five times the 1997 amount. The EPA's figures are for all sources of mercury exposure combined.

[202] Such as the witches' brew of other toxins in those vaccines.

[203] As reported in "The Not-So-Crackpot Autism Theory," *New York Times*, Nov. 10, 2002. Five days later, the *Times* issued a correction on the article, but not on this point. The director at Johns Hopkins, Neal Halsey, objected to the title of the article and to the direct link of thimerosal to autism.

[204] Since the time of this statement, many "scientific" studies have been done. None will override the positions of the two sides of the argument. Fortunately, thimerosal has been, for the most part, removed from childhood vaccines; but unfortunately, that is not the end of the story.

[205] Usually with DMSA or DMPS

[206] See chart in *Evidence of Harm*. Standard medical protocol is to chelate only after acute poisoning. Chelation for chronic conditions is rarely, if ever, recommended by mainstream medicine. Diet and exercise are all-important. A medical doctor I interviewed for this book told me that these kids need to stay away from sugar. "Why?" I asked him. "Because it makes them agitated." I knew, but I wanted him to say it without any prompting from me.

[207] Page title: "What is Thimerosal? Is it safe when used in some vaccines?"

[208] See Testing in Chapter 9.

[209] *California Dental Association Journal*, March, 2006, pg. 226 states that 71 million amalgam fillings were placed into American mouths in 1999. Today, fourteen years later, an increased number of fillings are made of composite materials. Nevertheless, do the math. Assuming that the 71 million figure is correct and figuring for a five-day work week, my figure is pretty close. This does not include the amount of the material that is being drilled out every day.

Chapter 12, Chelation and Detoxification

[210] I understand that this is the same reasoning that our public health departments use in not telling us of the dangers of many things. The difference is, I had no conflicts of interest.

[211] There may be cases where you cannot wait on this. A good understanding is absolutely necessary, however, because mercury can be loosened from other tissues of the body, and if not eliminated, be redeposited in the brain.

[212] Many people do not do well with chlorella and will react to it with an allergic-like response. For this reason, among others, Cutler is against using it. Klinghardt writes that the allergic response could actually be to the metals that the chlorella is binding to and not to the chlorella, and that the solution may be to increase the dosage instead of decrease it. If you are considering using chlorella, you may want to test it out beforehand. This could be pretty dicey, so you definitely want to research this one closely. Also, there is the question of how pure the product is. This is another of Cutler's objections to it. Some chlorella product may itself contain heavy metals, depending upon where it was grown. It always pays to get products from the most reputable sources possible. Having said all that, as far as we know, chlorella is one of the best binders for mercury in the gut, and getting the metal out of the gut is one of the most crucial steps in the entire detoxification process. I am also reminded while writing this that some of what we considered to be the highest quality chlorella is produced in Japan. And who knows if the growing area has been contaminated by radiation released from the 2011 meltdown at the Fukushima power plant.

Chlorophyll is used by some people who cannot tolerate chlorella. Charcoal is also used as a toxin binder.

[213] By "loose mercury," I mean that which had been released through the dental work and that which was remaining in the blood.

[214] If glutathione count is low, supplementation or injection of this amino-acid complex is recommended by some. It is highly discouraged by others, including Cutler (see Resources). Deborah's glutathione count was very sufficient perhaps because she took so much vitamin C. (See Bill's story in Chapter 11.)

Cilantro, another chelator, we understand from Klinghardt, should not be used around the time of dental work. Apparently it can cause the loosened mercury to cross the blood-brain barrier and enter the brain. **Most other protocols I have seen do not mention this,** but we heeded it. (See Klinghardt in Resources.)

All these chelators, or detoxification agents, Deborah monitored according to the principles of detoxification. (See Chapter 8.) If they made her a little sick, that was accepted as normal, because that is the way one feels when poisons are stirred up until they can be eliminated. If they made her too sick, that was because she was not eliminating the poisons from the body as fast as she was releasing the poisons into her system, so she needed to back off. With cilantro, Deborah reached a point where she needed to back off and eventually discontinue use altogether. Cutler is very much against the use of chlorella. See previous notes.

[215] Myofascial, abdominal, and Rolfing were other methods of massage therapy Deborah used to help move the poisons out of the body. All were done in a

specific sequence. When she first began these treatments, she was still trying to avoid having to use DMPS. Later, at the time of the DMPS chelation, she continued with these treatments.

[216] From various sources, including Institute for Progressive Medicine handout.

[217] DMPS was synthesized in Kiev, Ukraine in 1956. It was (and is) used for industrial workers with elevated mercury levels.

[218] For this reason, Huggins and Levy advise against using DMPS. Cutler severely warns about using DMPS by injection and has a very specific protocol for that use. (Huggins and Levy, pg. 252; Cutler)

DMPS releases mercury from the tissues. If it is released faster than it can be expelled from the body, the mercury simply settles somewhere else in the body—AND SOMETIMES CAUSES MORE HARM THAN BEFORE. For that reason, other than for emergencies—that is, when an acute poisoning has taken place—IN MY UNQUALIFIED OPINION, DMPS SHOULD NEVER BE TAKEN IF AMALGAM FILLINGS ARE IN THE MOUTH.

In my limited reading about complications, I observed that most, but not all, of the complaints against DMPS were from injections, not intravenous drips. Injections are fast; IVs are slow. In *any* detoxification program, the rate of provocation needs to be balanced with the rate of discharge or a repoisoning is inevitable. To complicate matters, the effects of DMPS treatment, as with exposure to mercury in general, may not manifest themselves for months after treatment, or maybe even longer. Therefore, we would never agree to any DMPS chelation for chronic toxicity in which the protocol does not include several other components designed to release loosened mercury from the body. DMPS is nothing to play around with or take because someone—*anyone*—says it is a good idea.

[219] See Poison Control Center website: www.pcc.vghtpe.gov.tw/old/antidote-information.htm.

[220] Likely a classic case of re-toxification. See previous note.

[221] That does not mean that they come without significant risk. The risks of use are substantial, but I do not cover them in this book. I will only say here that from what I have read, both of personal testimony and from medical sources, DMSA will make one quite ill. Cutler discusses DMSA in detail.

[222] *Our Daily Meds* covers this topic very well and gives several examples. (See Resources.)

[223] An intravenous injection of 250 mg of DMPS. Urine is then collected for 24 hours afterwards to determine the levels of metals discharged. Deborah's intravenous drips were diluted and took about three hours. They may be safer but are by no means risk-free.

[224] Actually, the terminology is misleading. The medical industry and dental industry are industries. The white lab coats do not make these industries safer than any other industry.

[225] Chapter 6 explains why we came to this conclusion.

[226] DMPS is not FDA approved and treatment using it must be under the supervision of a physician specifically licensed to prescribe and use the product. It is approved in Europe. Some US medical doctors do DMPS treatments, but

most won't touch it. Many who do the treatments are involved in what is called "integrative medicine;" that is, medicine that takes into account "alternative" methods of treatment. That DMPS chelation is risky should be obvious because it releases mercury from the tissues, and that mercury has the potential to resettle elsewhere in the body.

DMPS may, or may not, be more dangerous than many common FDA approved chemical therapies. One major difference is that the compounds used for chelation of heavy metals are very inexpensive compared to patented medications. The DMPS drips Deborah had were about the same cost as a vitamin C infusion. Chapters 14 and 15 discuss the significance of this statement.

[227] The clinic where Deborah had chelation done makes little mention of chelation in its office literature or on its website, and makes less mention of metals toxicity. (As of 12-28-12.)

[228] Hightower, pg. 24.

[229] She does not say in her book how she treats patients with mercury poisoning or how they should be treated if abstaining from fish and having a proper diet is not adequate to turn the effects of toxicity around.

[230] Jean was also given an ointment containing DMSA that she rubbed on her son's tummy. She said it was effective and calmed him. Many other autistic children are (or were) given slow injections of DMPS or DMSA on a regular basis. The results of the treatment are mixed, largely depending upon how much time elapsed between exposure and treatment. (See *Evidence of Harm.*) Many parents and doctors have reported improvement in the children after treatment, but I reject the claims of those doctors who state that it is successful with all, or even most, of their clients.

[231] In my opinion, this was going far too fast. The effects of a DMPS session are not known for some time; therefore, I think she should have gone slower. But it was her body and her call, and I respect her for that.

[232] Deborah is no stranger to tears, but this was different. The tears were not connected with any thought or feeling. Yet she could feel it coming on like a wave and then it would hit. It would last for ten minutes or up to a couple of hours. This was a physical reaction to detoxification and perhaps evidence that mercury was in the brain.

[233] As Klinghardt suggested, Deborah took the chlorella as far apart from the time she took vitamin C as possible. Clay is a binder, so she also timed it to be taken as far apart from the others as possible.

[234] If you are on blood sugar medications, I think you want to consult with your physician before taking this. Deborah tried just a dab of it on her skin and it dumped her blood sugar. Granted, she is very sensitive.

[235] Cutler (pg. 76) has very positive things to say about ALC. Deborah thinks the recommended dosages are far too high, however.

[236] Since we do not know where in the body the metals have attached, or in what form they are, we do not know the precise way in which they can be excreted. Mercola discusses this, but I think oversimplifies it greatly. Deborah tried to cover all the bases.

[237] While writing this book I interviewed an MD who told me he had done more than a thousand chelation treatments. He told me, "We don't see the number go down to zero." Deborah's tests did.

[238] We first did an unprovoked test to establish a "baseline." We did not bother to test after every treatment, only some of them.

[239] That means that none was released through the urine at that time, NOT that there was (and is) no more mercury in the tissues.

[240] See Chapter 8, Detoxification.

[241] Klinghardt explains this.

[242] By the way, Deborah has not been able to tolerate any oils for decades (instant headache). She fills the need for oils by eating sunflower and pumpkin seeds that she grinds in a coffee grinder.

[243] One of the medical doctors I interviewed for this book told me that he is now seeing many patients who have had joint replacements and now have heavy metals toxicity.

[244] You may want to check their sources as well as the experiences of others who have used the treatments.

[245] Although it is a good idea to have a professional monitor our progress, no one knows what is going on in the body as well as the patient. No matter what the doctor says is safe, the patient will be the one to suffer if things do not work out as planned. By saying this I am underscoring the need to understand the process and to also understand that no matter how well planned, bad things can happen.

[246] Most of what is called news is not news at all. The portion that is not entertainment is largely a purposeful attempt at shaping public opinion. Article was posted at http://www.cbsnews.com/8301-204_162-57545129/chelation-brings-slight-benefit-in-heart-disease-study-but-experts-unconvinced/ .

Chapter 13, The Repair Phase, Mercury Conclusion

[247] "Liver Chi," by Chi's Enterprises, has been the best by far of all herbal treatments Deborah has tried for her liver. This Chinese herbal combination contains Schisandra chinensis, Bupleurum chinense, and Smixax glabra. This is only part of Deborah's regimen and is effective probably because she does the entire regimen. (Read the rest of the book.) After the enzymes were well within the normal levels, Deborah's body told her to cut back on the herbal combination. She now uses it only occasionally.

[248] Deborah was told by her doctor that she should do these annually, but we disagree. She will not do any more unless there is good reason to do so.

[249] The skin is in fact an organ, and at that a major one when it comes to detoxification. (Forget the physiology textbook, the skin behaves like an organ, why not call it one?) My point in saying this is to underscore the effectiveness of sweating and of clay baths, etc. The healthful effects of mud packs and clay baths have been known for millennia.

[250] Like the tobacco "controversy," it will need to play out over time so that those who would be hurt financially by a quick reversal can reposition themselves. Before the boom came down on tobacco, those who trade in that way of death were given time to develop markets abroad and were enormously successful in doing so. Disgusting, but true.

[251] ATSDR website "Public Health Statement for Mercury."

[252] FDA website "About Dental Amalgam Fillings." They claim, however, that it is not enough to be problematic.

[253] Fredericks, pg. 216; Cutler, others

[254] For this book, I interviewed a few medical doctors who have treated heavy metals poisoning for many years. When I asked one, who runs a clinic, why there was so much confusion in medical circles about chronic metals poisoning, he said this: "Most doctors don't deal with it. They don't know."

[255] For example, see "Psychological, Allergic, and Toxicological Aspects of Patients with Amalgam-Related Complaints," *California Dental Association Journal*, March, 2006, pg. 226.

[256] Within the body, methyl mercury is secreted into the bile by the liver and exits with the feces—if the liver is functioning properly. If the liver is overworked, as it is when processing refined sugar, mercury can be reabsorbed into the body. See Clarkson, pg. 2, and the discussions of liver function in Chapters 4 and 14.

[257] "Demethylation of methyl mercury by micro flora in the gut is a key, probably rate-determining, process in the removal of methyl mercury from the body." "The fiber content of the diet has already been shown to affect the excretion rate of mercury." (Clarkson, pg. 10.)

Part III, Chapter 14, Smokers' Circle and Sugar

[258] Hippocrates: an ancient Greek, known as the Father of Modern Medicine.

[259] Hearing on the Regulation of Tobacco Products, House Committee, April 14, 1994

[260] To be metabolized, refined sugars need a combination of enzymes and various other nutrients. If these are not supplied with the food we eat, those needed nutrients will be taken from somewhere within the body, even from body tissues. This kind of depletion of stored nutrients stresses the body, and the effects of it can show up as any number of conditions of ill health.

[261] A sixth grade teacher recently told us that her students could be divided into three equal categories. About a third of them could only respond to the present stimulus. They had no ability to retain a thought and add another thought to it. Another third could ponder something, taking in additional information, and the last third could go either way at any particular time.

[262] ADD is now a protected disability under the Individuals with Disabilities Education Act (from "ADHD Drugs and Cardiovascular Risk," *New England Journal of Medicine*, April 6, 2006, pg. 1,446 (verified, TS); Section 300.8 c 9 (i)) of the Act.

[263] All these quotes are from books on nutrition written by medical doctors from renowned institutions. Just go to any library, pick up some books by medical doctors on nutrition, read what they say about sugar, and you'll find all the doozies like this that you can handle. Thankfully, some MDs don't agree.

[264] See *Our Daily Meds*, pg. 97, or just talk to the school nurse.

[265] Includes "pre-diabetes"

[266] The word "tempting" is often used in connection with sweets. Do we not know exactly what we are doing?

[267] *New York Times*, April 19, 1913

[268] *US News and World Report*, March 28, 2005. Sugar in all these stats is defined as any caloric sweetener. Some have argued that the amounts may refer to the amounts shipped, not actually consumed. In principle, does it make a difference? Another smokescreen from the sugar and unhealthy food industry is to speak in terms of "added sugar" instead of total sugar content.

[269] *Agricultural Outlook*, March 1997 (an FDA publication). In more recent years about half of this amount is corn sweetener.

[270] Teenage boys are reported by many government agencies to be the largest consumer group. Soft drinks are the #1 source of sugar consumed.

[271] That is, immediate and complete withdrawal from sugar. Actually, very few people have a small habit.

[272] These thrive on sugars.

[273] "What Can I Eat," from the American Diabetes Association website, as posted Nov. 11, 2012.

[274] From the American Diabetes Association website, Nov. 11, 2012.

[275] www.yahoofinance.com   Look up GM.

[276] Stats are from The World Health Organization and Yahoo Finance.

[277] If you want to get depressed, spend some time on the World Health Organization website and read about some of the issues developing countries are now facing due to the importing of industrialized food.

[278] http://www.cdc.gov/nchs/fastats/lcod.htm   from the US Center for Disease Control and Prevention. As posted Nov. 11, 2012.

[279] Lee Iacocca, the former chairman of Chrysler, had quite a battle over this one when his first wife died of diabetes. She asked him to promise her to put diabetes on her death certificate. See the first edition of his autobiography, *Iacocca*.

[280] http://diabetes.niddk.nih.gov/DM/PUBS/statistics/   from the US Department of Health and Human Services, National Diabetes Information Clearinghouse, National Diabetes Statistics. As posted Nov. 11, 2012.

[281] http://ndep.nih.gov/media/CVD_FactSheet.pdf   from the National Diabetes Education Program. As posted Nov. 11, 2012.

[282] Contrary to the American Diabetes Association stance, if you get away from a sugared-up, junk carbohydrate diet there is a lot you can do about it. You are not a victim. See also Julian Whitaker's book, *Reversing Diabetes*.

[283] http://www.cdc.gov/diabetes/consumer/eatright.htm CDC website, 11-5-12.

[284] See the story on the next page under the sugar chart. From *Banting's Miracle*, by Seale Harris, MD. (See Resources.)
All the sources I have read do not give a statistic on the frequency of diabetes before sugar was refined because statistics were not so available until more recent times. They simply state that diabetes was very rare. Sugar was first economically refined in the late 1870s.

[285] The count is on a different scale. The normal range is typically stated at 4.8 - 5.6, although some sources state different numbers, even going as low as 4.0 for normal.

[286] Although the fasting blood sugar level may be the most important number, that number can often be inaccurate if taken at a clinic. When we go to get our blood drawn, whether we know it or not, it is likely that we pump an excessive amount of adrenaline, nullifying the accuracy of the test.

[287] "Normal" is eating your typical diet, having your typical stress level, and being in your normal daily routine. "Abnormal" may be when you're stressed out, fasting, etc.

[288] http://diabeticmediterraneandiet.com/what-is-normal-blood-sugar/ As posted Nov. 11, 2012.

[289] www.providence.org/oregon/health_resource_centers/cardiacdiabetes.htm As posted Nov. 11, 2012.

[290] From *Journal of the American Medical Association* via http://www.webmd.com/heart-disease/news/20110503/heart-bypass-surgery-rate-is-declining As posted Nov. 11, 2012.

[291] Eventually the Chinese rebelled, and that's when the wars started.

[292] Nearly the entire concept of "health care," at least in the media, has been turned into an avoidance of individual responsibility. Unfortunately, many people have bought into this kind of thinking. Unknowingly they have become a commodity, which in the end can only result in oppression.

Chapter 15, Why Our Medical System So Frequently Cannot Help Us

[293] The Bayh-Dole Act of 1980 all but married the interests of the pharmaceutical companies with federally funded (taxpayer funded) medical research by allowing the researchers to profit from their discoveries. The scientists can do what they do best and the businesses can do what they do best, and the two now work together as a team to "help" you and me. It may be that all separation of federally funded research from business interests has been removed. The huge number of newer pharmaceutical products together with marketing so effective that many Americans all but believe they will die if they don't take their meds has removed the lid on "health care" costs.

[294] One drug alone was promoted by its manufacturer to "health care" professionals with 9,000 dinners, meetings, and other events. Another company did the same with 7,600 similar events. For details, see "Spending Hits the Wall," by Jonna Breitstein in *Pharmaceutical Executive*, September, 2002 (quoted by Petersen, pg. 171).

[295] So we have a blending of science and marketing, or what one pharmaceutical executive called "a marketing approach to research." See "When Worlds Collide: The Unleashed Power of Marketing/R&D Collaboration," in *Pharmaceutical Executive*, Sept, 2002 (from Petersen, pg. 184). See also: "Sounding Board: Buying Editorials," in *The New England Journal of Medicine*, Sept. 8, 1994, and "Scope and Impact of Financial Conflicts of Interest in Biomedical Research," in the *Journal of the American Medical Association*, January 22, 2003 (both verified, TS).

This latter article gives the following statistics: About 25% of biomedical research at academic institutions receives research funding from industry. The lead authors in 1 of 3 articles published hold relevant financial interests in the study. Two thirds of academic institutions hold equity in "start-up" businesses that sponsor research performed by their facility. After examining 1,140 studies, the authors of this article found that industry-sponsored studies were significantly more likely to reach conclusions that were favorable to the sponsors than were non-industry studies. (Duh!)

[296] For a detailed account of how this system works, see the Franklin v. Parke-Davis suit. You can get the links to the court documents on Wikipedia. Franklin was a whistleblower. Petersen devoted Chapter 7 in her book to this much-publicized case.

[297] For the last 25 to 30 years, the traditional income streams for American physicians have been drying up. Current salaries can no longer pay for the lifestyle that many medical doctors had become accustomed to. Nor can those salaries pay for the cost of student loans for new doctors. Therefore, in many cases, physicians are dependent upon the pharmaceutical companies for a considerable part of their livelihood. Abuse and fraud are rampant. In a House committee in 2007, Associate Deputy Attorney General Ronald J. Tenpas testified, "We are not seeing isolated instances of misconduct but repeated practices within the industry that have resulted in significant losses to federal health care programs." (See also Petersen, pg. 249.)

[298] According to a 2003 study done by Verispan, a consulting group, 82% of doctors would go to an event if they were offered cash to do so (Petersen, pg. 66). Verispan has since been acquired by SDI.

[299] "Pharmaceutical Promotions—A Free Lunch?" by D. R. Waud in *New England Journal of Medicine* 327:351-3, 1992 (verified, TS). This is a 20-year-old article. I list it because the content is essentially the same as the other articles mentioned in this section which are much newer. (See next notes.)

[300] See "Institute of Medicine Calls for Doctors to Stop Taking Gifts From Drug Makers," *New York Times*, 4-29-2009, pg. A22.

[301] "A National Survey of Physician-Industry Relationships," Campbell et al., *New England Journal of Medicine*, April 26, 2007. The physicians were in six specialties: anesthesiology, cardiology, family practice, general surgery, internal medicine and pediatrics. 94% *reported* having some type of relationship with the pharmaceutical industry.

[302] All these things and many more like them are allowed in the verbose AMA Code of Ethics. See http://www.ama-assn.org/ama/pub/physician-resources/medical-ethics/code-medical-ethics/opinion8061.page.

[303] Could there be a more classic case than the 2,000 page Affordable Care Act? Who read that bill before signing it? Speaker Pelosi's famous quote: "We'll have to sign it to find out what's in it" tells us that this practice has been well entrenched for decades.

[304] Many physicians have gotten fed up with this system and have renounced it. Obviously, they can pay a very high price for doing so. So they retire. From what I have observed in researching this book, it is only retired individuals, or soon to be retired individuals, who are making a stink about it. Like a former, or "lame duck," president or congressman making comments on policy, what they say does not hold much sway.

[305] Petersen says 20 years (pg. 179); I have seen 13 years in other sources.

[306] With great frequency, a drug is tweaked slightly and repatented as a new drug. Example: Claritin/Clarinex. See Petersen for many examples.

[307] The fact is, with such high up-front costs, these companies cannot afford to make a new drug that is *not* habit-forming.

[308] And no wonder. Guess who paid for writing and printing the book?

[309] Petersen, pg. 280.

[310] From "Mercury Concentrations and Metabolism in Infants Receiving Vaccines Containing Thimerosal," by Michael E. Pichicero, et al., published in *The Lancet*, the premiere British medical journal, on November 30, 2002. The "study" was also quoted on the CDC webpage.

[311] FDA "About Dental Amalgam Fillings," on FDA website May 8, 2013.

[312] A routine medical exam is a procedure. If that procedure does not address the cause of ill health, but rather addresses the symptoms, it is ultimately not in the patient's best interest.

[313] My own mother saw that her doctor had checked a box that did not apply to her on a form he was filling out. She told him, "I don't have that!" He replied, "I know, but I have to check that box in order to get paid." From what others have told me, this practice is rampant. What does this practice do to medical statistics?

[314] I imagine the exclusions in a physician's malpractice insurance policy would make for interesting reading.

Unhealthy Secrets

[315] In the years I have been working on this book, I have noticed a change on websites concerning this matter. It appears that the procedure is not the darling it once was.

[316] http://ukpmc.ac.uk/abstract/MED/17179057 ;
http://ukpmc.ac.uk/abstract/MED/19251007/ ;
http://gut.bmj.com/content/53/2/277.abstract ;
http://www.giejournal.org/article/S0016-5107(01)70155-1/abstract . All as posted October 28, 2012. The studies accessible on the web have been sporadic. What is currently available may not be available later.

[317] The skill of the person performing the procedure is all-important. Some facilities and individuals have a much better record than others. Read the UK study.

[318] One of the problems with the different colonoscopy risk studies is that they are based upon different criteria, so it is almost impossible to compare them.

[319] Routine colonoscopies are supposedly prescribed to keep us from dying from colon cancer. If your doctor or the medical establishment was really interested in helping you stay away from colon cancer, would they not emphasize above all else a diet free of refined foods?

[320] The standard medical doctor's line is something like: "Some people experience a little discomfort." People I have talked to who have had the procedure used different language. Here is what some told me: "Now I know what a woman's labor pains must be like." "It was excruciating!" "I've never known any pain close to that."

[321] These were (or are) all very popular drugs, and patients taking them, many entranced by advertising, had no idea what they were getting themselves into. For specifics, see *Our Daily Meds* or just go to Wikipedia.

[322] *New York Times*, March 23, 2010 (See printout.)

[323] Isaiah 29.16

[324] In the US, health insurance was relatively uncommon until after World War II. When President Eisenhower left office, he gave a famous farewell speech in which he expressed his concern about what he called the "military/industrial complex." He was gravely concerned about the power wielded by that system. If you read the speech (just do a web search on the term and it will come up), you can replace the term "military/industrial complex" with "medical/government complex" or "medical/agribusiness/government complex" and the speech is every bit as applicable and alarming.

Chapter 16, An Unhealthy Spell

[325] W.E. Vine, *Vine's Expository Dictionary of New Testament Words*

[326] See discussion of colonoscopy in Chapter 15 and related notes.

[327] By "soul," I am referring to our thoughts and feelings—our mind and emotions. By "spirit," I am referring to our conscience, our intuition, and our consciousness of God. Just as surely as God—the creator and sustainer of all things—is spirit, there is also a spirit world that is contrary to Him. With God, there is no unrighteousness. Darkness and confusion are the hallmarks of the spiritual world that is contrary to God.

Chapter 17, Germ Theory, Dead Food

[328] *Encyclopedia Britannica*; *New World Encyclopedia*; Bernard, Claude, *An Introduction to the Study of Experimental Medicine,* 1865. First English translation by Henry Copley Greene, published by Macmillan & Co., Ltd., 1927; reprinted in 1949.

[329] This story is taken from several sources, including: *The Milk Book: How Science is Destroying Nature's Nearly Perfect Food*, by William Campbell Douglass; the *Los Angeles Times* (several articles from the mid-1970's); *The Untold Story of Milk*, by Ron Schmid; and court records of Alta Dena Dairy v. County of San Diego 271 Cal. App. 2d 66.

[330] Having had fresh milk directly from the cow that has not been processed at all, I think of that milk as being raw milk. For the purpose of this account, however, I have used the term "raw" as a synonym for "unpasteurized and unhomogenized" for brevity and because Alta Dena Dairy used the term that way.

[331] Many health advocates today say that all milk is bad, that humans were never meant to eat the stuff. It seems to me that people who speak ill of milk in this way have ignored thousands of years of human history.

[332] At one point, Alta Dena filed an $80 million suit. I could not find record of the verdict (the verdict is not mentioned in *The Milk Book*), but it was almost certainly mixed, meaning it cost Alta Dena. Many such verdicts are "sealed." In other words, the public is kept in the dark, not only as to the outcome, but also about the details of the case.

[333] This is a very brief sketch of the raw milk controversy and of the Alta Dena Dairy story. You can substitute Alta Dena's name with the names of many other dairies across the country, and the story would be the same. Unfortunately, the battle for unpasteurized milk has been all but lost in the US. (However, after more than a 20-year absence, I did see some on a store shelf recently, in June,

2013). I am thankful for those who, in an honest way, try to keep the thought of whole foods alive.

[334] For sources of raw milk, see Resources at the end of the chapter.

[335] "Organic" milk is common now. In the author's opinion, to call milk "organic" that has had the vitality cooked out of it is misleading.

[336] The great majority of our food is manufactured on the largest scale by the largest companies leaving out the small operators, many of whom have (or more commonly, *had*) great reputations for producing quality foods. It is the same business/government model that drove out the "Mom and Pop" retail stores. This does not happen simply because of economy of scale. See the long note in the chapter on "organic" foods.

[337] Dr. Kellogg (see Chapter 8) was adamantly against pasteurized milk. He had many treatments for his patients using whole, raw milk. See pg. 319 of his book, *Autointoxication or Intestinal Toxemia*, 1919.

[338] Is it a surprise that acidophilus is usually cultured in milk and contains many of the kinds of bacteria that thrive in raw milk?

[339] The definitions of the terms "natural" and "artificial," etc., in the US and in other counties varies and is always changing. Sometimes "natural" can mean "derived from natural sources." In other words, orange flavoring does not have to be derived from oranges. Maybe it can be derived from cow manure if the chemists can link the chemical chains to do the job.

[340] This is the doozie. Since the petroleum industry is so advanced, most of these compounds are derived from petroleum or a petroleum product. In the petroleum industry there are a lot of waste products, and you and I are ingesting not a few of them. Whatever is cheapest will be what is used. If we have a surplus of old truck tires and cannot find anything to do with them, we might extract _____from them. And at any one time, it may be perfectly legal. This is an entirely fictitious example (I hope), but don't think that this kind of thing, in principle, does not happen.

[341] Or, as Mark Twain put it: "There is something fascinating about science. One gets such wholesale returns on conjecture out of such a trifling investment in fact." *Life on the Mississippi*, chapter 27.

[342] In August?

[343] In the Alta Dena days, due to volume, raw milk was inexpensive. Not so now.

Chapter 18, Soil and Digestion; Adulterated Food

[344] *A Guidebook to California Agriculture*, edited by Ann Foley Scheuring, 1983, pg. 275. This is a 1983 figure, obviously there are far more today.

[345] Applying tobacco juice (an early pesticide) is one thing—at least it is organic; applying disodium methylborboltate is quite another. (I made the name up, but you get the idea.)

[346] For many reasons. First, much of the world's richest soil has been covered over by development. Some other factors are: lack of proper crop rotation, lack of use of cover crops to enrich the soil, lack of fallow years, erosion of nutrient-rich topsoil, poisoning the soil, etc. Soils that contain more organic matter are richer in nutrients and are darker. Bleached-out looking soils have far fewer life-forms and are nutrient deficient.

[347] If you don't think that your digestive system is overworked, fast for two or three days. Usually the first day of a fast is a little rough—your body is always telling you: "Hey! Where's the food!" But the second day is quite different—commonly you feel great and have an abundance of energy. Where does that energy come from? From giving your digestive system the day off. Your body is rejoicing.

[348] There are exceptions. We must be able to digest them, and we cannot have an abundance of yeast, fungus, candida, or other parasites stealing the nourishment.

[349] (They didn't eat sesame seeds, but the seeds they ate did the same thing for them as sesame seeds did for me.)

[350] I am writing about the principle of nutrition here, not about magic fruits.

[351] See the World Health Organization website.

[352] See Monsanto Canada Inc. v. Schmeiser. *The Wall Street Journal* had an interesting article on this 2004 case of a farmer who was sued by a mega-corporation for allegedly using their seed without paying royalties. It is a very interesting case from many standpoints. Also, search the web for *The Future of Food,* to see a short documentary.

[353] GMO seed is sometimes developed so that it cannot reproduce. Since the seed cannot reproduce, the farmer cannot save seed for the next season. Such "terminal" or "terminator seed" requires the farmer to purchase new seed for every crop he plants.

[354] GMO crops are classified as "food" and therefore do not require FDA approval. At this time, the industry is almost entirely unregulated.

[355] One of the real dangers is that seed banks of what these corporations call inferior seed are purposefully being destroyed. (At universities, in government agencies, and in private businesses that have been absorbed by larger businesses.)

[356] *The Food and Drugs Act, A Study*, 1906, by Arthur P. Greeley

[357] See *Foods and Their Adulteration*, by Harvey W. Wiley, 1907

[358] The book was *Folk Medicine*, by D. C. Jarvis. See court records of 338 F.2nd 157 – United States v. Bottles "Sterling Vinegar and Honey Aged in Wood…"

[359] See court records of 984 F.2nd 814 61 USLW 2491, United States of America v. Traco Labs, Inc. No. 92-1172.

[360] *Los Angeles Times* article titled "Raw Food Raid," July 25, 2011. A surveillance camera video of the bust was posted on www.youtube.com/watch?v=ifvp3Fxi7Uo .

[361] This story comes from three sources: *The Family Ranch*, by Linda Hussa, 2009, pg. 54; an article by Michael Pollan published in the *New York Times Magazine*, March 31, 2002, titled "Power Steer;" and "History of Meat Grading in the United States," by J.J. Harris, et al, Texas A&M University.

[362] In effect it was mandated—by the new grading system.

[363] I happened upon this story by leafing through a copy of the *Yearbook of Agriculture, 1913*, published by the US Department of Agriculture. The book states that although the practice would kill the cattle in short order, if the sawdust was fermented, the cattle could ingest some of it. I have also read of cattlemen feeding beet tops to cattle to fatten them just before slaughter. Cattle were designed to eat grass, not leafy vegetation, so the cattle would choke on the beet

tops. "No problem," said the rancher, "You cow hands just reach down their throat and pull the stuff out if you see them choking." The workers didn't think that was a good idea, so they were given tongs to do the job. I got this gem from *The Irvine Ranch* by Robert Glass Cleland, 1962.

[364] In the mid-1930s, the slaughterhouse age of steers was about 3-4 years old. Now, largely by feeding them corn, it is 14-16 months. From "Power Steer."

[365] Corn is heavily subsidized by taxpayer dollars as is the heart disease industry. This is part of the unhealthful alliance between the food and medical industries with government.

Chapter 19, "Organic" Food; What it is; What it is Not

[366] I found this out while researching for a better way to control codling moth. See UC IPM Online, Codling Moth.

[367] I wish I was making this up. Plastic pellets are commonly used as "roughage" (to speed digestion) in feedlots. The cows cannot pass them, so cannot survive very long on that diet.

[368] For one thing, tax laws greatly favor large businesses over small businesses. Historically, all a conglomerate has had to do in order to avoid paying any income tax is purchase some little business or businesses. If they have a bad year, they can spin off a few of these to make up the shortfall in income. So the conglomerates play a shell game with each other by moving around these little businesses like chess pieces. In this environment, it is almost impossible for a small business to survive once a conglomerate sets its sights on it. This is just one of many such rules that make it difficult for small businesses to survive.

Once the big boys get the business, they almost always tweak it according to their business model and away from the founder's business model. In the food industry, this usually involves adding sugar or other unhealthful ingredients.

[369] Some fruits, bell peppers, tomatoes, and other vegetables commonly are. Start looking and feeling and you can usually tell which are and which are not.

[370] As we seek to live a healthier life, we are confronted with our tendency toward destructive habits both individually and collectively. In humankind—who can aspire for the good and wholesome things—obviously something has gone desperately wrong. It cannot be healthy to ignore the larger issue.

Chapter 20, Vitamins, Minerals, Supplements

[371] This refers to water soluble vitamins and minerals. Those vitamins that are fat-soluble, such as vitamins A, D, E and K, I'm not sure about.

[372] Many other "health care" bills were lumped into this one law.

[373] Article by Richard Passwater in *Whole Foods Magazine*, August, 2005. (Not related to Whole Foods grocery stores.) The FDA claimed that primrose oil was a food additive and as such was unapproved. They lost in court.

[374] *Health at Gunpoint: The FDA's Silent War Against Health Reform*, by James J. Gormley, 2013, pg. 72

Chapter 21, Some Principles of a Healthy Diet

[375] See Chapter 14.

[376] Many (if not all) nuts and seeds are now pasteurized, which kills a lot of the nutritional benefit. We try to stick with those least processed, but admittedly that is getting harder and harder to do. The FDA recently (I think it was in 2009) started requiring the pasteurization of almonds. Before we knew about this new regulation, my son and I both observed that something had happened to the almonds for the worse. We simply were not getting nearly the nourishment out of them that we had previously.

[377] See Chapter 8.

[378] Many fungicides contain a mercury compound.

[379] Vegan books tend to ignore the blood sugar issue or pay very little attention to it. All I have seen assume that the reader can metabolize sugars and various carbohydrates correctly (such as grains and beans), which is not the case with a significant number of people.

[380] Murray, pg. 77, says "up to 50%." He bases the figure on the consensus of testimony at FDA hearings in the 1970's.

[381] See the story of USDA Choice in Chapter 18.

[382] Both unhealthy varieties of oils and overheating the good ones. Overheating changes the chemical composition of the fats.

[383] Some say two full movements a day. They may be right.

[384] Many people in the "alternative" realm have hurt themselves in this way.

[385] Fungi, such as mushrooms, harbor other fungi. If you have a fungus problem, see Chapter 22, Prescription Drugs, Fungus.

Part IV, Chapter 22, More Stories, Lessons Learned

[386] Some pressure points may only be an eighth of an inch in diameter, and you often need to dig around to find them.

[387] By the way, college athletes, though an asset to a university, are commonly forsaken by the university if they get injured. We know this now.

[388] People who normally do not take drugs may react to them more than people whose bodies are accustomed to the kind of assault that these products make on the body.

[389] By the way, her regular doctor was quite angry with her that she went to the ER and still insisted that she did not need B-12. She switched doctors, which was not an easy thing to do with her "Health Maintenance" Organization.

[390] Without taking this step, that is, without setting out to learn how to care for ourselves in a better way, all "helps," no matter how good, are not that beneficial in the long run.

[391] Acyclovguanosine

[392] See *Wall Street Journal*, June 10, 2012.

[393] The worst case was probably in 2011 when natural thyroid was all but taken off the market.

[394] When I say "Lord," I mean more than "God." God is our creator, and He certainly cares for His creation. The Lord is God in covenant relation with man. God is a covenant making God; and the Bible is the story of the covenants God has made with man. See Genesis, chapters 6 and 17; Exodus, chapters 3, 19, and 20; Jeremiah, chapter 31 (quoted in Hebrews 8); and Luke, chapter 22.

[395] It is precisely the same as defragmenting the hard drive on your computer. For those not familiar, it simply means that all data is filed away neatly. With proper sleep, random thoughts are connected together properly and are filed in the proper files in our minds. In both cases, the "desk" is cleared of clutter creating a clean and clear environment in which to work.

[396] Diabetes damages far more than the pancreas. The entire body has been thrown into a diseased state. If the disease is not arrested, by the time it has gone its course, it is unlikely that insurance premiums alone will be able to pay for all the drugs, medical tests, hospital bills, hearing aids, bypass surgeries, and whatever else it will take to keep you going.

[397] I see no value in taking the standard deception of, "Oh, it's in your genes, you can't help it." What those who say such things really mean is, "Act like a victim and help yourself to some chocolate pie."

[398] Those who say that the bowel always cleans itself adequately are mistaken. The colonic tube does not lie.

[399] A medical doctor once told me that a saltwater solution preparation may be helpful. Bad idea; it corked me up big time. No lasting harm was done in this case (just a lot of discomfort for several hours), but I have heard a bad story or two of people who followed a protocol without checking it out adequately first.

[400] Until they had billed Medicare for all the "health care" she had received?

[401] You can use cornstarch baby powder if you want to, but all you want is the cornstarch, not the dietherolglovalbulberate. (I think you know what I mean.)

[402] This book is about having a healthy lifestyle, and keeping shoes off as much as possible (as long as you do not need the protection and the environment is clean) is part of a healthy lifestyle.

[403] See *Physician's Desk Reference* concerning your medication(s) and take the warnings seriously.

[404] One of her prescriptions was M _____, a popular drug used to treat diabetes. Apparently it (like many other pharmaceuticals) can deplete the body of vitamin B-12. See the story on diabetes meds earlier in this chapter.

[405] Also, many people with adrenal problems cannot tolerate being in the sunshine for very long without having severe hot flashes.

[406] She also used it fresh for a while.

[407] This is a common scenario with medicinal herbs. When there is a crisis, you may need a lot more, then gradually work down to a maintenance level or stop treatment completely. Many herbs should only be taken for a short time. Heed the warnings.

[408] I find it amazing that the medical folks missed this one—and don't care about it either. If you heal yourself of the problem and tell your doctor, he will probably do what Deborah's doctor did, that is, give a blank look as if he did not understand. It is not in the medical textbooks, therefore it cannot be valid.

[409] Some medical doctors object to this term, saying that it is meaningless. I have a book written by a renowned doctor at the Mayo Clinic who says this. Apparently he and others who say the same are unfamiliar with Mr. Webster.

[410] My condition was probably just chest muscle spasms; my friend had a mild case of pleurisy.

[411] If you don't know already, I will tell you how a diabetic is treated in a hospital and how the elderly diabetics are cared for in nursing homes. You feed 'em ham and potatoes for dinner, with cheesecake for dessert, then shoot 'em up with insulin to make up the difference. That is standard medical facility procedure, at least in California. Deborah and I have seen this in *many* places. And, according to my friend, the patient does not even have to be diabetic to get the insulin!
I wish I was exaggerating.

This being the case, we never trust the dietitian at the hospital. Their training and procedures are fixed in a large body of laws, and they cannot, and will not, deviate from protocol. We have plenty of experience on both sides of the family with this.

Their orders are to serve a sugared-up typical American diet. The dietary adjustments they make for a diabetic, if they make any at all, are to substitute the sugar with chemical sweeteners. We have yet to see anything close to a healthy meal served in a hospital though we have visited several facilities. Some may, I don't know, but from all we have seen, we have reason to think that at least in many facilities the dietitians do not know what a healthy meal is.

So, if the case calls for it, be prepared to take your own food. If you can.

Chapter 23, It's Not Starbucks' Fault

[412] Includes the newly defined "pre-diabetics." See Chapter 14.

[413] The rest of the story goes like this: The little produce market was later purchased by business people who decided to expand the operation and get into more profitable products. They started carrying wine, cheese, and many other items. They even put in a butcher shop. And they opened five other stores. They forgot where they came from, however, and let their "unprofitable" produce slip. In a short time they were out of business.

[414] "Health care" is greatly subsidized by our tax dollars. It is in fact a government/industry enterprise and has been so for decades. What we pay for in insurance premiums does not come close to covering the tab.

Appendix I

[415] Otherwise, you may want to get a showerhead filter and replace it every three months or so.

[416] Reverse osmosis filters work well but may be taking too many necessary minerals out and consequently depleting our bodies. Some filtering systems add various minerals. This needs to be determined on a case by case basis. Taking a multimineral supplement may be beneficial.

Appendix II

[417] Refined sugar was not economical until the late 1870s.

[418] These metabolize almost as quickly as refined sugar.

[419] An excellent protein source. With nuts and seeds, always look at the label to see the ratio of protein to carbohydrates, sugars and fats. You want lots of protein, and minimal or no sugars. Fats are great—these are healthy fats—and carbs should be minimal. Of course, get them raw and unsalted. Chew them well. Soak them in water if you have anything close to constipation. You can also

grind them with a coffee grinder, add water or vegetable juice and have them for a meal. They are great as a spread on celery.

[420] Note: Grains, as they existed before the 1870s, are probably no longer available. Grains are a great source of protein, but if the gluten component is out of balance with the germ and bran, as it is in modern grains, grains are limited in their value as a healthy food. Negative reactions to gluten were rare thirty years ago; now they are common. What was most healthy has become not so, at least for many people. Perhaps consumption of most modern grains should be reduced and largely replaced with non-starch vegetables and seeds or nuts.

[421] In order to live optimally with this disease, animal flesh is probably needed. Although not necessary from a blood sugar standpoint, I think that beef should be grass fed and limited; chicken is much easier to digest. Also wild caught fish is much better than farm raised (on grains).

[422] Typically smaller squashes with more skin are better. The skin is not starchy.

[423] Almost all grocery store breads contain fine ground bleached flour and/or unhealthful chemical additives.

[424] Try it both ways and compare how much energy you have. You will see the difference. Roasting changes the chemical makeup of the foods.

[425] The glycemic index does not take into account other factors besides glycemic response, such as adrenal and insulin responses. That in itself makes the index largely impractical as a guide. Also, the index varies greatly by the precise type of food, the ripeness of the food, the processing and storage of the food, and the cooking or cooking method. Most of all, glycemic response is different in different people, and even in the same person at different times of the same day. In other words, the glycemic index may (or may not) be useful for a very general idea of glycemic response, but it is not close to adequate as a dietary guide and in fact can be quite misleading if used as such.

Appendix IV

[426] Many other "health care" bills were lumped into this one law.

[427] *Wall Street Journal*, May 7, 2010

Resources, Mercury!

[428] Huggins lost his dental license because of being outspoken against the use of mercury in his trade and for making certain claims about the connection between mercury and MS and other diseases. In his book, he states that he has MS himself, but has had it in remission for a long time. (If you have MS, get his book!)

Understand that those in the medical profession, such as Klinghardt, Huggins, and Levy who break ranks with mainstream medicine are targets of all kinds of accusations.

Glossary of a few key terms used in this book

American Medical System: That economic system of pharmaceutical companies, medical schools, hospitals, clinics, medical products companies, and medical practitioners as represented by the American Medical Association and its many related "nonprofit" organizations, as well as the American Dental Association and its related "nonprofit" organizations, which lobby for their interests and thereby form US government health policy.

Diabetic: A person who typically has high blood sugar levels. A high blood sugar level is anything over the norm of 80-120 mg/dl. Diabetes is a very serious disease. It is a leading cause of death in the US, mostly by way of heart disease and stroke. A rare disease 130 years ago, before the economical refining of sugar, it is rampant now. It is almost always caused by the excessive consumption of sugar, either by the diabetic or by his ancestors or both. Usually both.

Glucose intolerance: The inability to ingest sugar or simple carbohydrates without having a negative reaction to them. Typically, those reactions will bring on the symptoms of hypoglycemia. A person who is glucose intolerant will not necessarily have a blood sugar count that is high or low, but will have an abnormal insulin response, which results in hormonal imbalance. Glucose intolerance is an accumulative condition. It means that the glands and organs are stressed and may in fact be damaged.

Health care: Taking care of our health.

"Health care": That *system* of business and political/government interests that, by compromising with the basic principles of health for the sake of gain, moves us away from taking care of our health. One glaring example within the "health care" system is the diabetes industry, which is described in Chapter 14.

Hypoglycemic, hypoglycemia: A person who has a condition of low blood sugar. Frequently the condition can be more accurately called "**hyperinsulinism**," a condition where the pancreas produces too much insulin thereby *usually, but not always*, dropping the blood sugar level below the norm. The condition is commonly accompanied by adrenal irregularities, hypothyroidism, and/or any of a host of other maladies involving the endocrine system and organs. In perhaps the majority of cases, none of these maladies show up on standardized medical tests. Severity of the condition in individuals varies greatly. Chronic hypoglycemia or hyperinsulinism is very common and if not controlled will typically eventually result in diabetes. Hypoglycemia also refers to the state in which a diabetic finds himself when his blood sugar plummets. A medical doctor will typically only acknowledge the latter.

Pre-diabetic: A diabetic. We, and many medical doctors (although a minority of them), object to the term. A diabetic is a diabetic is a diabetic. High blood sugar is high blood sugar.

Science: An objective, logical, and systematic means of experimentation and fact-finding by which we can arrive at a (usually limited) understanding of a matter. When financial interests govern the scope or results of scientific research, true science ceases to exist. When marketing marries science, the resulting offspring is science fiction.

Sugar: In this book I am usually referring to refined sugar, including all caloric sweeteners such as corn sweetener, etc. In the context, sometimes I am also referring to natural sugars or simple carbohydrates and starches, which are converted into sugar almost immediately upon ingestion. The context will make that distinction clear enough. For the purpose of this book, and for the reasons stated herein, I have often put all the types of sugars together— glucose, fructose, maltose, lactose, etc. Sugar (actually glucose) is the fuel into which all foods must be converted in order to be used as fuel for the body.

Wise, wisdom: The ability to discern the inner qualities of a matter; good sense. There is a tremendous difference between wisdom and learning. We may learn and understand a lot of things but that does not make us wise. Wisdom comes from an awe of, and fear of, our Maker. To not respect the perfection of the creation is the utmost of foolishness.

Bibliography

Books and Articles:

A Guidebook to California Agriculture, edited by Ann Foley Scheuring, 1983

American Medical Association Code of Ethics, AMA

Amalgam Illness: Diagnosis and Treatment, by Andrew Cutler, PhD, 1999

American Journal of Dental Science, by The American Society of Dental Surgeons, 1845

An Introduction to the Study of Experimental Medicine, by Claude Bernard, 1865, first English translation by Henry Copley Greene, published by Macmillan & Co., Ltd., 1927

Autointoxication or Intestinal Toxemia, by J. H. Kellogg, MD, 1919

Back to Eden, by Jethro Kloss, 1939

"Balancing Risks and Benefits: Primum non Nocere Is Too Simplistic," article by Halsey and Goldman, *Pediatrics*, 2001, 108:2, pgs. 466-467

Banting's Miracle, by Seale Harris, MD, 1946

California Dental Practice Act with Related Statutes and Regulations, by the Dental Board of California, 2012 edition

Colon Hygiene, by J. H. Kellogg, MD, 1915

Diagnosis Mercury: Money, Politics and Poison, by Jane Hightower, MD, 2009

Empty Harvest, by Bernard Jensen and Mark Anderson, 1990

Encyclopedia Britannica

"Epidemiological and Clinical Study and Historical Background of Mercury Pollution on Indian Reservations in Northwestern Ontario, Canada," paper by Harada, M. Fujino, et al., published in the

Bulletin of the Institute of Constitutional Medicine, Kumamoto University, Kumamoto, Japan

"Evaluating Mercury Exposure: Information for Health Care Providers," US Agency for Toxic Substances and Disease Registry (the ATSDR is a part of the Department of Health and Human Services)

Evidence of Harm: Mercury in Vaccines and the Autism Epidemic: A Medical Controversy, by David Kirby, 2005.

Foods and Their Adulteration, by Harvey W. Wiley, 1907

Health at Gunpoint: The FDA's Silent War Against Health Reform, by James J. Gormley, 2013

Herbally Yours, by Penny C. Royal, 1993

"History of Meat Grading in the United States," paper by J.J. Harris, et al, Texas A&M University

How to Live with Diabetes, 5th edition, by Henry Dolger, MD, and Bernard Seeman, 1985

Hypothyroidism: The Unsuspected Illness, by Broda O. Barnes, MD, 1976

Iacocca, by Lee Iacocca, 1986

Is Low Blood Sugar Making You a Nutritional Cripple? by Ruth Adams and Frank Murray, 1970

It's All in your Head: The Link Between Mercury Amalgams and Illness, by Dr. Hal A. Huggins, 1993

Kitchen Medicine, by Ben Charles Harris, 1968

Know Your Nutrition: The Complete Guide to Good Health Through Natural Living, by Linda Clark, 1973

"Limiting Infant Exposure to Thimerosal in Vaccines and Other Sources of Mercury," article by Neal A. Halsey, MD, *Journal of the American Medical Association*, Nov. 10, 1999

Mercury Contamination from Historic Gold Mining in California, by Charles N. Alpers and Michael P. Hunerlach, USGS Fact Sheet FS-061-00

National Organic Program, Part 205 of the *Electronic Code of Federal Regulations,* US EPA

Natural Detoxification: A Practical Encyclopedia, by Jacqueline Krohn and Frances Taylor, 2000

New Low Blood Sugar and You, by Carlton Fredericks, 1985

Our Daily Meds, by Melody Petersen, 2008

Physicians' Desk Reference, 2010

"Pink Death in Iraq," article by E. Hughes, in the *London Sunday Times,* Sept. 9, 1973

"Power Steer," article by Michael Pollan, published in the *New York Times Magazine*, March 31, 2002

Prescription for Nutritional Healing, by Phyllis A. Balch, James F. Balch, MD, 4th edition, 2000

"Principles of Ethics and Code of Professional Conduct," by the American Dental Association, revised April, 2012

"Public Health Statement, Mercury, Cas#: 7439-97-6," by the US Agency for Toxic Substances and Disease Registry, 1999

Reversing Diabetes, by Julian Whitaker, MD, 2001

Silent Spring, by Rachael Carson, 1962

"Symptoms and Differential Diagnosis of Patients Fearing Mercury Toxicity from Amalgam Fillings," article by S. Stenman and L. Grans, 1997 (Published on PubMed)

The American Medical Association Family Medical Guide, Jeffrey Kunz and Asher Finkel, editors, 1987

The Bible

The Case Against the Little White Slaver, by Henry Ford, 1914

The Family Guide to Symptoms, Ailments and Their Natural Remedies, by Carlson Wade, 2000

The Family Ranch, by Linda Hussa, 2009

The Food and Drugs Act, A Study, 1906, by Arthur P. Greeley

The Healthy Liver and Bowel Book, by Sandra Cabot, MD, 1999

The History of the Crime Against the Food Law: The Amazing Story of the National Food and Drugs Law Intended to Protect the Health of the People Perverted to Protect Adulteration of Foods and Drugs, by Harvey W. Wiley, 1929

The Irvine Ranch, by Robert Glass Cleland, 1962

The Milk Book: How Science is Destroying Nature's Nearly Perfect Food, by William Campbell Douglass, 1994

The New Method in Diabetes, by J. H. Kellogg, MD, 1917

"The Three Modern Faces of Mercury," by Thomas W. Clarkson, Department of Environmental Medicine, Univ. of Rochester School of Medicine, Rochester, NY, 2002

The Way of Herbs, by Michael Tierra, 1998

"Thimerosal Content in Some US Licensed Vaccines," chart by the Institute for Vaccine Safety, Johns Hopkins Bloomberg School of Public Health, publication updated May, 2012

Tissue Cleansing Through Bowel Management, by Bernard Jensen, DC, PhD, 1981

"Toxic Effects of Mercury on the Cardiovascular and Central Nervous Systems," by a panel of authors in the *Journal of Biomedicine and Biotechnology*, 2012

"Toxicological Effects of Methyl Mercury," article by the National Research Council, Washington DC, National Academy Press, 2000

"Understanding Thimerosal, Mercury, and Vaccine Safety," by US CDC, last updated March 2012

Uninformed Consent, by Hal Huggins, DDS, and Thomas E. Levy, MD, 1999

Vines Expository Dictionary of New Testament Words, by W. E. Vines, +/- 1904

Yearbook of US Department of Agriculture, 1913

Periodicals consulted:
Agricultural Outlook
California Dental Association Journal
Journal of Biomedicine and Biotechnology
Journal of the American Dental Association
Journal of the American Medical Association
New England Journal of Medicine
Pharmaceutical Executive
Reuters Health
US News and World Report

Newspapers consulted:
Los Angeles Times
New York Times
New York Times Magazine
Wall Street Journal
Washington Post

Websites frequently consulted:
American Dental Association
American Diabetes Association
American Medical Association (AMA)
National Diabetes Education Program
PubMed
US Centers for Disease Control and Prevention (CDC)
US Department of Agriculture (USDA)
US Department of Health and Human Services
US Environmental Protection Agency (EPA)
US Food and Drugs Administration (FDA)
US Geological Survey (USGS)
Wikipedia (sources, if used, always checked)
World Health Organization
Yahoo Finance

Acknowledgements

Thanks to God for my dear wife, Deborah. Uniting us has been His means for drawing us both to Himself.

Thanks to my wife, Deborah. Deborah has been a source of inspiration to me through all of her afflictions. She did not give up or give in to what she knew was wrong. Although it is tough having her private life broadcasted, she has been willing to do so for the sake of others. Thank you Deb, you are one of my heroes.

Thanks to Viola Ingalls, Bernard Jensen, and Carlton Fredericks. All these stood against the tide, and by doing so gave Deborah the basis of knowledge needed to be restored to better health.

In learning a new way of living we had some good examples early on whom I want to acknowledge:

Thanks to the Dale and Lonny Mandon, who by example taught us something of healthy eating.

Thanks to Kathy Jones, who told Deborah to use cornstarch instead of talc for diaper rash, to use lanolin or glycerin instead of mineral oil, and to avoid food colorings, etc.

Thanks to that dear lady—her name now long forgotten—who told Deborah to use chamomile tea for our son's colic and advised against the use of medications.

Thanks to the Stueve family, founders of Alta Dena Dairy, for providing unpasteurized milk and for fighting so hard to keep it on the store shelves. Though that battle was lost, sanity may yet return.

Thanks to David Bundy, DC. My, what we learned from you!

Thanks to Andrew Pallos, DDS, for his patience and caring.

Thanks to Allan E. Sosin, MD, for allowing me to interview him for this book.

Thanks to Jane M. Hightower, MD, for answering some of my questions.

Thanks to those medical doctors whom I interviewed for this book who wished to remain anonymous. I greatly appreciate you all!

Thanks to Andrew Cutler for writing his great work and for corresponding with me about it and about this book.

Thanks to the International Academy of Oral Medicine and Toxicology (IAOMT) for allowing me to print its "Recommended Procedures and Guidelines for Amalgam Removal" in the book.

Thanks to Marie Flowers of Dental Amalgam Mercury Solutions (DAMS) for her work and for allowing use of their photo.

Thanks to the many anonymous friends and acquaintances who shared your stories with me for this book. For that I am most grateful. The book is more rounded and helpful because of you.

Thanks to Joanna Oyzon at the Heritage Park Library in Irvine for her assistance.

Thanks to our son, James, for his most helpful comments on the manuscript, especially on the organization of the material.

Thanks to Milford Brenneman, Gary Shippy, John Stanley, Lisa O'Bryan, and Sam Asiedu-Kumi for their comments on the manuscript. All of you were very helpful.

Thanks to Linda Seed and Rebecca Twitchell, my editors, who both did a great job. Any remaining errors or awkwardness in the text are mine.

Thanks to everyone who has encouraged us by living in a healthy way, whether it be in spirit, soul, or body, and especially to those who have endeavored to be healthy in all three.

And last, but certainly not least, thanks to so many dear friends who have prayed for us or simply wished us well. We hope that we have also been a source of encouragement to you!

Index

By the Same Author:

Letters to My Feathered Friends
Observations, Meditations and Thanksgivings

A collection of seventy-six bird poems and stories with
complementing color photographs.
142 pages, soft cover

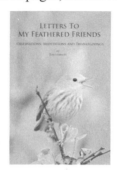

The Last of the Prune Pickers
A Pre-Silicon Valley Story

Not long before the Santa Clara Valley of California was known for silicon, the Valley was largely covered with orchards. There were orchards of pears, apricots, cherries, walnuts, and the king of them all: prunes. Most of the orchards were part of small family farms, and there were thousands of them. This is the story of what preceded those farms, how they came into being, and how they thrived. It is also the story of one of the last of those farms, of the farmer, and of some of the young boys and girls who had the privilege of working for him.

239 pages with 50 photos, soft cover

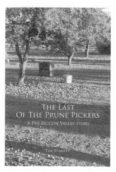

Order at 2timothypublishing.com